Thieme

Diseases of the Chest

Imaging Diagnosis Based on Pattern Classification

Toshiharu Matsushima

Toshiharu Matsushima, MD, PhD, FCCP
Professor Emeritus
Kawasaki Medical School
Director of Respiratory Center
Kurashiki Daiichi Hospital
Junpukai Foundation
Okayama, Japan

Kenji Eguchi

Kenji Eguchi, MD, PhD
Professor and Chairman
Division of Medical Oncology
Director of Tokai Oncology Center
Tokai University School of Medicine
Kanagawa, Japan

Masayoshi Kuwabara

Masayoshi Kuwabara, MD, PhD
Director of Lung Cancer and Chest
Diseases Center
Kusatsu General Hospital
Shiga, Japan

601 illustrations

Thieme
Stuttgart · New York

Library of Congress Cataloging-in-Publication Data is available from the publisher.

Important note: Medicine is an ever-changing science undergoing continual development. Research and clinical experience are continually expanding our knowledge, in particular our knowledge of proper treatment and drug therapy. Insofar as this book mentions any dosage or application, readers may rest assured that the authors, editors, and publishers have made every effort to ensure that such references are in accordance with **the state of knowledge at the time of production of the book.**

Nevertheless, this does not involve, imply, or express any guarantee or responsibility on the part of the publishers in respect to any dosage instructions and forms of applications stated in the book. **Every user is requested to examine carefully** the manufacturers' leaflets accompanying each drug and to check, if necessary in consultation with a physician or specialist, whether the dosage schedules mentioned therein or the contraindications stated by the manufacturers differ from the statements made in the present book. Such examination is particularly important with drugs that are either rarely used or have been newly released on the market. Every dosage schedule or every form of application used is entirely at the user's own risk and responsibility. The authors and publishers request every user to report to the publishers any discrepancies or inaccuracies noticed. If errors in this work are found after publication, errata will be posted at www.thieme.com on the product description page.

This authorized and revised international edition

Rüdigerstraße 14, 70469 Stuttgart, Germany
http://www.thieme.de
Thieme New York, 333 Seventh Avenue,
New York, NY 10001, USA
http://www.thieme.com

Printed in Germany by Grammlich, Pliezhausen
ISBN-10: 3-13-143571-2 (GTV)
ISBN-13: 978-3-13-143571-2 (GTV)
ISBN-10: 1-58890-562-4 (TNY)
ISBN-13: 978-1-58890-562-8 (TNY)

1 2 3 4 5 6

Preface

About 6 years ago I was approached by International Medical Publishers, Ltd., with a plan to produce a book that, rather than simply providing examples of the image findings of respiratory diseases, would serve as a guide to the imaging diagnosis of chest diseases through analogy using image findings. I suggested that one method could be the classification of chest image findings into patterns that would enable inference of the disease groups involved. Based on this proposal, I drafted a review of the thinking behind the classification of chest image patterns and how this classification could be accomplished. Following that, the most suitable specialists in their field were selected by a team of three editors to provide explanations of the different patterns. The task was completed in about 2 years.

Chest imaging diagnosis is a quantitative diagnostic technique, not a method for qualitative diagnosis. It simply indicates whether there is a shadow present and, if so, provides an understanding of the location, size, and characteristics of that shadow. It does not shed light on the true nature of the shadow. Imaging diagnosis is no more than a valuable tool that enables the classification of shadow characteristics into patterns as a first step to identifying diseases that must be differentiated before further tests are conducted to reach a definite diagnosis. Image findings alone cannot provide a final diagnosis and, as such, should never be used with this purpose in mind.

With the widespread use of chest CT, however, much finer analysis of shadow characteristics is now possible. The view is that CT has made it easier to classify patterns and achieve more precise disease or disease group inference. In this book, chest image findings have been simply classified into 20 pattern types. An attempt has been made to describe the characteristics of different patterns for easier classification, and to outline the diseases associated with particular patterns and the distinctive features of the accompanying shadows to enable analogical inference of the diseases involved.

We believe that the method proposed here for pattern classification is clear and simple. It may be easy in some cases to infer a disease by following the classification, while in other cases in may be difficult. There may, for example, be more than one pattern present at the same time. In such cases, further examinations and tests are required to clarify the situation. We have every confidence in the clarity of the chest radiographs, CT images, figures, and tables presented in this book.

It is our hope that this work will provide readers with a systematic and efficient method for evaluating radiologic images of the chest with a high degree of certainty, and a solid understanding as to why pathology appears as it does in radiographs and CT images.

Toshiharu Matsushima

Contents

Chapter 1

Introduction: Pattern Classification of Abnormal Shadows

●Author — Toshiharu Matsushima

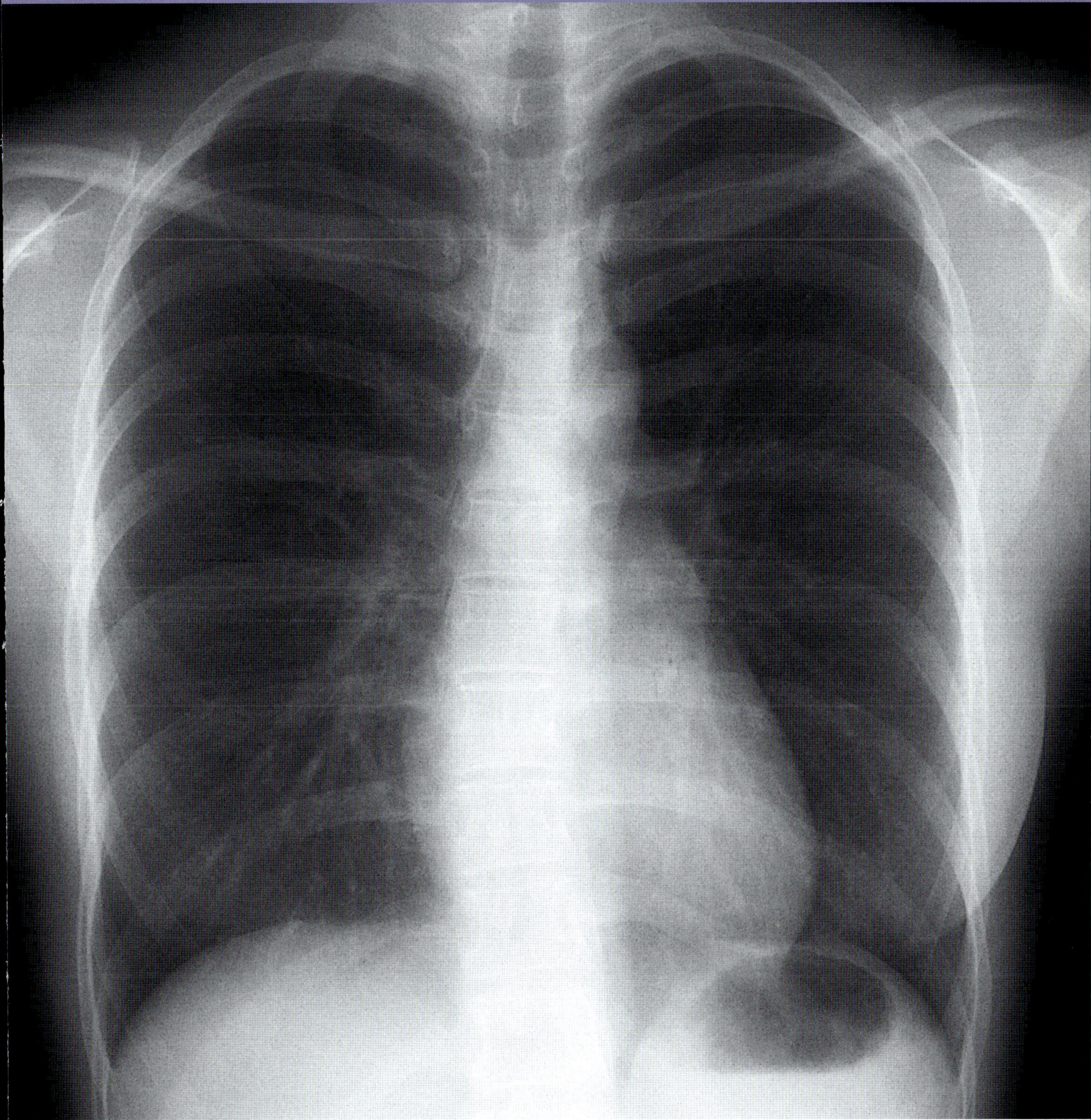

Keywords of this chapter:

Radiolucency
Pattern classification
Alveolar space disease
Consolidation
Atelectasis
Pulmonary interstitial disease
Granulomatous lesion
Fibrous lesion
Alveolar + interstitial disease
Hilar type (pulmonary edema pattern)
Peripheral type
(reverse pulmonary edema pattern)
Nodular shadow (tumor-like shadow)
Solitary nodule
Multiple nodules
Ring shadow
Cavity
Cyst
Abnormal linear shadow
Bronchial lesion
Hilar enlargement
Hilar lymphadenopathy
Increase and decrease of
pulmonary markings
Calcification

Pattern Classification

Toshiharu Matsushima
Respiratory Center, Kurashiki Daiichi Hospital, Junpukai Foundation, Okayama, Japan

Chest radiographs are based on differences in the radiolucency of thoracic organs and tissues. When radiolucency increases compared with normal lungs, owing to reduced hindrance, the image becomes blackish, while decreased radiolucency gives a whitish image. The latter case in particular is called abnormal shadow and is classified into several patterns related to the pathological background. How to interpret and classify chest radiographs is explained in this book. This chapter is an outline of pattern classification.

Pattern Classification Based on Radiolucency

When radiolucency rises compared with normal thoracic organs, film exposure increases and gives a blacker image. In extreme cases, radiolucency is the same as in extrathoracic air, and the image becomes completely black. If the content in the thorax is air-rich, the image becomes generally blackish as in cases of pneumothorax and emphysematous cysts.

Decreased radiolucency leads to under-exposure of the film and produces a whitish image. The heart and liver hinder permeability considerably and appear white on the film. In the same way, water retention in the thorax (hydrothorax, pulmonary edema) produces a whitish shadow.

Thoracic lesions can be divided into intra- and extrapulmonary lesions. The relationships between the shadows and the lesions are classified I through V in the table below. Group IV is listed in subclasses because it covers most of the lesions we encounter.

	Pattern classification		Found in:		
I	**Extrapulmonary lesions in thorax with increased radiolucency (pneumothorax)**		Increased radiolucency		Chapter 2
II	**Intrapulmonary lesions with increased radiolucency (emphysema, cavity, cyst, pulmonary embolism, etc.)**				
III	**Extrapulmonary lesions with decreased radiolucency (hydrothorax, pleural thickening, pleural tumor)**		Pleural disease		Chapter 3
IV	**Intrapulmonary lesions with decreased radiolucency**				Chapter 4
	A. Alveolar space disease	1. Consolidation	Alveolar shadow	Consolidation	-1
		2. Atelectasis		Atelectasis	-2
	B. Pulmonary interstitial disease	1. Granulomatous lesion	Interstitial shadow	Granulomatous sign	-3
		2. Fibrous lesion		Fibrotic shadow	-4
	C. Alveolar + interstitial disease	1. Hilar type (pulmonary edema pattern)	Alveolar Interstitial shadow	Pulmonary edema	-5
		2. Peripheral type (reverse pulmonary edema pattern)		Reverse pulmonary edema shadow	
	D. Nodular shadow	1. Solitary	Nodular shadow	Solitary nodular shadow 1, 2, 3	-6, 7, 8
		2. Multiple		Multiple nodular shadows	-9
	E. Ring shadow	1. Cavity	Ring shadow	Cavity	-10
		2. Cyst		Cystic shadow	-11
	F. Abnormal linear shadow	1. Bronchial lesion	Lesions of trachea and bronchus		-12
		2. Others	Abnormal linear shadow		-13
	G. Hilar enlargement	1. Hilar lymphadenopathy	Hilar shadow		-14
		2. Enlargement of main pulmonary artery			
		Note: Increase and decrease of pulmonary vascular markings			
	H. Calcification		*(Omitted because of little clinical relevance)*		
V	**Mediastinal lesions with decreased or increased radiolucency**		Mediastinal lesions		Chapter 5
	Mediastinal lesions				

Table. **Pattern Classification List**

I. Extrapulmonary lesions with increased radiolucency

(Blackish shadow on radiograph: Pneumothorax)

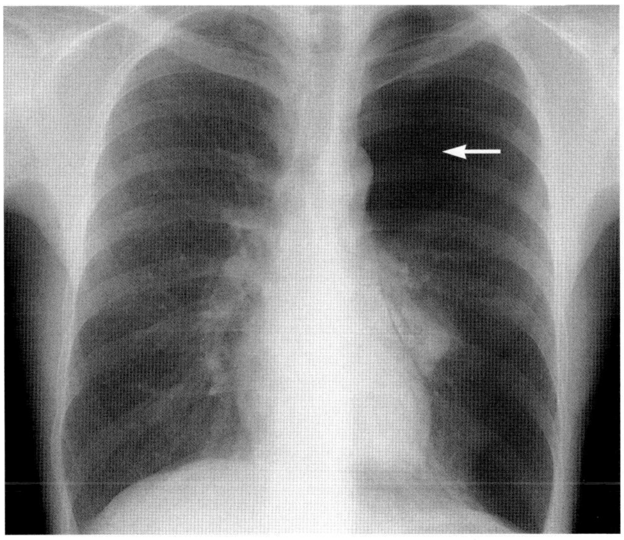

Figure 1. **Pneumothorax**

II. Intrapulmonary lesions with increased radiolucency

(Blackish shadow on radiograph: Emphysema, cavity, cyst, pulmonary embolism, etc.)

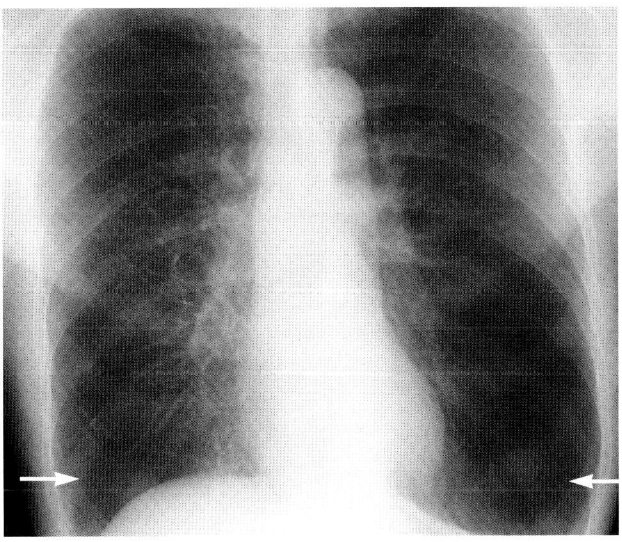

a

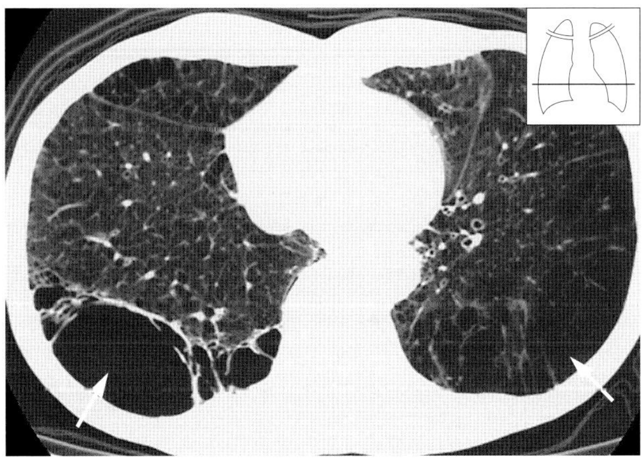

b

Figure 2 a–b. **Pulmonary emphysema (cyst)**

III. Extrapulmonary lesions with decreased radiolucency

(Whitish shadow on radiograph: Hydrothorax, pleural thickening, pleural tumor)

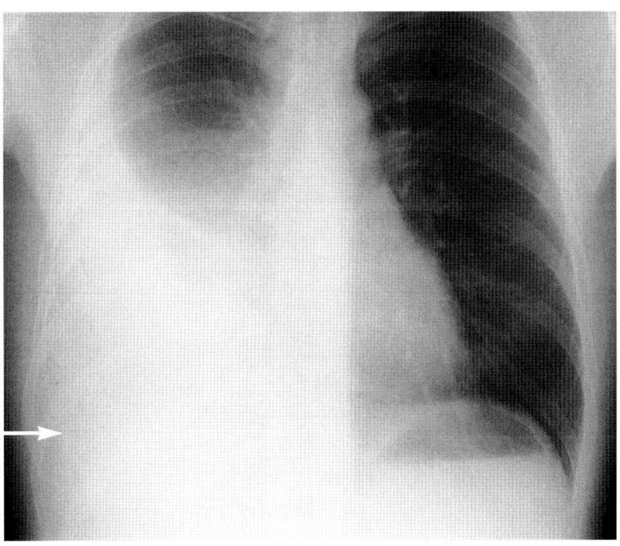

Figure 3. **Hydrothorax: Pleural effusion**

IV. Intrapulmonary lesions with decreased radiolucency

(So-called abnormal shadow, whitish shadow on radiograph)

A. Alveolar space disease: This pattern indicates probable presence of lesion in the alveolar space

1. Consolidation (retention of exudation and cell infiltration in the alveolar space causes decrease of radiolucency)

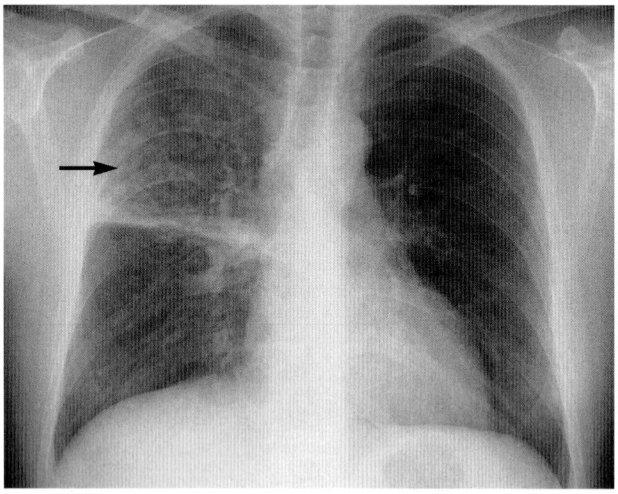

a

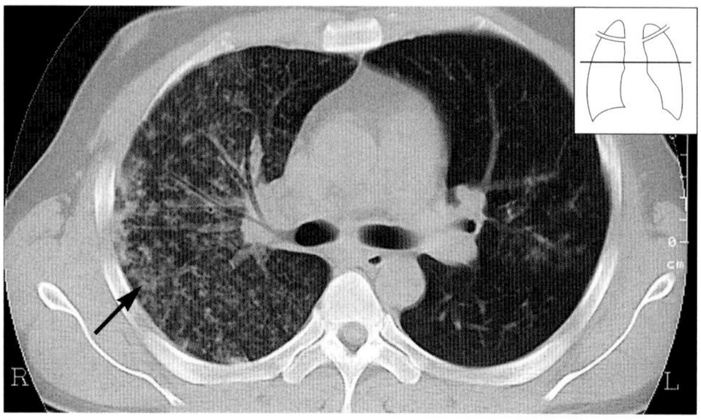

b

Figure 4 a–b. ***Mycoplasma*** **pneumonia in the right upper lobe**

2. Atelectasis absorption of air in the alveolar space (causes reduced radiolucency and reduction of lung volume)

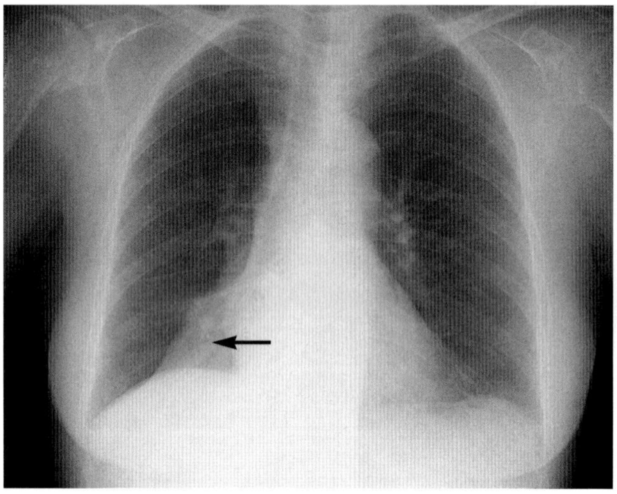

a

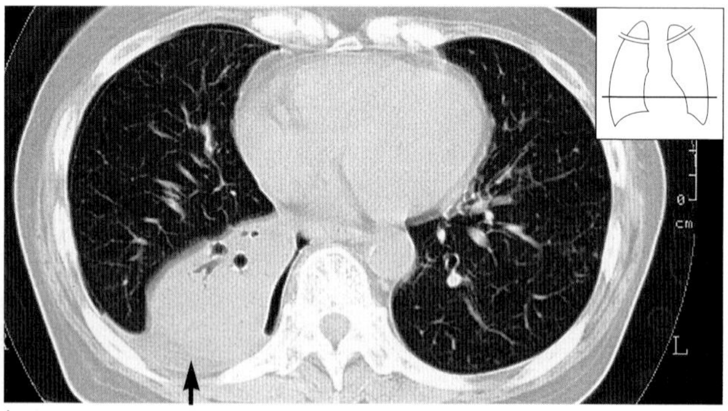

b

Figure 5 a–b. **Atelectasis in the right lower lobe**

B. Pulmonary interstitial disease

This shadow indicates probable presence of lesion in the pulmonary interstitium

1. Granulomatous lesion: The shadow indicates granuloma in the interstitium, and is not accompanied by volume reduction

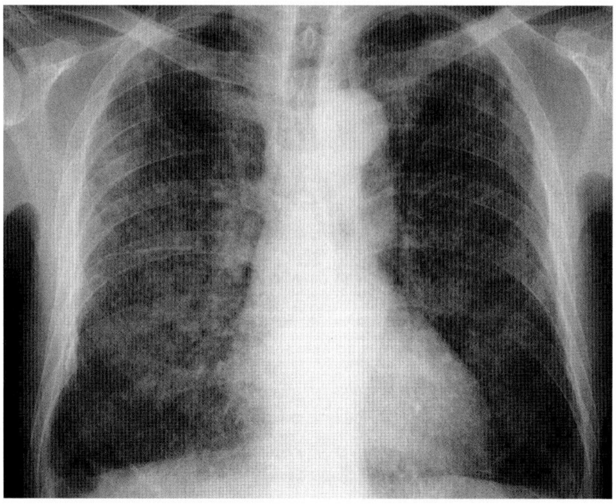

a

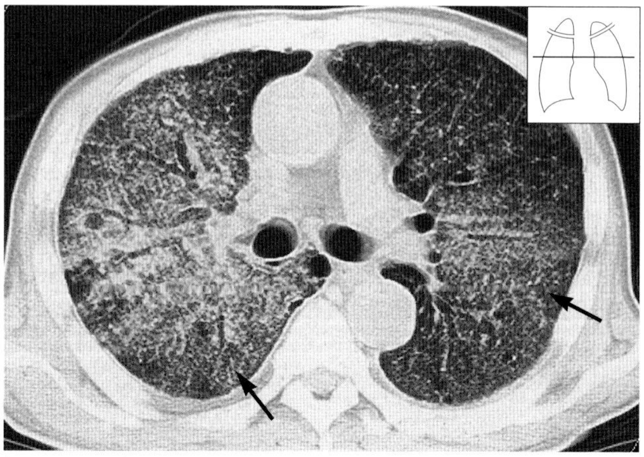

b

Figure 6 a–b. **Miliary tuberculosis**

2. Fibrous lesion (shadow presumed to be caused by widespread fibrous formation in interstitium, usually accompanied by contraction of pulmonary volume)

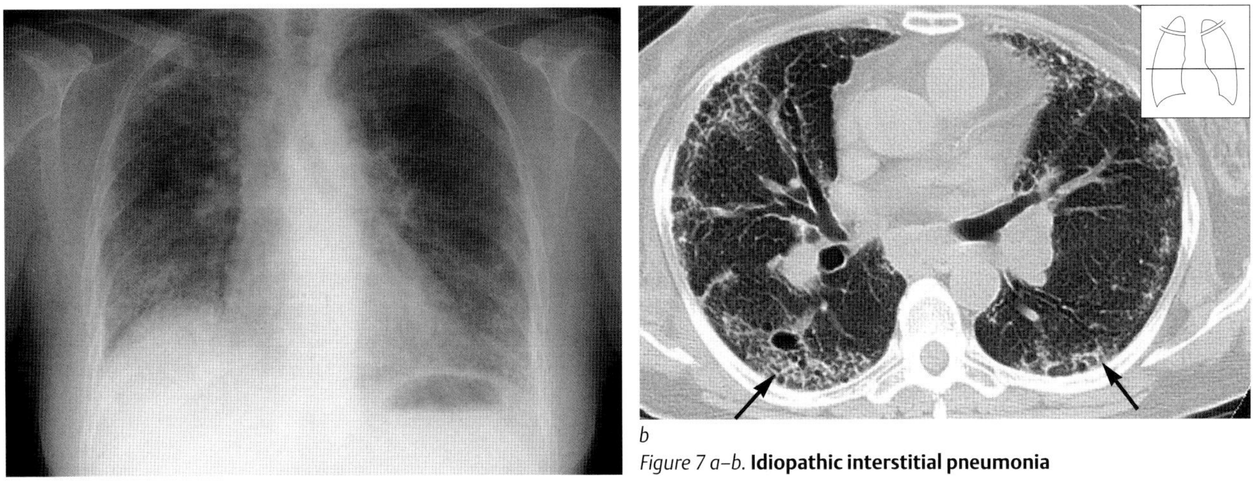

a

b

Figure 7 a–b. **Idiopathic interstitial pneumonia**

C. Alveolar + interstitial disease: Shadow presumably caused by the presence of lesions in both pulmonary interstitium and alveolar region

1. Hilar type (pulmonary edema pattern): Shadow is seen in perihilar zone, clear peripheral shadow

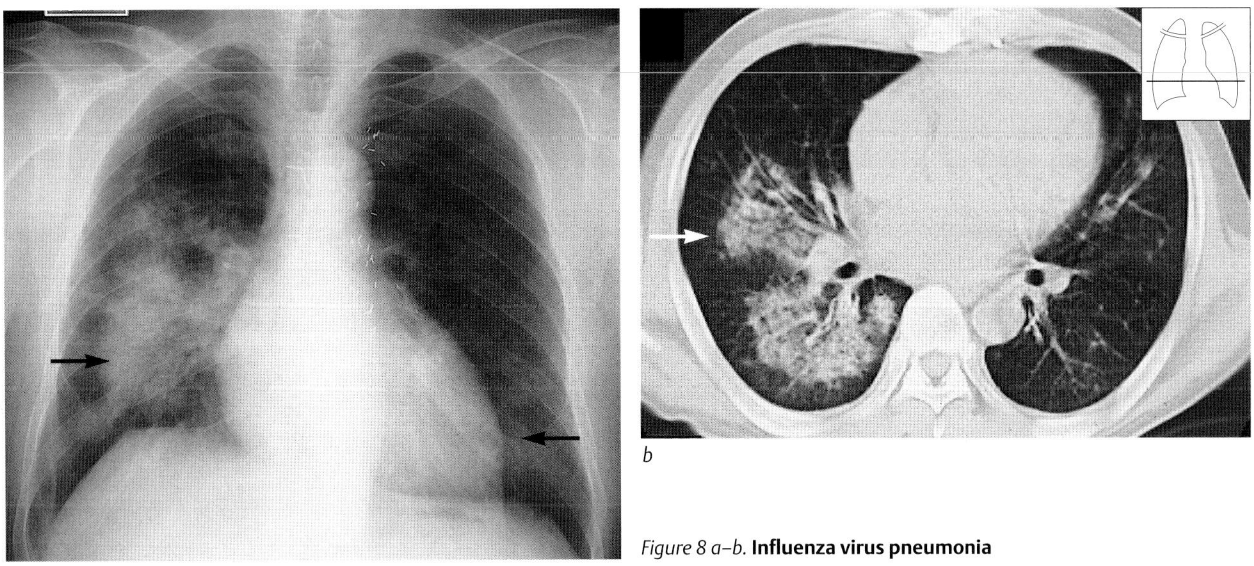

a

b

Figure 8 a–b. **Influenza virus pneumonia**

2. Peripheral type (reverse pulmonary edema pattern): Diffuse shadow in peripheral zone, clear perihilar shadow

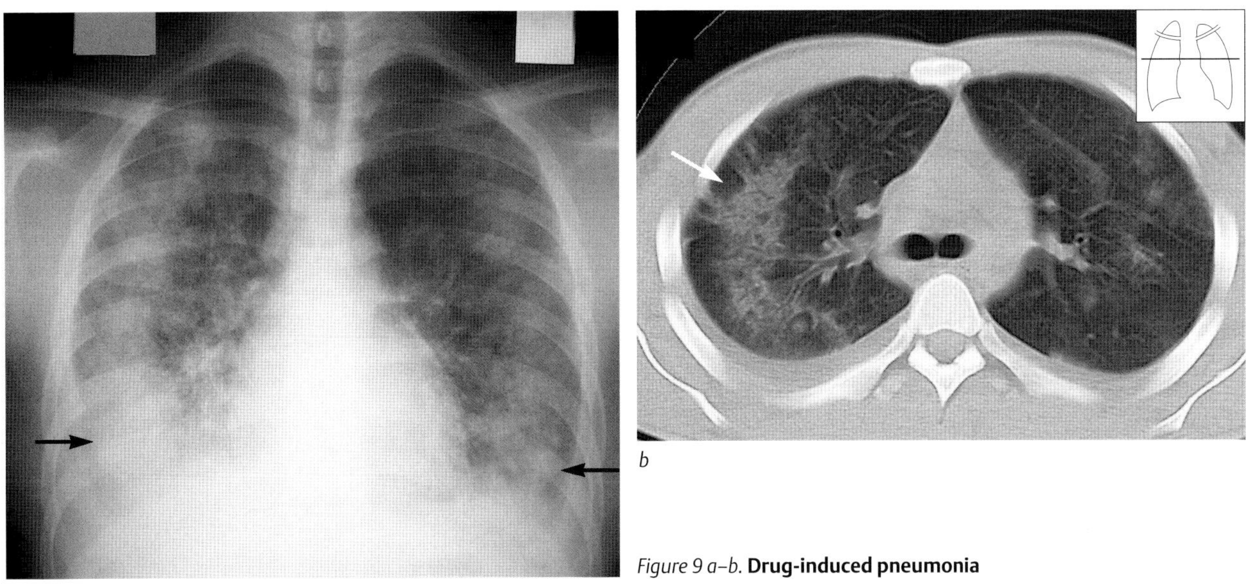

a

b

Figure 9 a–b. **Drug-induced pneumonia**

D. **Nodular shadow (tumor-like shadow)**: Shadow of spherical mass is seen

1. Solitary nodule (solitary nodular shadow; a small shadow is usually called a coin lesion, while a bigger shadow is called a mass lesion)

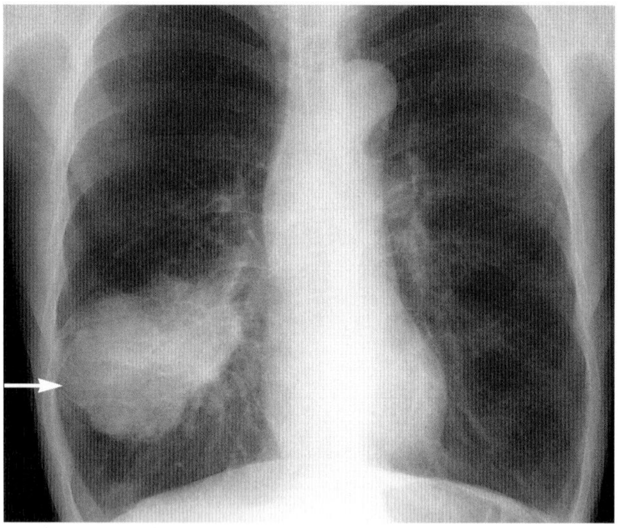

a

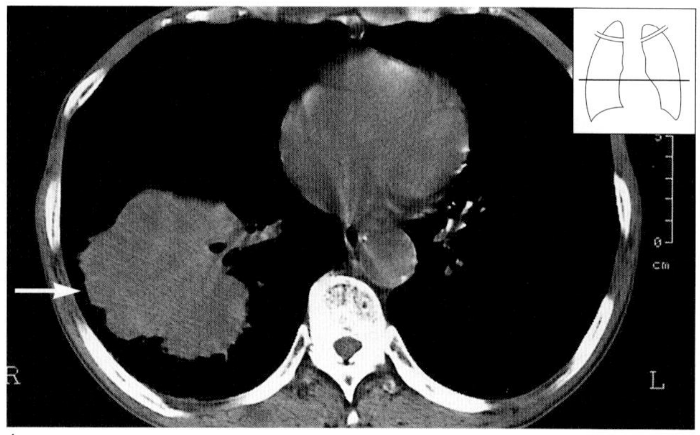

b

Figure 10 a–b. **Lung cancer**

2. Multiple nodules (two or more nodular shadows are seen in bilateral lungs)

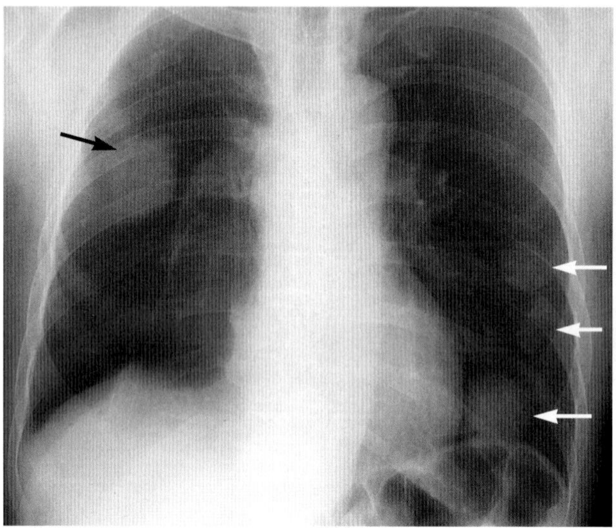

a

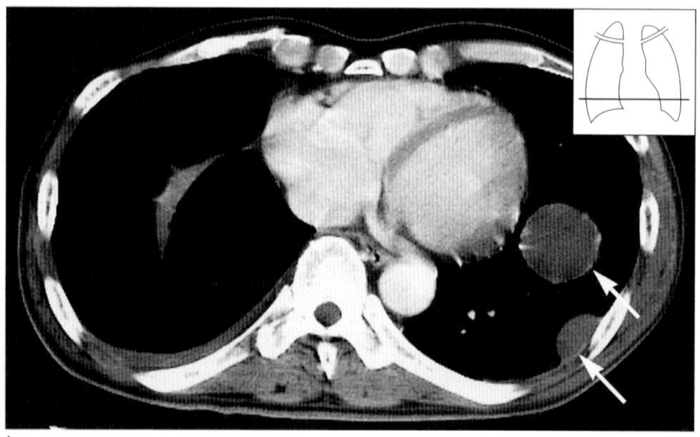

b

Figure 11 a–b. **Metastatic lung cancer**

E. **Ring shadow**: Space containing air surrounded by linear or band-shaped shadow

1. Cavity: Space containing air formed by detached necrotic tissue; This term refers to thick-walled lesions in radiographs.

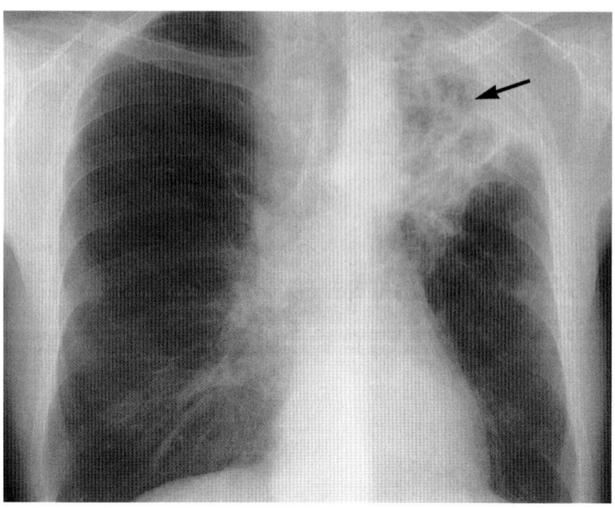

a

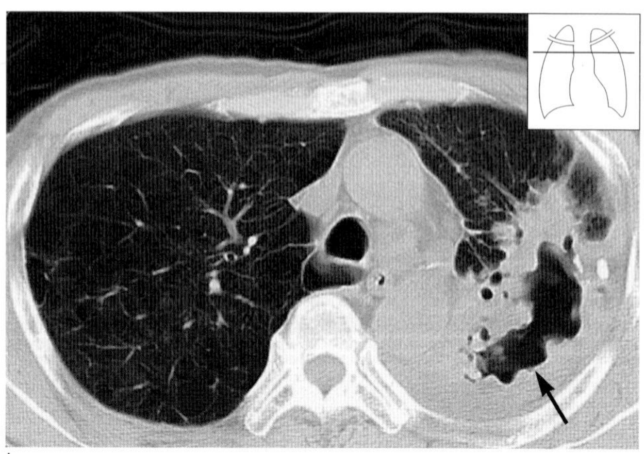

b

Figure 12 a–b. **Aspergilloma**

2. Cyst (air space surrounded by thin walls)

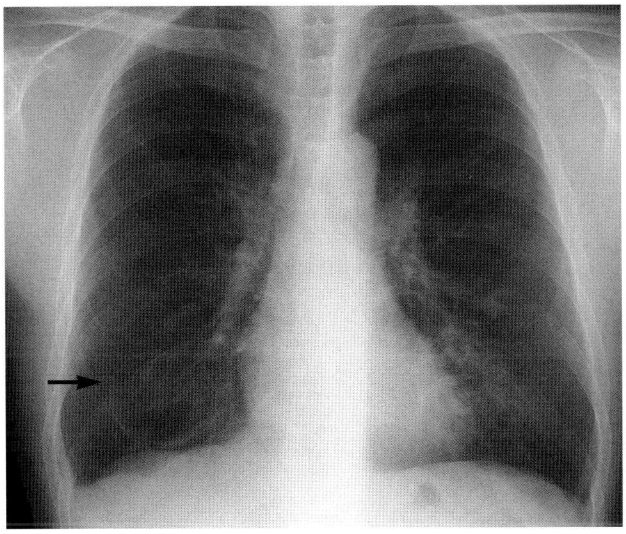

a

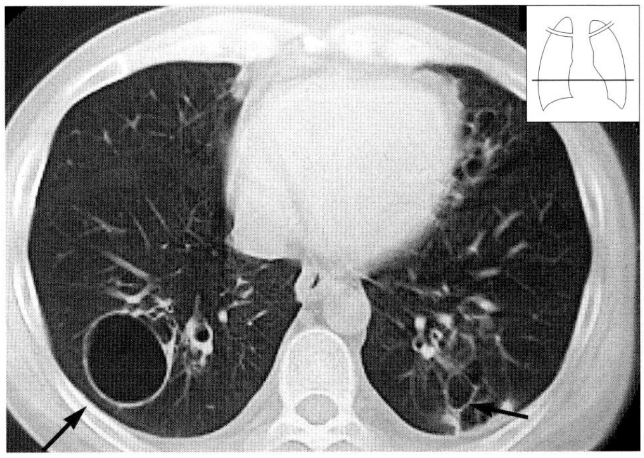

b

Figure 13 a–b. **Cystic bronchiectasis**

F. Abnormal linear shadow : Lines not usually observed

1. Bronchial lesion: Various linear shadows caused by thickening of bronchial walls

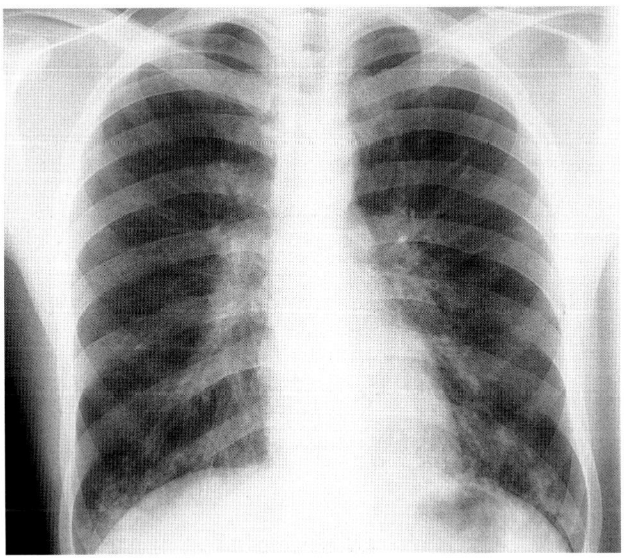

a

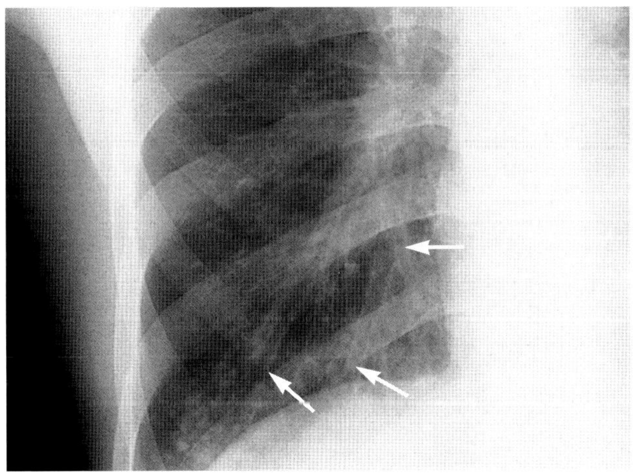

b

Figure 14 a–b. **Bronchiectasis. (b) Magnified imaging**

2. Other linear shadows due to various causes

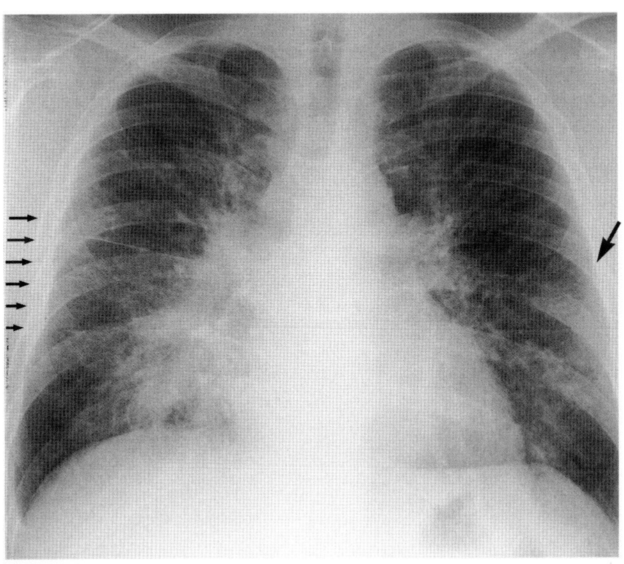

a

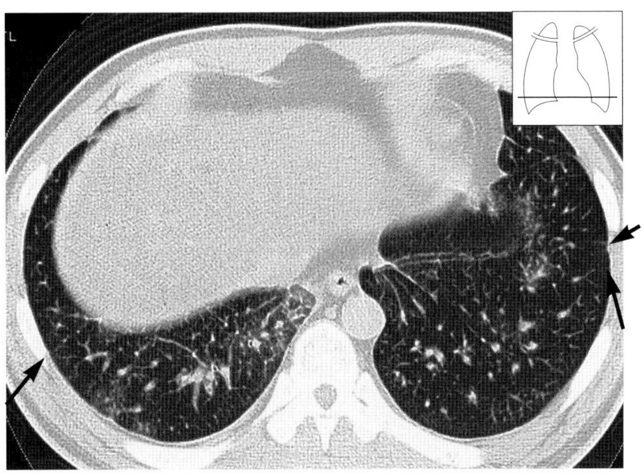

b

Figure 15 a–b. **Lymphangitic carcinomatosis from gastric cancer**

G. Hilar enlargement

1. Hilar lymphadenopathy: Swelling of hilar lymph nodes with enhanced shadow

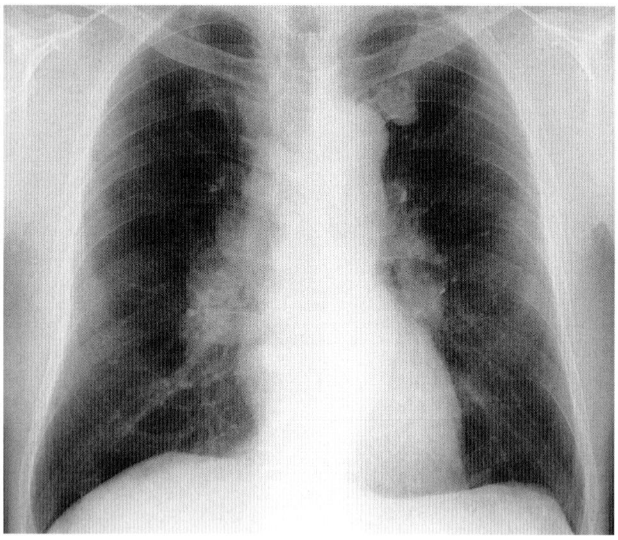

a

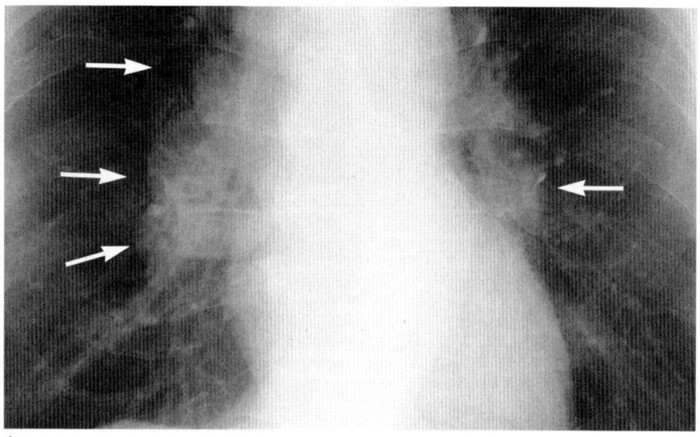

b

Figure 16 a–b. **Sarcoidosis. (b) Magnified imaging**

2. Hilar vascular enlargement (pulmonary artery shadow, etc.)

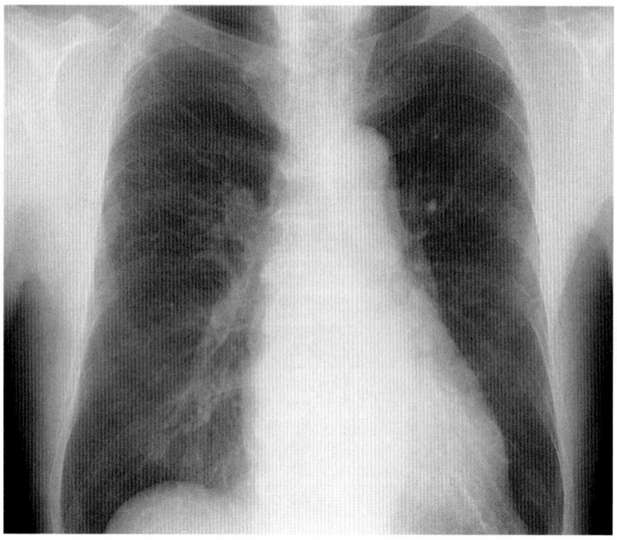

a

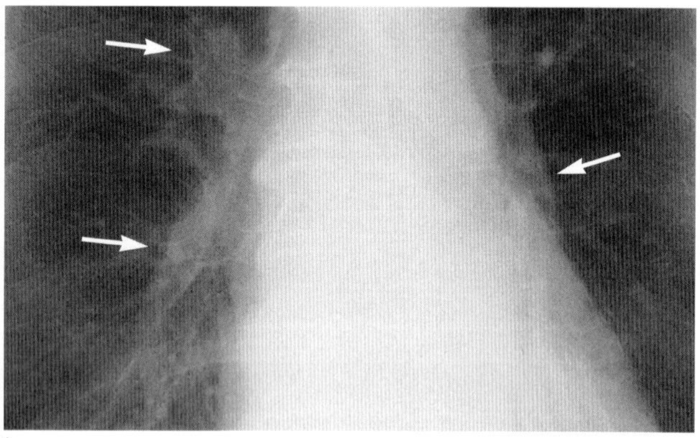

b

Figure 17 a–b. **Pulmonary hypertension. (b) Magnified imaging**

Note: Increase of pulmonary markings through vascular and bronchial lesions

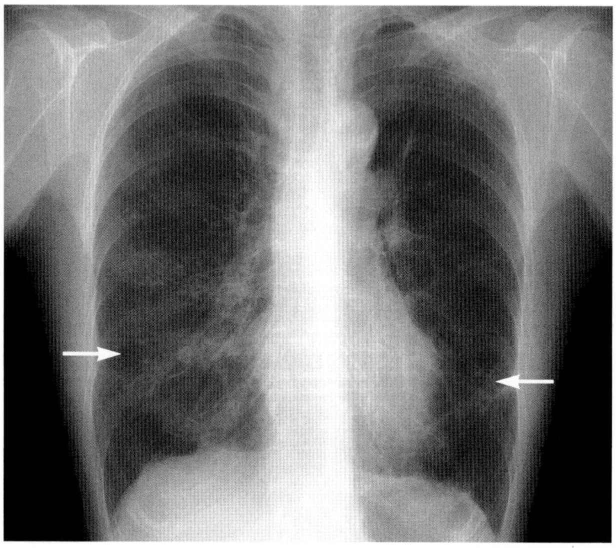

a

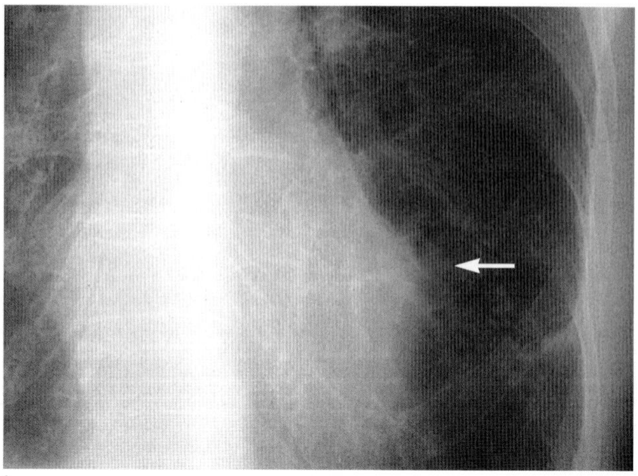

b

Figure 18 a–b. **Chronic bronchitis (enhanced markings). (b) Magnified imaging**

Note: Decrease of pulmonary markings

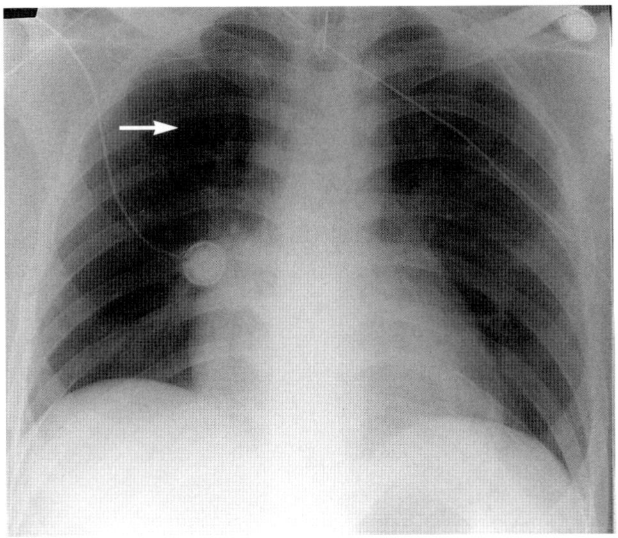

a

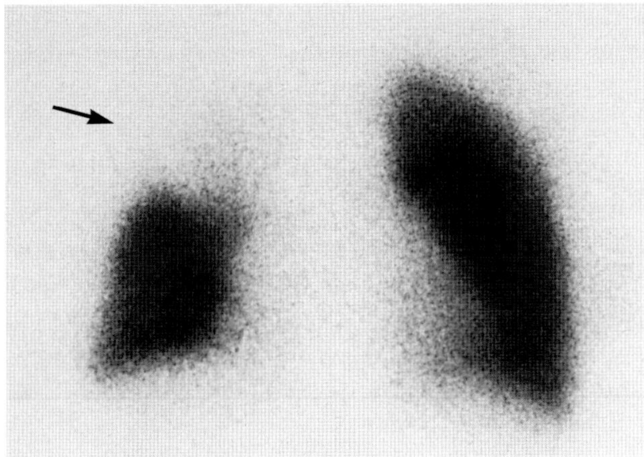

b

Figure 19 a–b. **Pulmonary embolism: decreased pulmonary markings. (b) Scintigram**

H. Calcification: Abnormal calcified shadow in the lung and the mediastinum

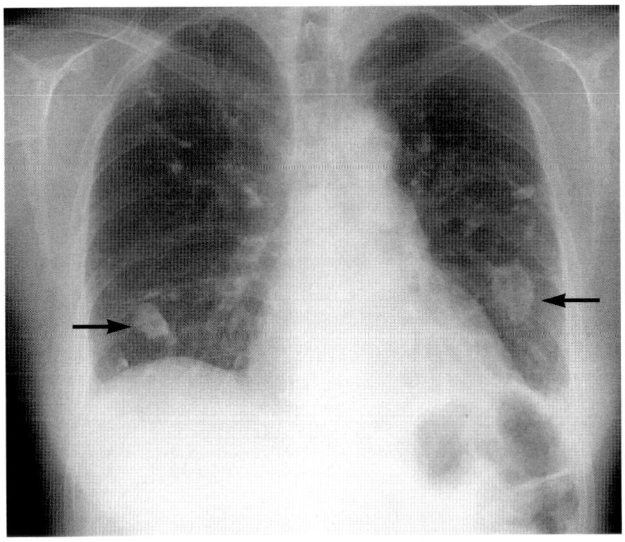

a

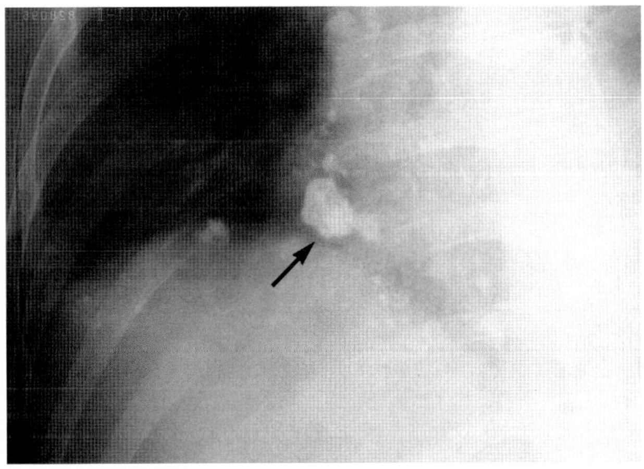

b

Figure 20 a–b. **Calcification of old tuberculous lesion. (b) Magnified imaging**

V. Mediastinal lesions with decreased or increased radiolucency

Abnormal shadow in the mediastinum

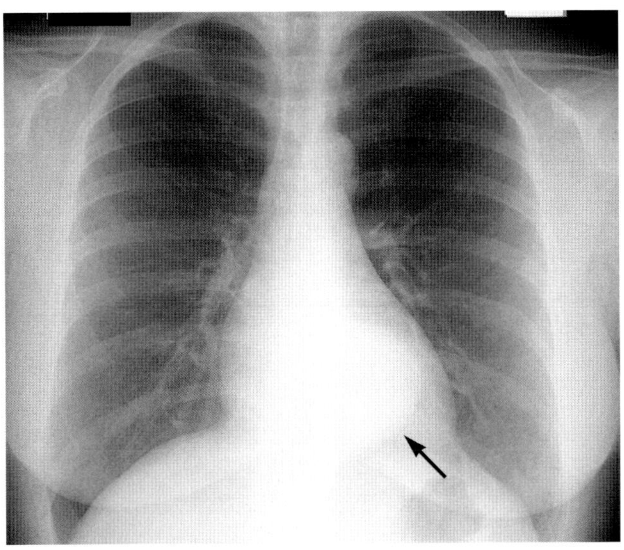

a

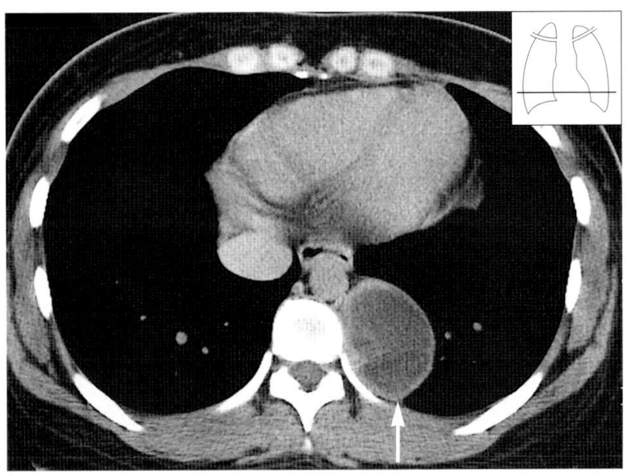

b

Figure 21 a–b. **Mediastinal tumor: neurilemmoma**

Chest CT

Chest computer tomography (CT) shows latent lesions and smaller abnormalities more effectively than conventional chest radiographic examinations. Properties of a shadow are shown in greater detail. At present CT has made progress in various directions including 3-D CT, detailed observation of lesions and functional analysis of organs. Clear identification of the relationships between pathological and morphological changes is regarded as the ultimate objective of CT. If this objective is established, it will stand as a landmark in the study of airway diseases. One of the purposes of this book is to elucidate in detail the significance of CT versus conventional radiographs. Chest CT shows a cross-section of the thorax, which is quite unlike the morphology based on classical anatomy. Following are a series of CT images of the lungs of a healthy person in 1 cm slices at 2 cm intervals. Transverse lines show corresponding height in chest radiograph.

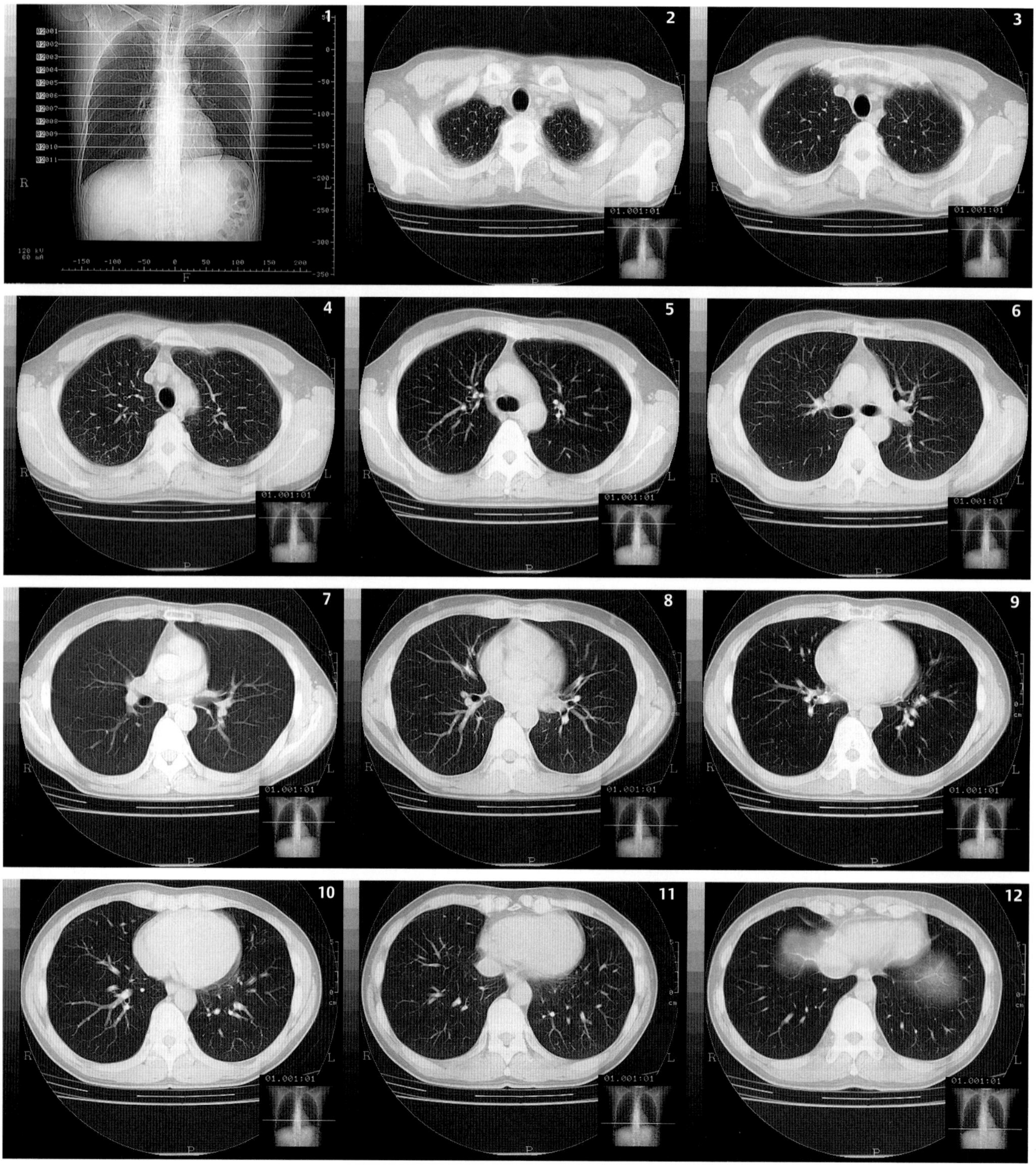

Figure 22. **Chest CT of normal lungs**

Comparison of chest CT with corresponding position in conventional chest radiograph

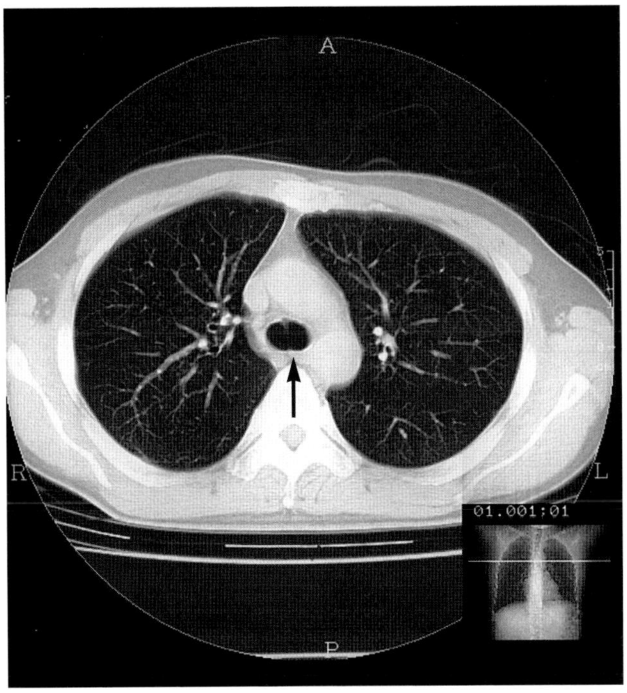

a. Level of bifurcation of trachea

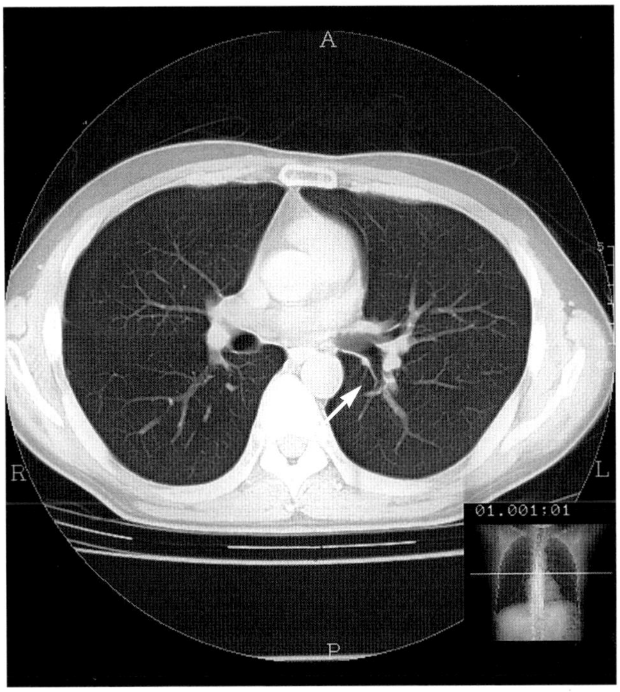

b. Level of bifurcation of left side B^6

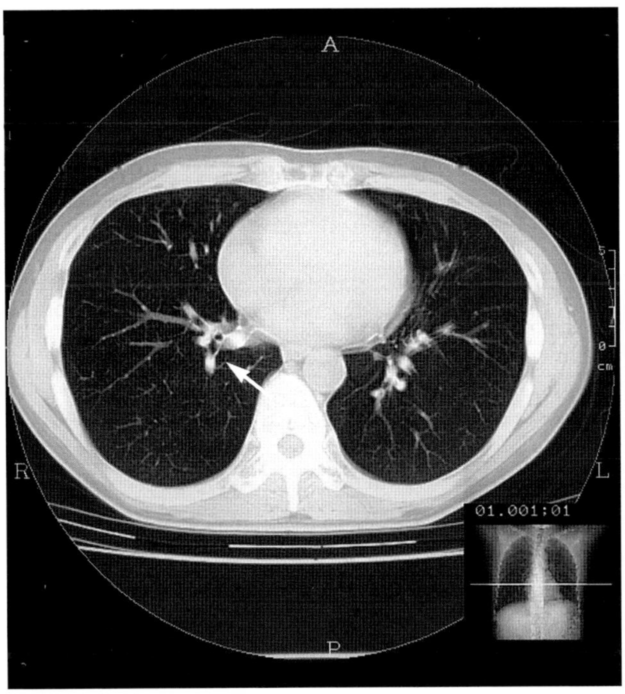

c. Level of bifurcation of right basal bronchus

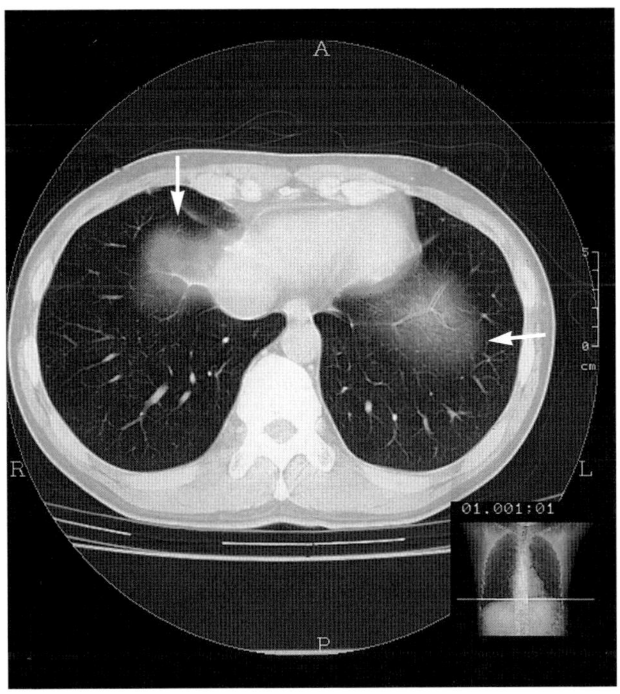

d. Level at which the diaphragm appears

Figure 23 a–d. **Chest CT**

Thinking process of Pattern Classification

This book tries to explain how to understand abnormal shadows based on pattern classification and to seek ways to their diagnosis. Chest radiograph interpretation is merely an observation, the same as looking at pictures showing general outlines of organ abnormalities, and does not go into their origins. It is not permissible to make a final diagnosis based on radiographs alone. In other words, imaging diagnosis of the chest can not be a qualitative diagnosis. We must proceed to the next step of definitely confirming or rejecting conceivable differential diagnoses suggested by pattern classification by means of pertinent diagnostic methods. Parallel applications of chest CT have widened the information obtained from conventional chest radiographs. The authors will show this fact in the course of this book.

In utilizing pattern classification, we stress the importance of pathological and morphological changes in the background of imaging.

First, the alveolar space and its supporting tissue of interstitium were considered and three types of lesions were differentiated: namely those of the alveolar space, interstitium or both. Lesions of the alveolar space decrease radiolucency through the presence of retention, or through lack of air, which correspond to pneumonia and atelectasis, respectively. When the interstitium was regarded as the main site of lesions, they were classified into granulomatous and fibrous lesions by shadow characteristics. This distinction is not always clear-cut. When the lesions affect almost equally both the alveolar space and interstitium, as in the case of pulmonary edema, they may be classified into the pulmonary edema pattern and the reverse pulmonary edema pattern from chest radiograph findings.

Nodular lesions may be regarded as tumor-like lesions or large granulomatous lesions. This classification is important, as it is logical to assume that a solitary tumor is primary while multiple tumors are metastatic lung cancer. However, caution is indicated because this assumption is not always true. This sign has gained in importance with the increase of lung cancer cases. Moreover, diagnosis based on radiographs only is difficult. Auxiliary diagnostic methods should be utilized.

Relatively large ring shadows, such as those caused by cavities and cysts, are frequently observed. As they are classified by wall thickness, the classification does not always agree with the pathological one. These lesions are caused by various diseases, some of which are serious or rare. We must remind you that the presence of a cavity suggests tuberculosis.

We sometimes observe abnormal linear shadows, especially Kerley's lines, which give important hints for diagnosis. They include many important bronchial lesions which are sometimes indicated in radiographs by the condition of the bronchial wall.

Enlargement of hilar shadows was exemplified by hilar lymph nodes and dilated blood vessels. I should also mention the so-called enhancement of pulmonary markings. The interpretation of pulmonary vascular markings in chest radiograph findings needs experience and is not very easy.

Shadows caused by pleural lesions are usually readily visible, but their differential diagnosis is not always easy. Diagnosis of mediastinal lesions has made great progress through the introduction of CT. But the difficulty of definite diagnosis, together with the lack of diagnostic methods, remains a problem.

I have tried to conduct pattern classification with the above-mentioned thoracic shadows. I expect the authors of each chapter will amplify the explanations for the reader.

Chapter 2

Radiographs of extrapulmonary and intrapulmonary lesions with increased radiolucency

Increased radiolucency

[Pattern classification I & II]

●Author — Atsushi Nagai

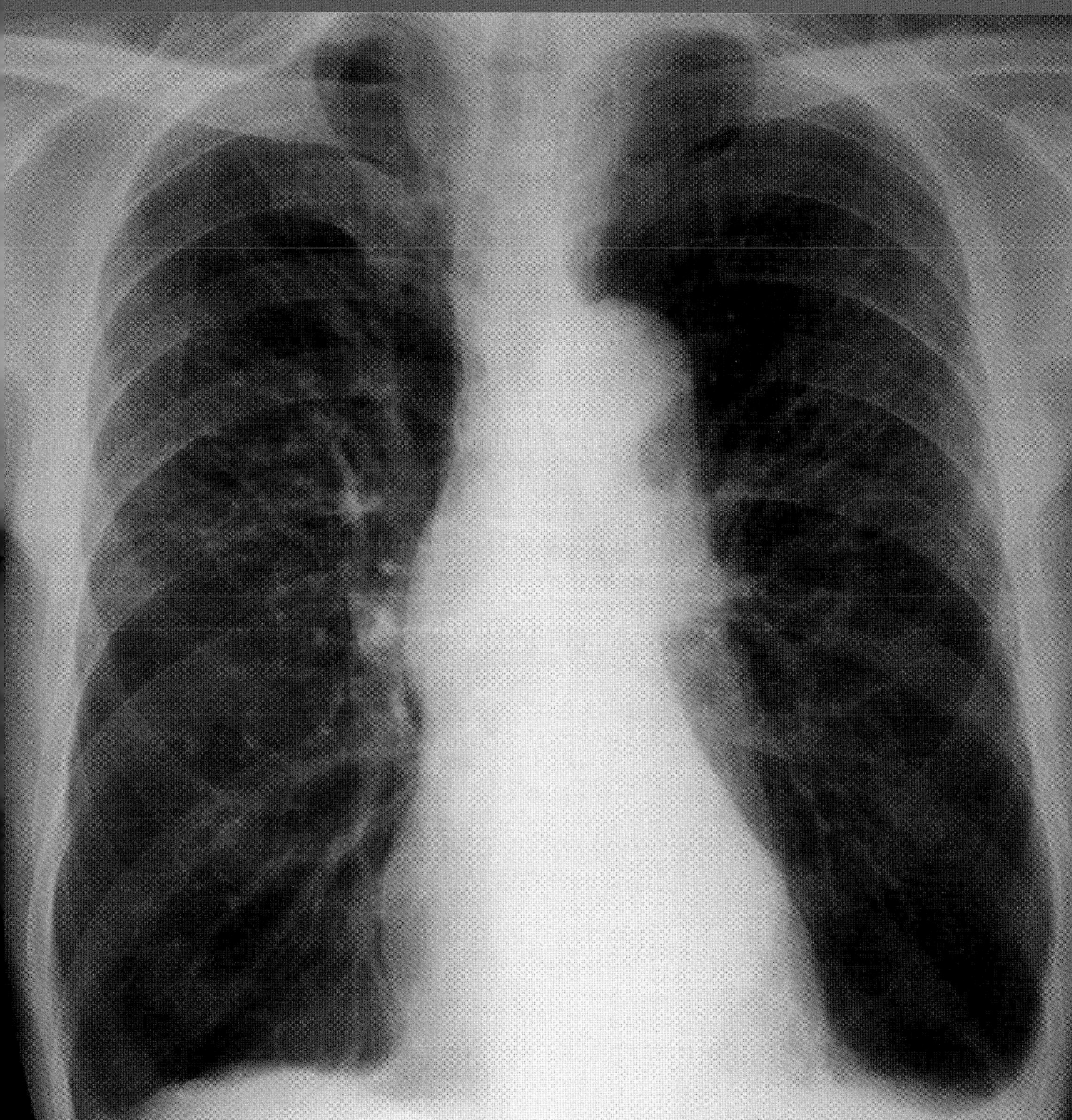

Keywords of this chapter

Dyspnea
Rhonchi
Low attenuation areas
Smoking
Chronic obstructive pulmonary disease (COPD)
Pulmonary emphysema
Alpha-1 antitrypsin deficiency
Ventilation-perfusion scintigraphy
Pneumothorax
Cyanosis
Bronchoscopic examination
Ultrasound

Increased radiolucency

Atsushi Nagai
Director of Tokyo Women's Medical University Hospital, Tokyo, Japan

Increased radiolucency is seen in diseases in which gases account for a larger ratio than tissue. The fundamental pathology is an increase in the volume of intrapulmonary air due to airway obstruction and/or reduced or interrupted blood flow due to pulmonary vascular obstruction. This chapter deals with the essential points concerning differential diagnosis of diseases indicating these findings.

Case 1 64-year-old male

Chief complaints: Dyspnea on exertion, palpitations
Medical history: Hives from the age of about 62
Smoking history: 25/day for 38 years
Present illness:
The patient had been healthy, but after he began suffering from palpitations and dyspnea from about a year ago he received a medical examination at a hospital specializing in cardiovascular diseases. He underwent cardiac examination and was told there were no abnormalities. Following this, he received regular medical examinations that indicated no abnormalities. However, as the palpitations and shortness of breath on exertion continued, he underwent thorough examination at this department.
Physical findings:
The findings were height 169 cm, weight 53 kg, body temperature 36.1°C, blood pressure 140/88, pulse 78/min, respiration rate with costo-abdominal respiration 16/min, no edema or cyanosis observed. No clubbed finger. Sternocleidomastoid muscle on the neck somewhat noticeable, with beer barrel shaped thorax and tapping producing a drum sound. Auscultation of the thorax indicated reduced respiratory sound and wheezing was heard, with rhonchi during forced expiration.
Laboratory data:
Arterial blood gas analysis indicated mildly reduced PaO_2 levels while respiratory function tests showed severe obstructive ventilatory impairment which was not improved by bronchodilation agents. A precise investigation of respiratory function showed a low value for pulmonary diffusing capacity (D_{LCO}), and increased static lung compliance.
Imaging findings:
In a plain chest radiograph (P. 13), in the bilateral lung field vascular shadows have disappeared, and increased radiolucency can be seen. The diaphragm is in a lower position while the thin, vertical cardiac contour is seen as a tear-drop heart shape.

A lateral chest radiograph (*Fig. 1*) shows enlarged retrosternal space (→) with the diaphragm low and flat and an angle of 90° or more between the sternum and diaphragm (➤).

High-resolution chest CT (*Fig. 2*) shows low-attenuation areas in all slices with enlarged air spaces (➤) occupying most of the lung, clearly indicating tissue loss in the alveolar parenchymal area.

These findings are observed in chest CT at both TLC and RV lung capacities.

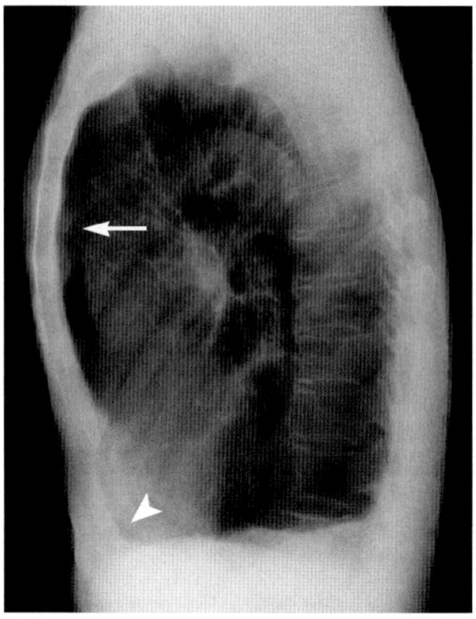

Figure 1. **Chest radiograph**

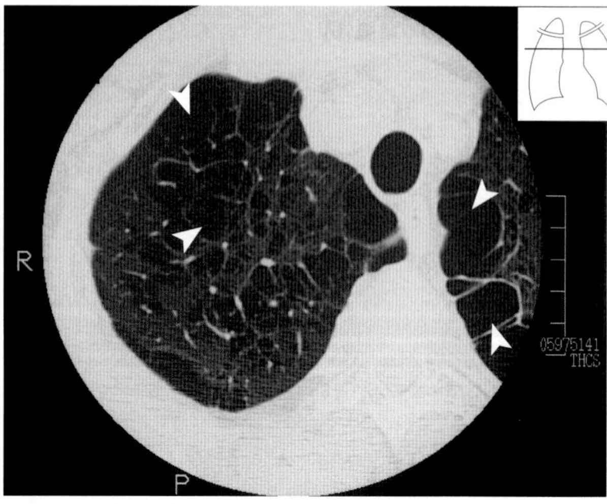

Figure 2. **High-resolution CT**

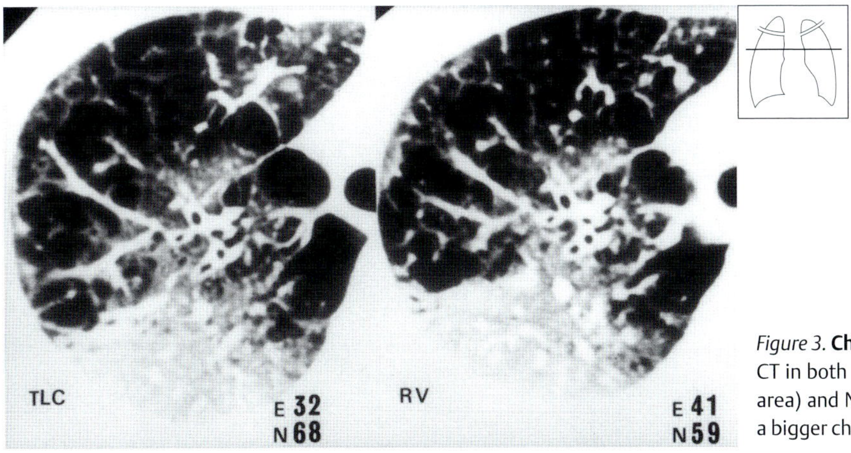

Figure 3. **Chest CT**
CT in both TLC and RV. The ratios of area for E (emphysematous area) and N (normal area) are indicated. Lung capacity indicates a bigger change in the normal area.

Diagnosis

Due to habitual smoking and dyspnea during exertion, chronic obstructive pulmonary disease was suspected. Respiratory function tests showed reduced pulmonary diffusing capacity and precise function tests showed increased pulmonary compliance, indicating the possibility of pulmonary emphysema. Chest radiographs showed findings of overinflation and the major change in pulmonary construction of enlarged air spaces, a distinctive indication of emphysematous change, was observed, leading to a diagnosis of pulmonary emphysema.

Conclusions of this case: Pulmonary emphysema

This case was an elderly male with a history of smoking, with dyspnea on exertion. Respiratory function tests indicated obstructive ventilatory impairment, and there were findings of overinflation and abnormal enlargement of air spaces on chest radiographs, from which pulmonary emphysema was diagnosed.

Pathomorphologically, pulmonary emphysema is defined as a disease in which air spaces are enlarged and the walls that create the air spaces are destroyed. Depending on the distribution of the lesions, the disease is classified as centrilobular emphysema, panlobular emphysema or paraseptal emphysema (*Fig. 4*). Among these, the two types that cause clinical problems due to abnormal pulmonary function are centrilobular emphysema, which destroys tissue architecture predominantly in the respiratory bronchiole, and panlobular emphysema, in which lesions are distributed throughout the entire pulmonary acinus.

Centrilobular emphysema is often seen in smokers, while panlobular emphysema is often seen in patients with Alpha-1 antitrypsin deficiency. Differentiation of these two types of emphysema using chest radiographs is possible up to the moderate stage of the disease at the most. Once the disease has progressed to the stage where there are severe lesions, architectural destruction is the only thing that can be observed throughout the lung field.

Definite diagnosis requires agreement with the pathomorphological definition. Clinically, when symptoms, a history of smoking, nonreversible obstructive ventilatory impairment and reduced pulmonary diffusing capacity are suspected, and when plain chest radiographs show findings of overinflation and reduced vascular shadow, many cases are diagnosed as pulmonary emphysema. In recent years, since low attenuation areas in chest CT indicate emphysematous lesions, the trend has been towards the use of CT examination. Chest radiographs and pulmonary function tests enable accurate diagnosis of emphysema up to and beyond the moderate stage of the disease.

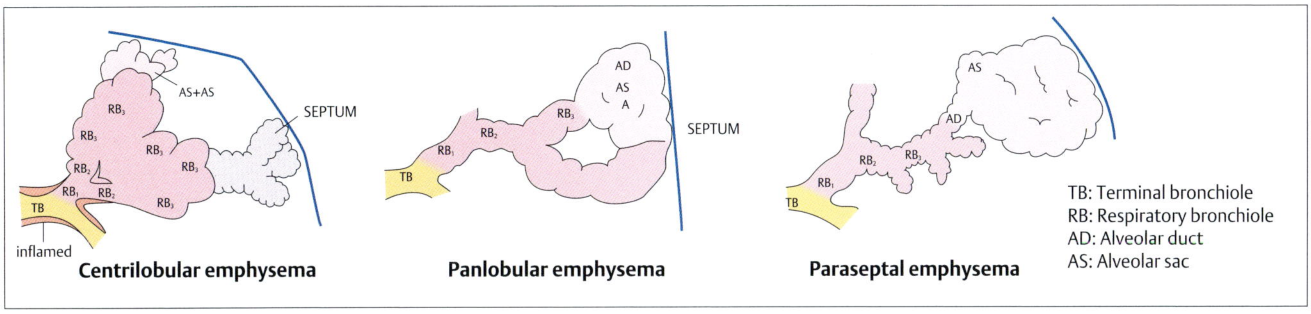

Figure 4. **Schematic diagrams of pulmonary emphysema**

Differentiation of diseases indicating increased radiolucency

Increased radiolucency indicated on chest radiographs is due to 1) reduction or loss of extrapulmonary soft tissue, 2) loss of lung parenchyma, 3) pulmonary overinflation, and 4) reduced intrapulmonary blood flow. In almost all cases, the addition of CT examination enables the cause to be inferred. If no abnormalities are confirmed with CT examination, consider conducting bronchoscopic examination for endotracheal lesions, ventilation-perfusion scintigraphy for vascular lesions, angiography and other examinations. The *Table* below indicates cause and diseases, and *Figure 5* indicates diagnostic procedure.

	Causative disease	
	Bilateral lung field increased radiolucency	Unilateral lung field increased radiolucency
Increased volume of air in lungs	Chronic pulmonary emphysema Bronchial asthma (during attack) Pulmonary cysts Acute bronchiolitis Bronchiolitis obliterans organizing pneumonia Tracheal foreign body Laryngeal tumor Endotracheal tumor	Giant bulla Lung cancer Metastatic lung cancer Bronchial tuberculosis Bronchial atresia Bronchial foreign body Compensatory hyperinflation Swyer-James syndrome
Reduced pulmonary blood flow	Pulmonary embolism Congenital heart disease (Diseases with left/right shunt and reduced pulmonary blood flow)	Pulmonary embolism Vascular invasion due to central lung cancer, lymph node swelling Aortitis with pulmonary artery involvement Pulmonary artery loss of hypoplasia
Increased volume of extrapulmonary air		Pneumothorax
Decreased soft tissue	Following bilateral mastectomy Leptosomatic body type	Following unilateral mastectomy Congenital absence of pectoral muscles (Poland syndrome)

Table. **Increased lung field radiolucency classification and major causative diseases**
(Taken from the reference literature, partially changed)

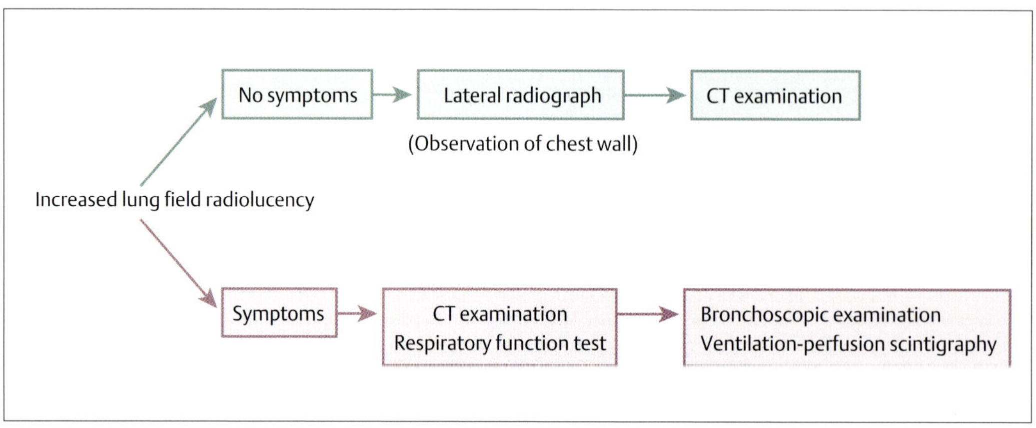

Figure 5. **Diagnostic procedure**

Case 2 Pneumothorax
32-year-old male

A plain chest radiograph shows complete disappearance of vascular shadow on the right lung, with formation of a mass in the hilum of the collapsed lung. There is enlarged intercostal space on the pneumothorax side, with shifting of the mediastinum to the opposite side, from which it can be inferred that escaped air has increased extrapulmonary pressure resulting in tension pneumothorax.

For some reason, tension pneumothorax occurs when a hole to the thoracic cavity functions as a one-way valve that lets air into the thoracic cavity during inspiration but does not allow it out during expiration. In many cases there is sudden intense respiration, cynanosis, tachycardia and perspiration, with reduced respiratory movement, and analysis of arterial blood indicates marked hypoxemia. Insertion of a thoracic cavity tube is required to immediately release the air.

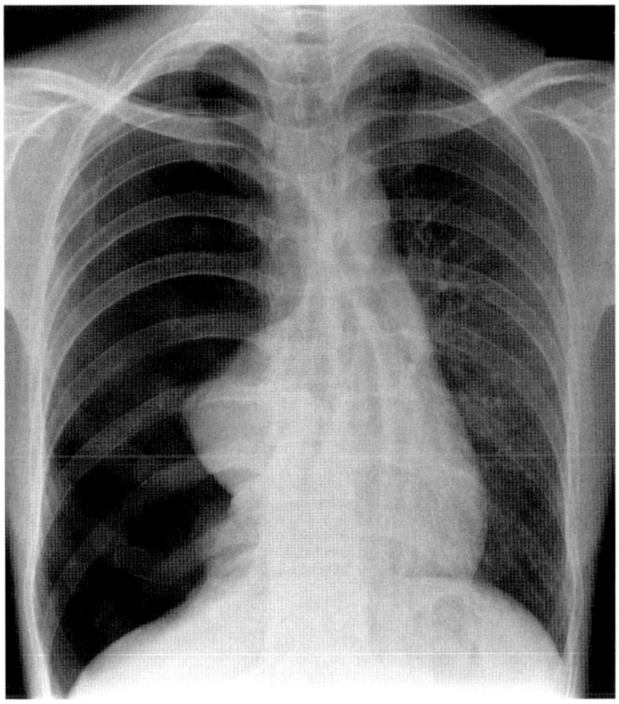

Figure 6. **Chest radiograph**

Case 3 Pneumothorax
67-year-old male

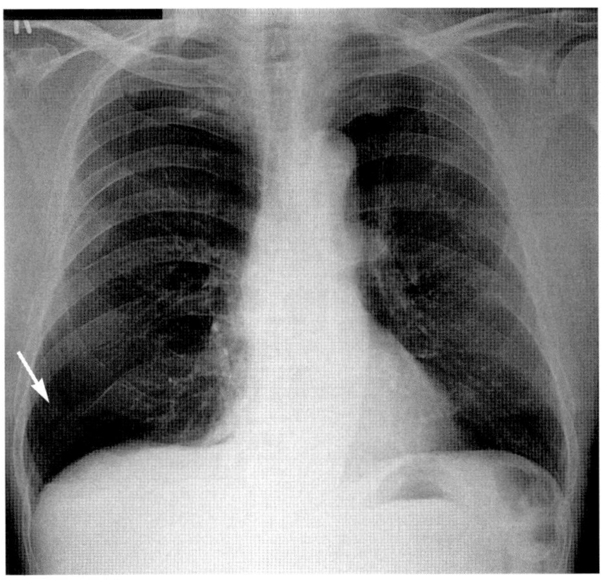

Figure 7. **Chest radiograph**

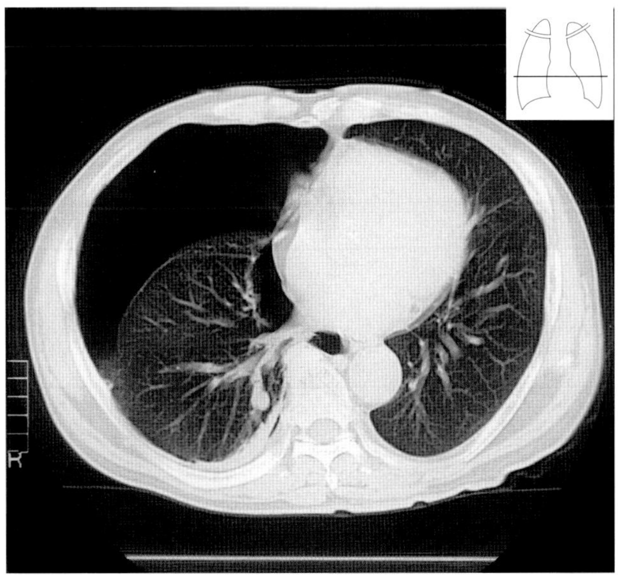

Figure 8. **Chest CT**

A plain frontal chest radiograph shows that avascularization has occurred in parts of the lower right lung field resulting in an area of increased radiolucency (→). Since the visceral pleural line (boundary of the collapsed lung) is visible, pneumothorax is suspected.

A chest CT shows moderate collapse of the lower lobe, indicating more clearly than can be inferred with a plain chest radiograph the severe collapse of the lung.

For chest examinations, CT is a more useful detection method and offers a clearer depiction of the severity of the disease. At the same time, CT is also useful for detecting underlying diseases of the chest such as emphysematous lesions and cancer lesions.

Case 4 Pulmonary thromboembolism

52-year-old male

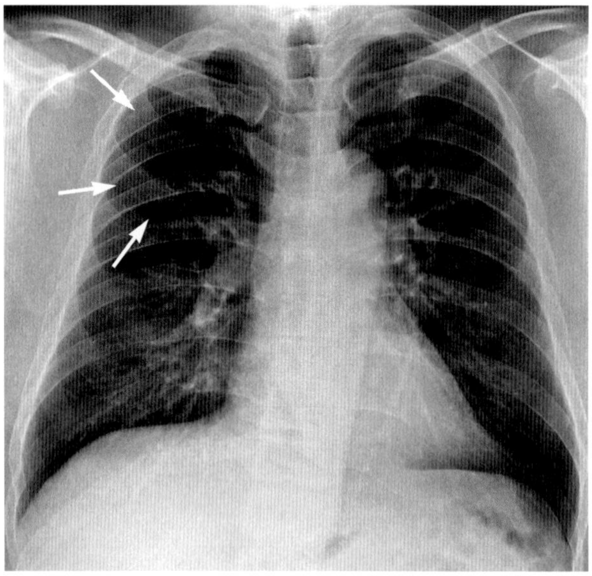

Figure 9. **Chest radiograph**

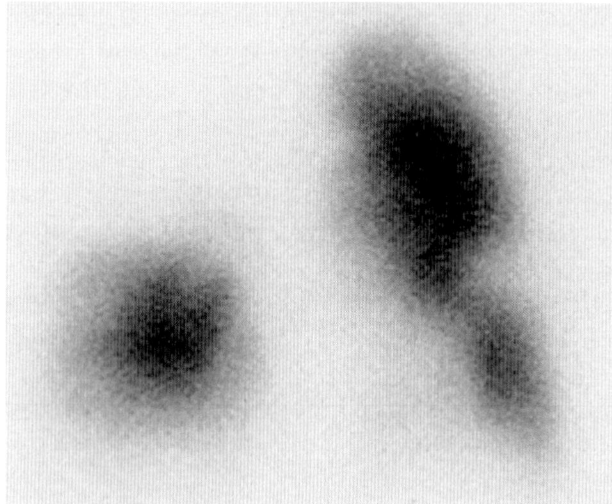

Figure 10. **Pulmonary blood flow scintigraph**

A plain frontal chest radiograph shows partially increased radiolucency in the right lung (→), with central pulmonary arterial dilation. There is no evidence of overinflation of the lung.

A pulmonary blood flow scintigraph shows reduced blood flow to the left lung.

Case 5 Bronchiolitis obliterans organizing pneumonia

45-year-old female

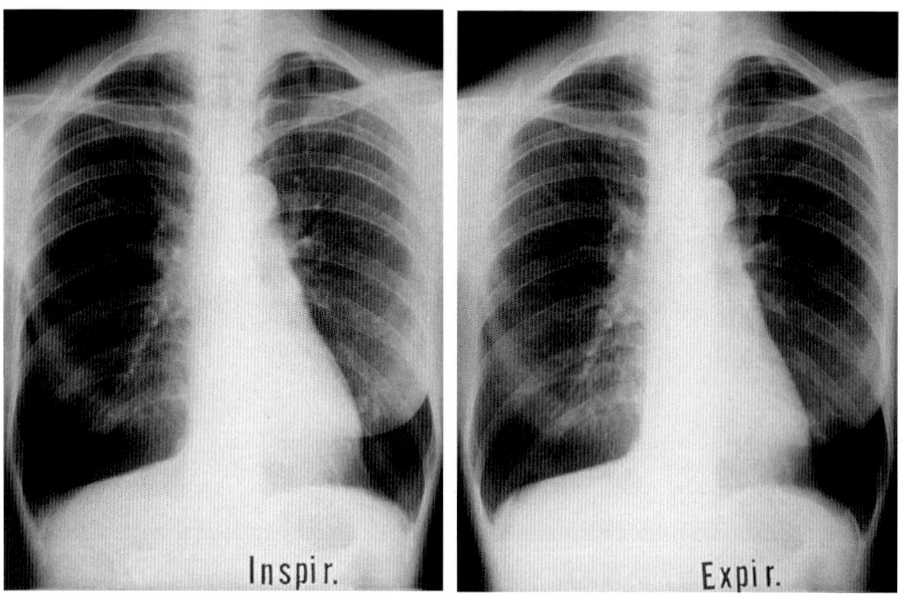

Figure 11. **Chest radiograph**

A plain frontal chest radiograph (*Fig. 11*) indicates increased radiolucency in the entire lung fields of both lungs, with the diaphragm located at the 11th intercostal space indicating overinflation, and no respiratory changes seen.

A bronchogram (*Fig. 12*) shows that from the segmental branch, at the respiratory tract periphery on multiple planes there is tapered stenosis and a semicircular image of occlusion. At the same time, almost no peripheral respiratory tract contrast is observed, suggesting that from the small bronchi to the bronchiole there is organic stenosis and obstruction over an extensive area.

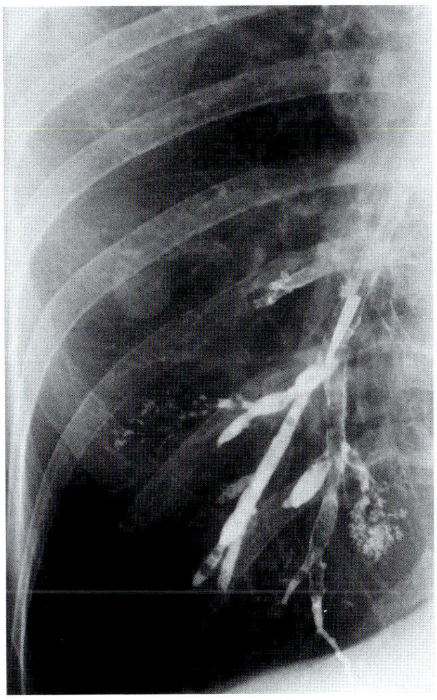

Figure 12. **Bronchial contrast**

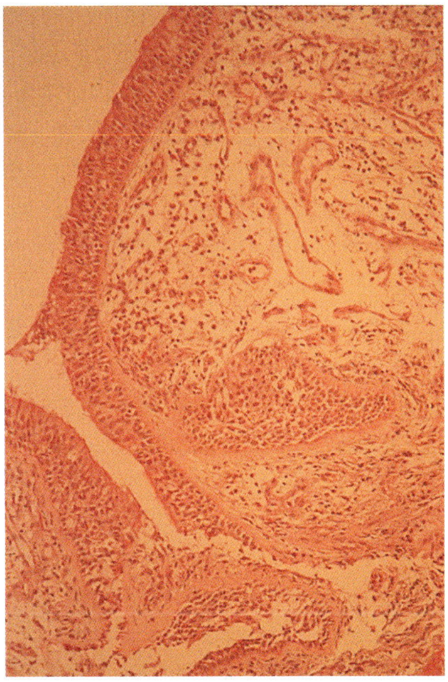

Figure 14. **Respiratory tract mucous membrane biopsy tissue**

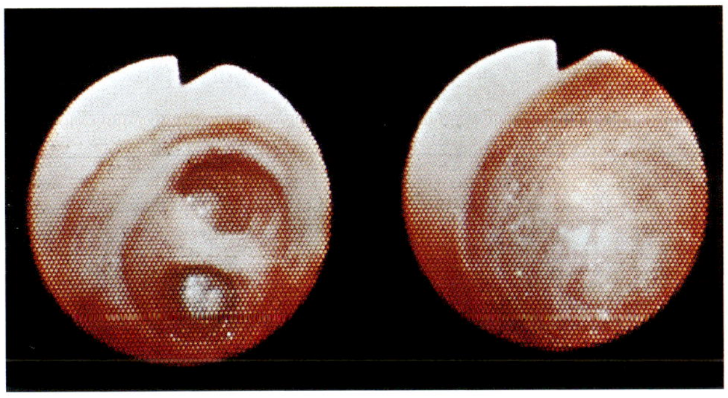

Figure 13. **Bronchoscopic findings**

A bronchoscopic examination indicated that at the B^9b bronchus, the 5th level respiratory tract is conical, with obstruction observed (*Fig. 13*).

In an examination of respiratory tract mucous membrane biopsy tissue, nonspecific inflammation from the lamina propria mucosae to the submucosa was observed (*Fig. 14*), resulting in a diagnosis of bronchiolitis obliterans organizing pneumonia.

Case 6 Mastectomy (mammary cancer)

72-year-old female

In the right lung there is thickening of the pleura over a wide area and calcification resulting in reduced radiolucency. In contrast, radiolucency of the left lung is uniformly increased. The disappearance of the pectoralis major muscle and mammary shadows is probably due to the mastectomy.

Radiolucency of the lung field is strongly influenced by chest wall characteristics. If the patient is thin, radiolucency increases for lung fields on both sides. For females, as in this case, radiolucency increases after a mastectomy, so it is important to pay full attention to chest wall characteristics when interpreting chest radiographs.

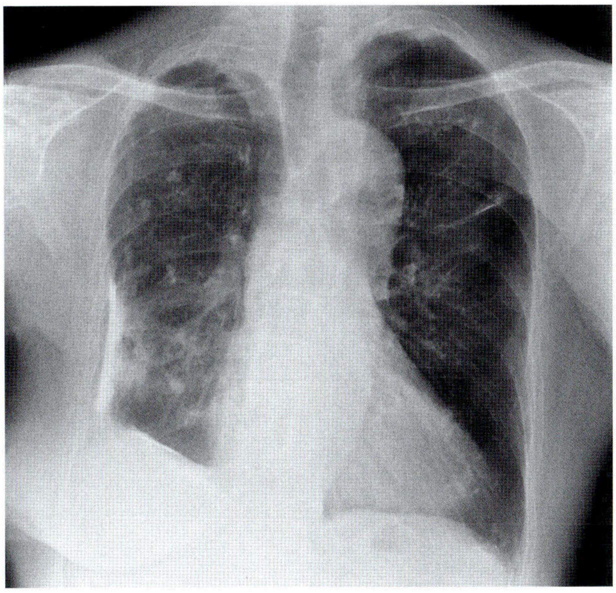

Figure 15. **Chest radiograph**

Conclusion

When looking at a radiograph with increased radiolucency, it is necessary to carefully confirm whether this abnormality is due to intrathoracic lesions or because of overexposure when filming or chest wall characteristics. To prevent increased radiolucency occurring due to chest wall characteristics or filming conditions, factors that can influence radiolucency must be confirmed. This includes checking that the radiographic examination was taken at the proper position, that there are no marked abnormalities in the thickness of the muscle or fatty layers, that the film is not overexposed, and that the roentgenogram is taken during proper deep inspiration.

Having taken into account the above points, in cases of suspected intrathoracic lesion, confirm whether it is unilateral or bilateral, whether increased radiolucency is uniform throughout the entire lung field, and discern whether in some areas it is localized.

In general, CT is used to differentiate between diseases that cause increased radiolucency. With CT at the lung window setting it is possible to detect bronchiole lesions and other factors that cause cystic diseases such as emphysematous lesions, and peripheral respiratory tract obstruction. On the other hand, when using a contrast agent with CT at the mediastinal window setting it is possible to infer the presence of lesions in bordering areas causing stenosis, and a thrombus causing decreased pulmonary blood flow. When respiratory tract or vascular stenosis (obstruction) is suspected, precise tests, such as bronchoscopic examination, ultrasound tests and nuclear medical tests are required.

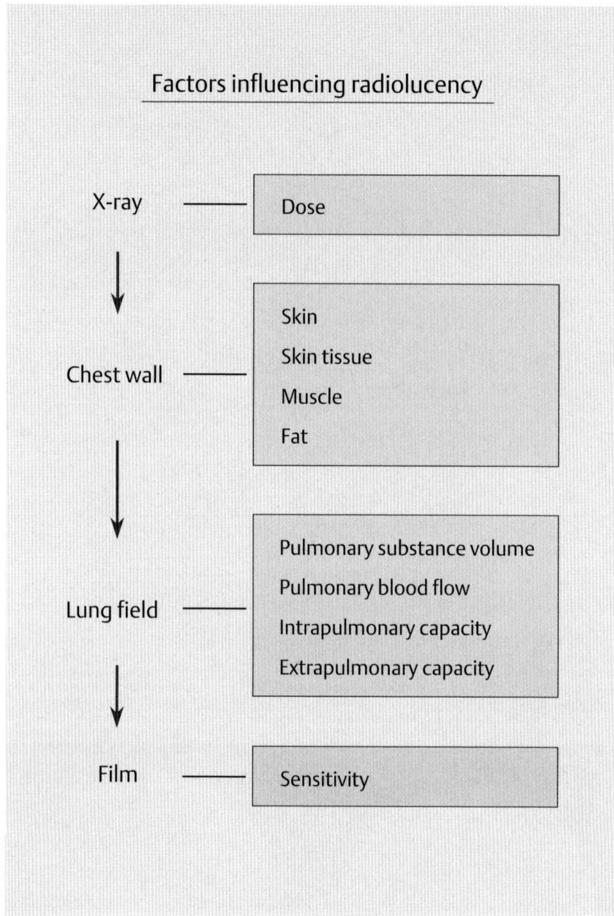

Figure 16.

References

1) Takashi Inoue: Increased radiolucency. Respiratory organ diagnosis using X-ray patterns (Atsushi Nagai, Minoru Kanazawa edition). Chugai Pharmaceutical Co. Ltd., Tokyo, 1999

Chapter 3

Radiographs of extrapulmonary lesions with decreased radiolucency

Pleural disease

[Pattern classification III]

●Author — Hiroshi Niwa

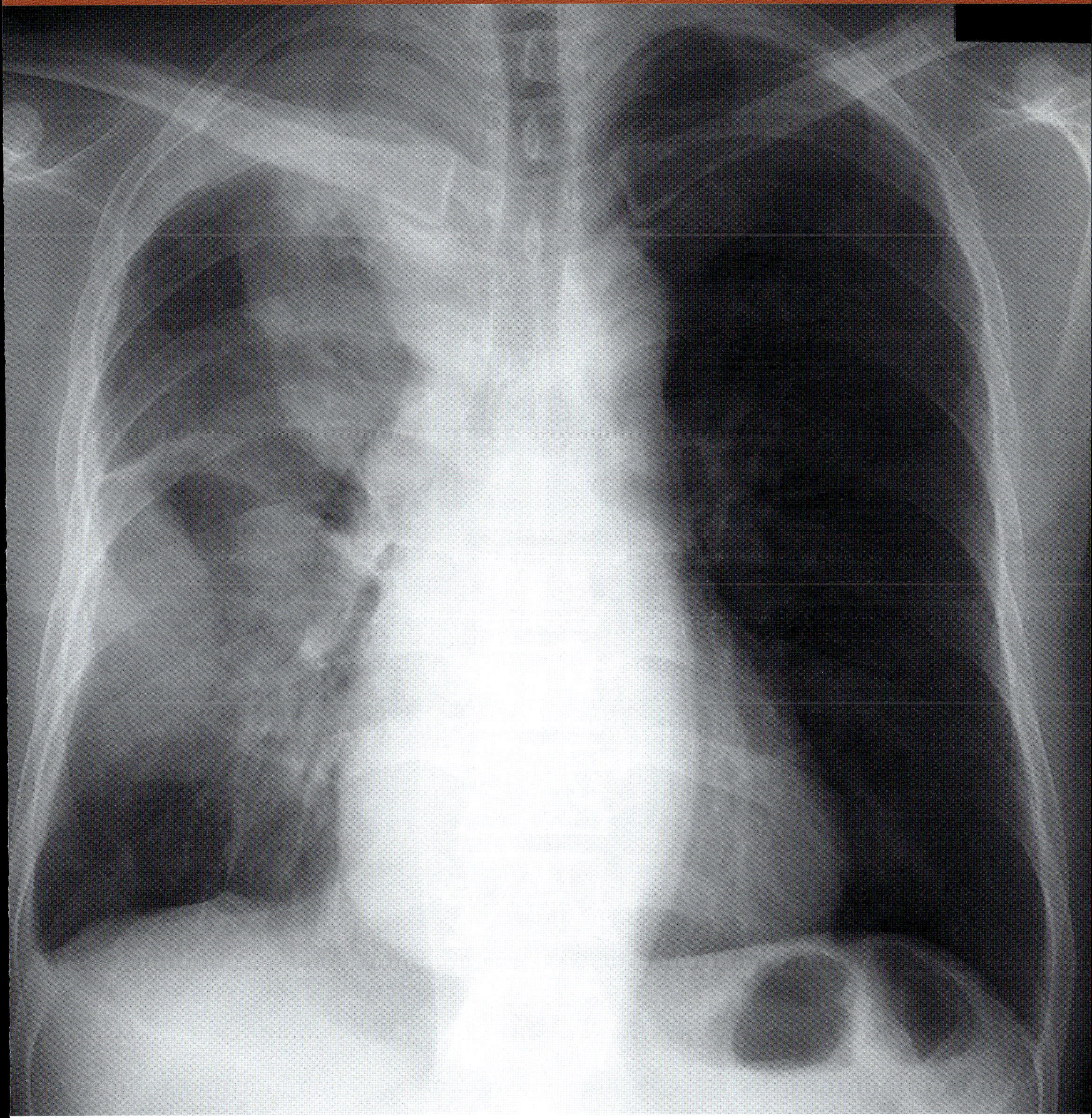

Keywords of this chapter

Malignant pleural mesothelioma
Fissural pseudotumor
Contarini's condition
Pleural plaque (asbestosis)
Solitary fibrous tumor
Loculated tuberculous empyema
Tuberculous empyema with a bronchopleural fistula
Chronic expanding empyema
Pleural effusion
Subpulmonic effusion
Encapsulated effusion
Split pleura sign
Pleural thickening
Fibrothorax

Pleural disease

Hiroshi Niwa
Respiratory Disease Center, Division of Thoracic Surgery, Seirei Mikatahara General Hospital, Hamamatsu, Shizuoka, Japan

The pleura is divided into the parietal pleura and visceral pleura. Pleural diseases occur in one or both pleura with most lesions developing in the pleural space. Since each pleura can not be observed separately except in cases of pneumothorax or conditions with fluid accumulation, it is important to assess its relationship with contiguous layers of the chest wall, lung, mediastinum, and diaphragm.

Case 1 Malignant pleural mesothelioma
53-year-old male

Chief complaints: Cough and dyspnea
Asbestos exposure: None
Smoking history: 30/day for 20 years
Present illness:
The patient had felt dyspnea since four months before. Cough and yellow sputum had started one month before. He had been febrile (37-38°C) since one week before. He visited a doctor, a chest radiographic examination revealed an abnormal shadow and he was referred to the respiratory disease center. He complained of a 7 kg weight loss. A chest thoracentesis revealed a straw-yellow jelly-like substance. The material was so thick it prevented assessment of hyaluronate and ADA levels.

Chest radiograph (frontal view) (p.21) revealed rind-like pleural thickening in the right chest and mass formation in the upper mediastinum and lateral chest. The open angle of the tracheal carina suggests a mass situated in the lower mediastinum.

Contrast-enhanced CT revealed a multi-locular cystic mass occupying the entire right pleural space. The cyst wall was enhanced (➤) and an inhomogeneous part (➞) was seen inside the mass (*Fig. 1*). The cyst was located in the mediastinal side and interlobar space. A large subcarinal mass pressed the left atrium toward the front side and stretched the right inferior pulmonary vein (➞) (*Fig. 2*).

T2-weighted coronal MRI revealed that a huge mass with increasing intensity was extending from the diaphragm to the apex. The mass in front of the lower thoracic vertebra protruded to the left side (➞) (*Fig. 3*). A multi-locular mass burying the entire pleural space was verified at thoracoscopic biopsy (*Fig. 4*). A pleuropneumonectomy combining resection of the pericardium and diaphragm was performed after the pathological diagnosis of epithelial type mesothelioma. Mediastinal lymphadenectomy was simultaneously performed.

Surgical specimen (*Fig. 5*): The whole lung was encased with thickened tumor derived from not only mediastinal and costal parietal pleura but also interlobar visceral pleura. There were white mass-like formations at the apex, interlobar space, and mediastinal side (➞).

Pathologically, the pleural lesion was diagnosed as epithelial type mesothelioma with mucous formation (*Fig. 6*). Although mesothelioma cells were also present

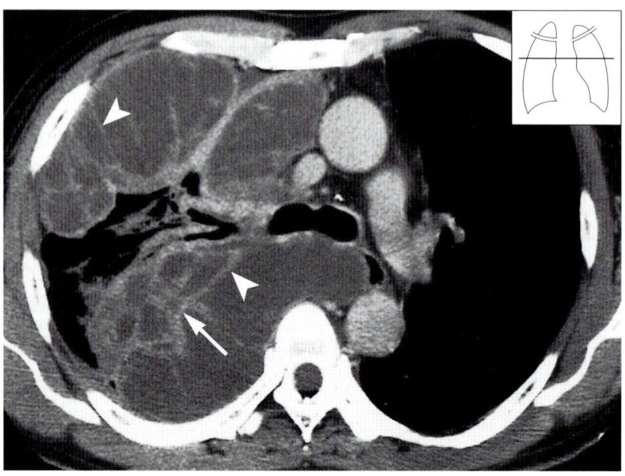

Figure 1. **Chest CT at the level of the tracheal carina**

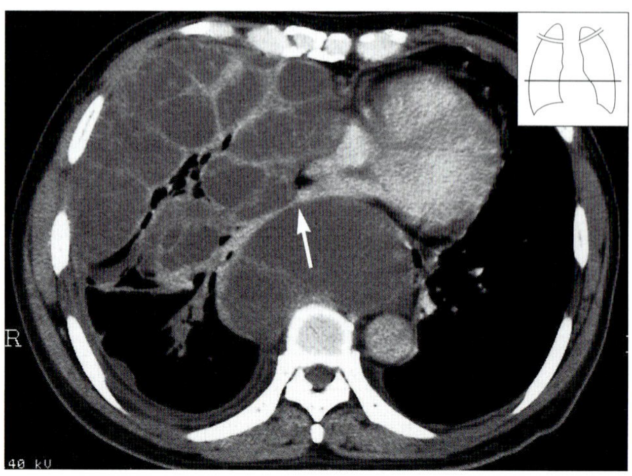

Figure 2. **Chest CT at the level of the left atrium**

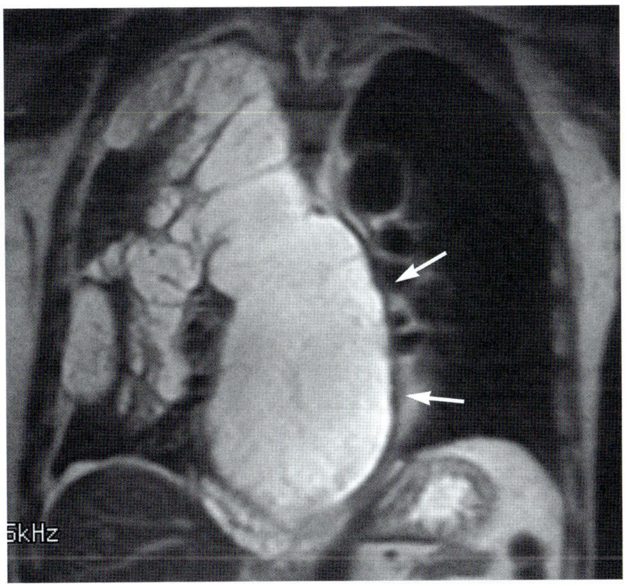

Figure 3. **Coronal T2-weighted MRI**

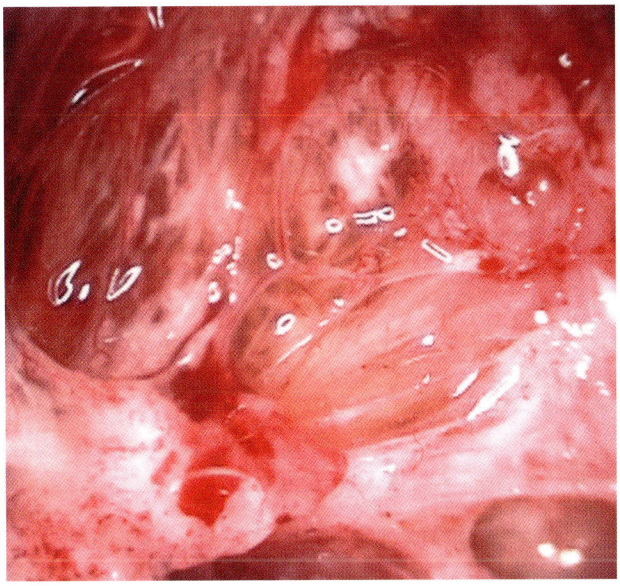

Figure 4. **Intrathoracic view at thoracoscopic biopsy**

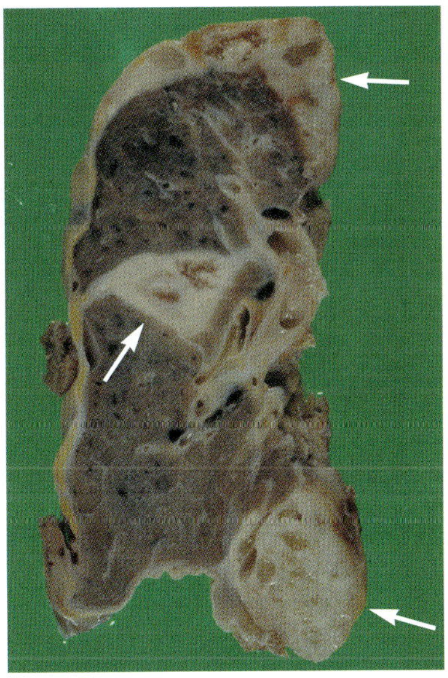

Figure 5. **Surgical specimen**

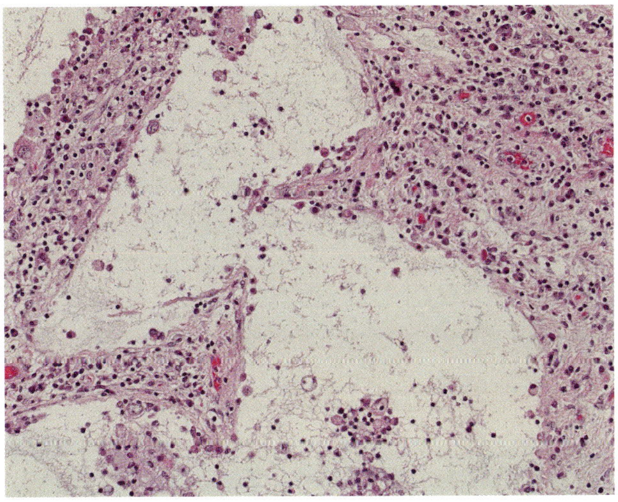

Figure 6. **Pathological finding**

in the lung extending through the lymph canal, no involvement was detected toward the outer side. The endothoracic fascia, pericardium, and diaphragm were not involved. Number 1 and number 7 lymph node metastases were observed. The diagnosis was T2N2M0 stage III mesothelioma. The patient is well without recurrence 6 years after surgery.

Summary of Case 1: Malignant pleural mesothelioma

The chest radiographic characteristics of malignant pleural mesothelioma are unilateral, diffuse, sheet-like or lobulated pleural thickening encasing the entire lung. Ordinarily, over 1 cm and irregular, or sometimes nodular, pleural thickening is found not only on the costal side but also on the mediastinal side. In cases of mucous producing cystic mesothelioma like this patient, CT demonstrates a low density mass with circumferential enhancement by contrast medium. There is often superficial invasion of the lung and extension into the interlobar fissure. Pleural effusion is observed in 80% of patients. Large fluid correction obscures the mass shadow in the chest radiograph. The tumor encasing the lung extends to the contiguous layers of the chest wall, pericardial space, contralateral thorax, and abdominal cavity. Tumor cells often extend into the lymph canal causing carcinomatous lymphangitis. Calcification is seen in 10% of cases and usually represents engulfment of calcified plaque. Rarely, it is the result of an osteosarcomatous component. Even if there is massive fluid correction, obvious mediastinal shift is not observed. The reason is that the lung–not the tumor–presses the mediastinum and the tumor develops along the configuration of the mediastinum.

Differential diagnosis of diffuse pleural thickening

Pleural thickening is diagnosed as diffuse on CT when it extends for more than 8 cm craniocaudally and 5 cm laterally, and the pleura is more than 3 mm thick. Important points for differential diagnosis are whether it is bilateral or unilateral, the presence of accompanying lesion in lung parenchyma or previous rib fracture, and the location and shape of pleural calcification (*Table*).

Differential diagnosis of pleural mass

Pleural lesions generally remain confined between the layers of the pleura and cause obtuse angles between the lesion and the chest wall (*Fig. 7*A). Pleural lesions, however, may be pedunculated, in which case they may prolapse into the pulmonary parenchyma, resulting in acute angles between the lesion and the chest wall (*Fig. 7*B) (Case 7). Pleural fibrosis may result in fusion of the parietal and visceral pleura leading to abnormal configurations of pleural lesions and/or loculation of pleural fluid which is low density with circumferential enhancement by contrast medium (*Fig. 7*C) (Case 8). Parenchymal lesions, if subpleural, abut the pleura resulting in acute angles between the lesion and the chest wall (*Fig. 7a*). Extrapleural lesions displace the overlaying parietal and visceral pleura, resulting in an obtuse angle between the lesion and the chest wall (*Fig. 7b*).

	Site	Location of lesion		Pulmonary parenchymal lesion	Location of calcification		Shape of calcification		Rib fracture
		Costal pleura	Mediastinal pleura		Visceral pleura	Parietal pleura	Sheet-like	Line or spot	
Old tuberculous pleurisy	unilateral	◎		◎	◎	○	◎		
Old hemothorax	unilateral	◎			◎	○	◎		◎
Asbestos fibrosis	bilateral	◎			○	◎		◎	
Pleural metastasis of malignant tumor	unilateral	◎		○					
Diffuse malignant mesothelioma	unilateral	◎	◎		○	○		○	
Collagen disease (RA)	bilateral	◎		○					

Table. **Differential diagnoses of diseases leading to pleural thickening**

◎ : frequent, ○ : less frequent

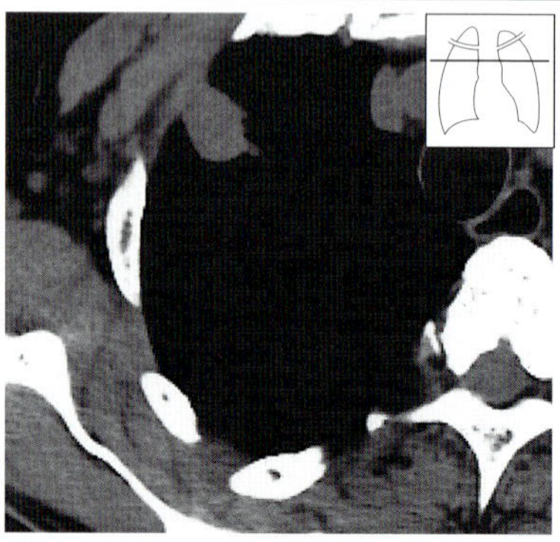

a. Intrapulmonary tumor (squamous cell carcinoma)

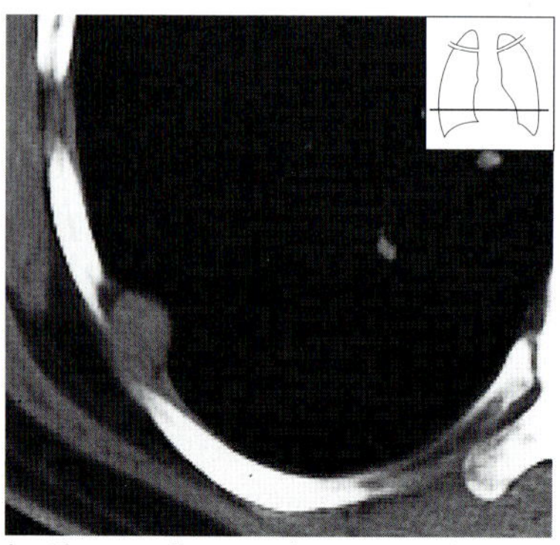

b. Chest wall tumor (neurinoma)

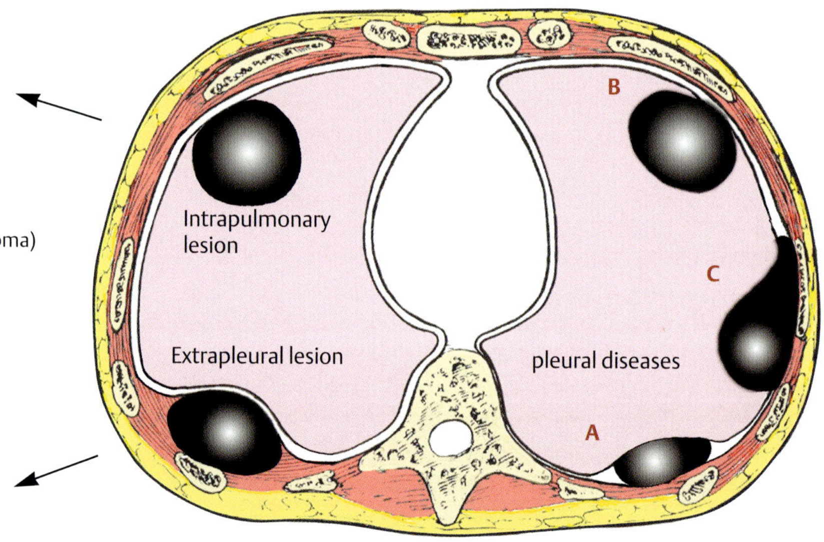

Figure 7. **Differential diagnoses of pleural mass**

Case 2 Idiopathic chylothorax

61-year-old female

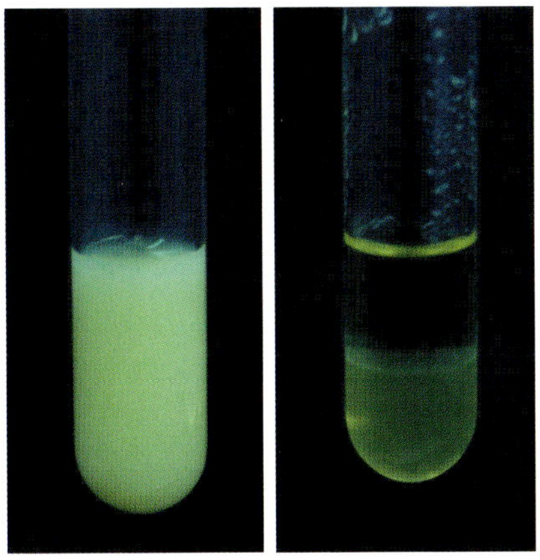

Figure 8. **Chyle taken by thoracentesis**

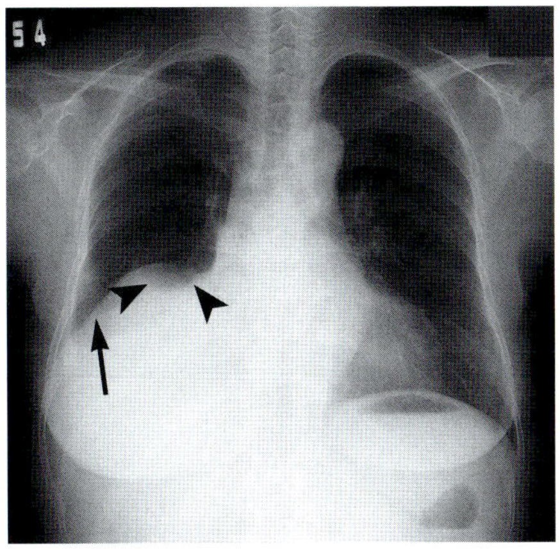

Figure 9. **Chest radiograph**

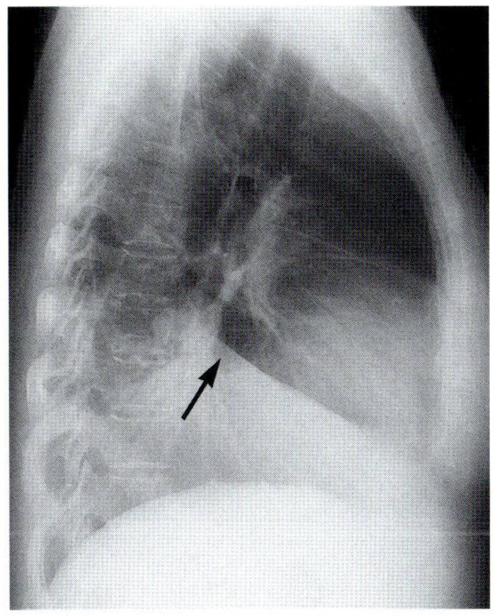

Figure 10. **Chest radiograph**

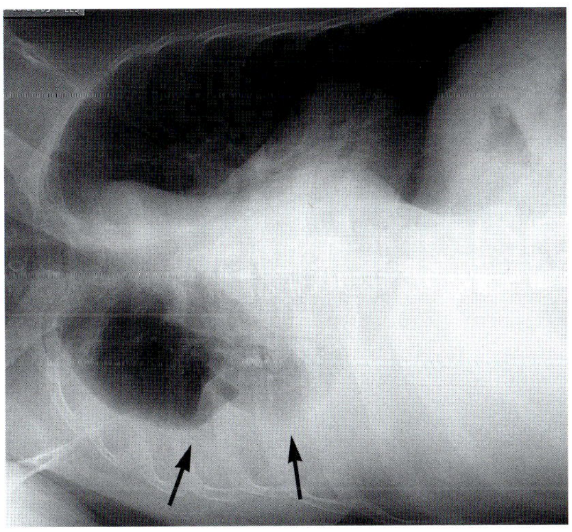

Figure 11. **Chest radiograph taken in decubitus position**

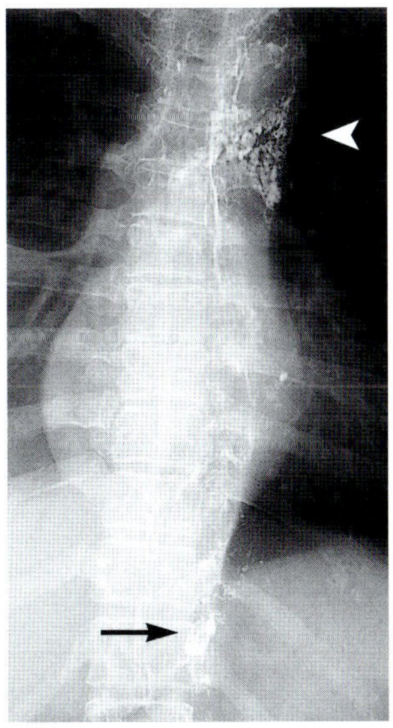

Figure 12. **Lymphangiography**

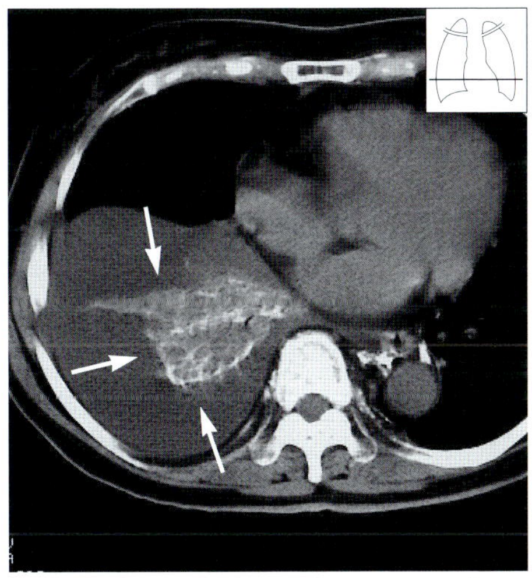

Figure 13. **Chest CT 24 hours after injection of contrast medium into lymph canal**

The patient was referred to the respiratory disease center due to an abnormal chest shadow. She suffered from common cold-like symptoms. Thoracentesis revealed a white milky fluid (TP 3.3 g/dL, T-cho 82 mg/dL, TG 84 mg/dL) (*Fig. 8, left test tube*). Since the turbidity was cleared by adding ethyl ether (*Fig. 8, right test tube*), the fluid was proved to be chyle.

Chest radiograph (frontal view) (*Fig. 9*) revealed elevation of right hemidiaphragm (→) and shrunken right lower lobe (➤). Subpulmonary fluid correction was suspected because of a sharp costophrenic angle.

Chest radiograph (lateral view) (*Fig. 10*) revealed shrunken right lower lobe and wedge shaped fluid correction between lower and middle lobe (→).

Chest radiograph (*decubitus view*) (*Fig. 11*) revealed fluid (→) moving downward to the right lateral side that proved to be subpulmonary fluid correction.

Lymphangiography (*Fig. 12*): The thoracic duct was not well defined at the level above the cisterna chyli (→). A bypass developed at the left side of the thoracic vertebra (➤). Although no outflow to the thoracic cavity was observed, disturbance of passage through the thoracic duct was considered. Chest CT after 24 hours (*Fig. 13*) revealed that contrast medium flowed backward to the shrunken lower lobe (→). In addition, no obvious outflow into the thoracic cavity was observed. It was considered that contrast medium flowed backward through broncho-mediastinal lymph canal to the lung parenchyma. Fat-rich chyle without high protein concentration, unlike this patient's, expresses a minus CT value.

Case 3 Interlobar fluid correction, tuberculous fibrothorax (Contarini's condition)

89-year-old male

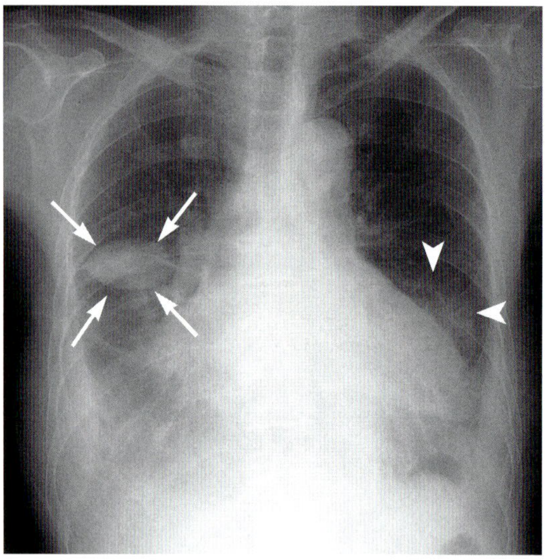

Figure 14. **Chest radiograph**

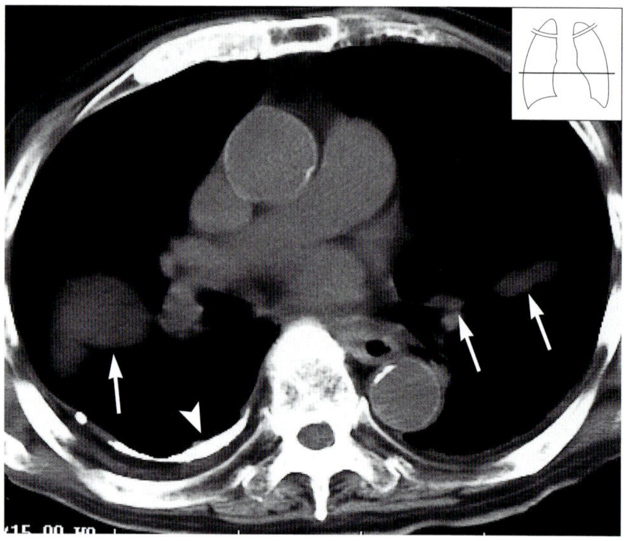

Figure 15. **Chest CT at the level of right pulmonary artery**

The patient complained of edema in bilateral legs and dyspnea. He had history of tuberculous pleurisy in his youth and acute myocardial infarction four years ago.

Chest radiograph (frontal view) (*Fig. 14*) revealed cardiomegaly and oval mass opacity (→) with a linear shadow linking to an interlobar fissure in the right middle lung field. An ill-defined faint mass was observed in the left middle lung field (➤). A bilateral dull costophrenic angle expressed fluid accumulation.

Chest CT (*Fig. 15*) revealed a round low density area at the right major fissure and a thin oval low density area at the left major fissure (→). Crescent shaped sheet-like pleural thickening and calcification were observed in the right lower back (➤). The diagnosis was bilateral interlobar fluid correction due to congestive heart failure and right tuberculous fibrothorax. Bilateral pleural effusion, which has a different etiology, is known as Contarini's condition.

Case 4 Tuberculous pleurisy and pericarditis

28-year-old male

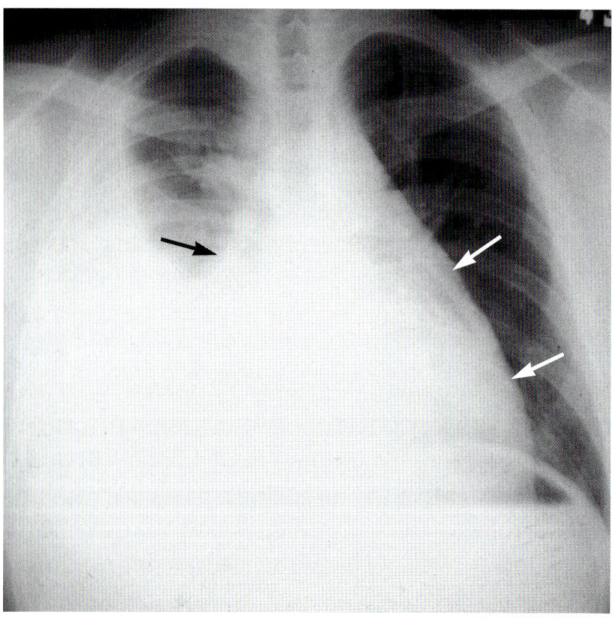

Figure 16. **Chest radiograph**

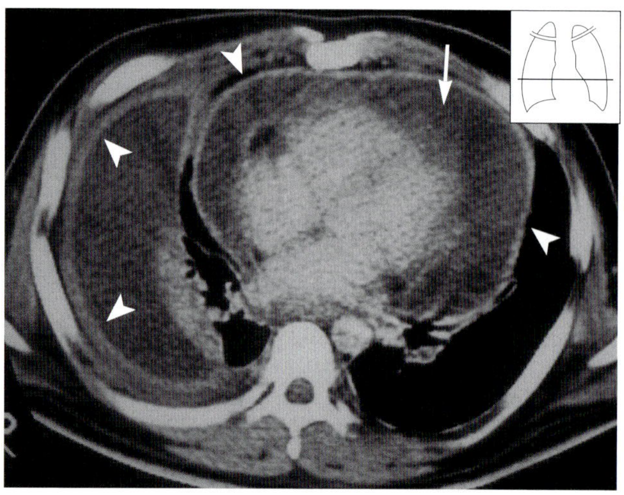

Figure 17. **Chest contrast-enhanced CT at the level of inferior pulmonary vein**

The patient had suffered from dyspnea for 2 months and visited a doctor because of orthopnea.

Chest radiograph (frontal view) (*Fig. 16*) revealed mas-

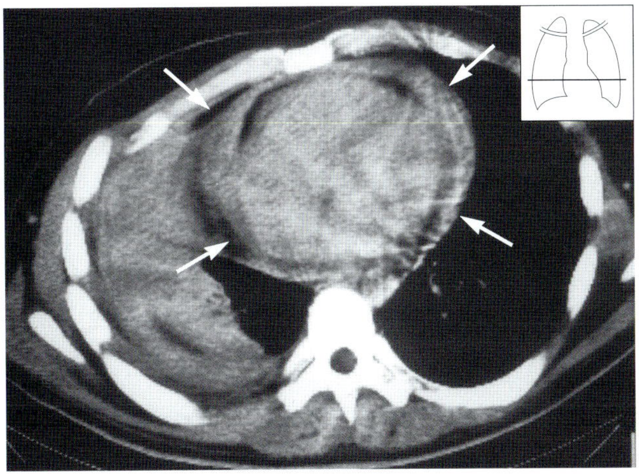

Figure 18. **Chest CT after treatment with antituberculous drugs**

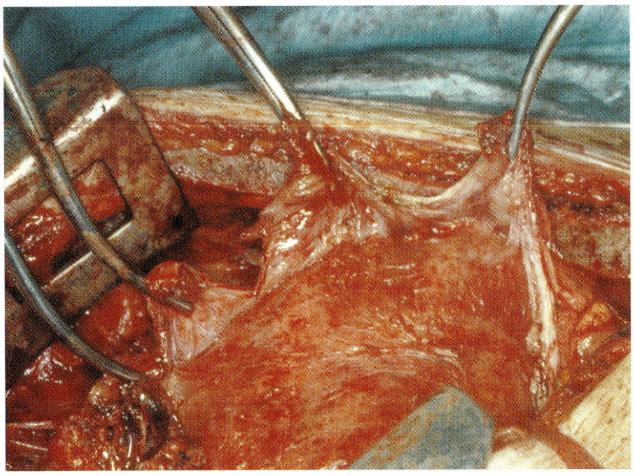

Figure 19. **View of decorticated pericardium at the thoracotomy**

sive right pleural effusion and bell shaped cardiomegaly (➞).

Chest CT (*Fig. 17*) revealed massive right pleural and pericardial fluid correction (➞). Slight thickening of the pleura and pericardium was observed (➤). Emergency pericardial drainage was performed and mycobacterium tuberculosis was detected by Ziel Neelsen's stain. A pericardial biopsy also verified tuberculosis.

Chest CT (*Fig. 18*) after treatment with both antituberculous drugs and steroids revealed advancing pericardial thickening (➞), so a pericardiectomy was performed (*Fig. 19*).

Case 5 Pleural plaque (asbestosis)

50-year-old male

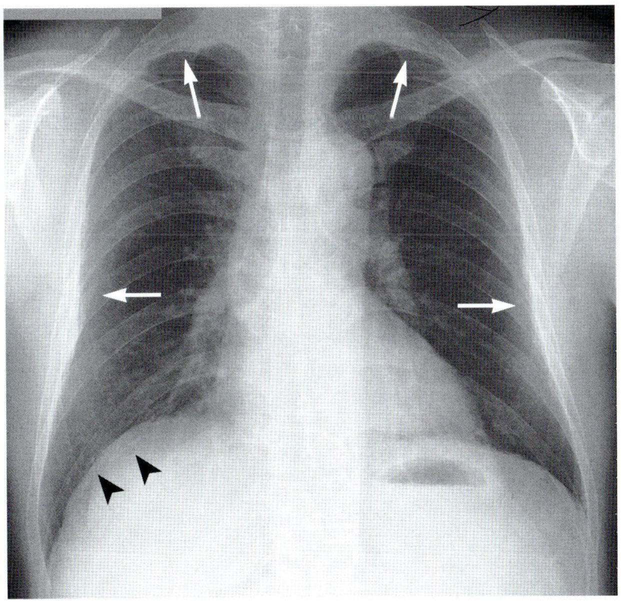

Figure 20. **Chest radiograph**

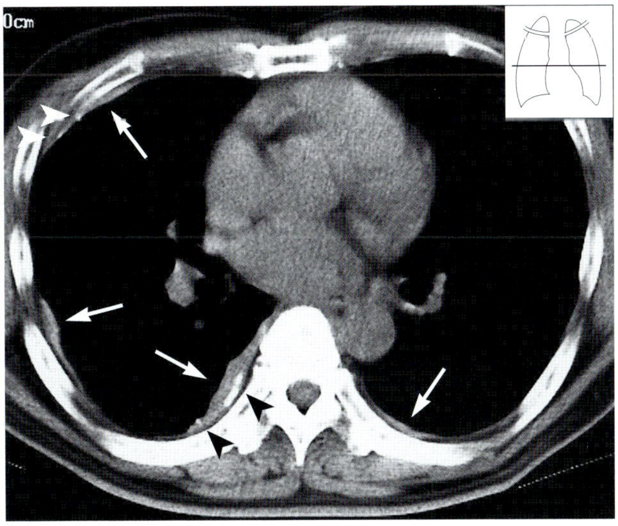

Figure 21. **Chest CT at the level of inferior pulmonary vein**

The patient had occupational asbestos exposure from the age of 20 to 35 years. An abnormal shadow was detected on a chest radiograph at mass screening.

Chest radiograph (frontal view) (*Fig. 20*) revealed pleural thickening in lateral chest and apex, known as apical cap, in bilateral lungs (➞). Thin line and small spot calcification was observed on the right diaphragm (➤).

Chest CT (*Fig. 21*) revealed solitary pleural thickening in the right anterior, lateral, and posterior chest (➞) with thin line or spot calcification (➤).

Case 6 Solitary fibrous tumor
52-year-old female

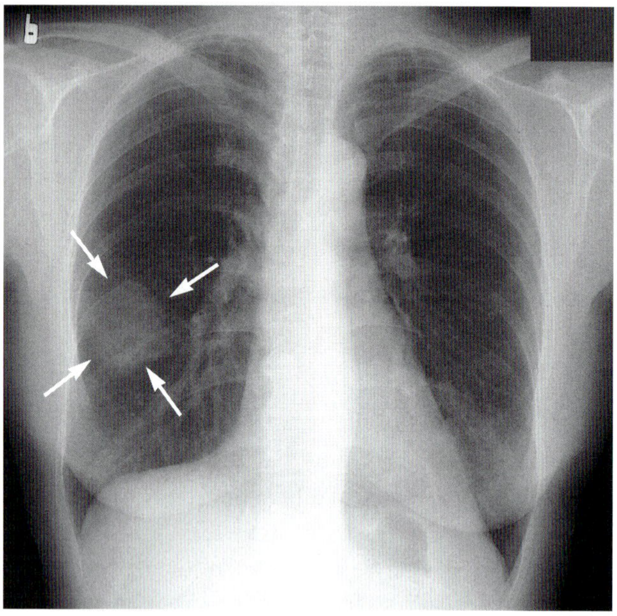

Figure 22. **Chest radiograph**

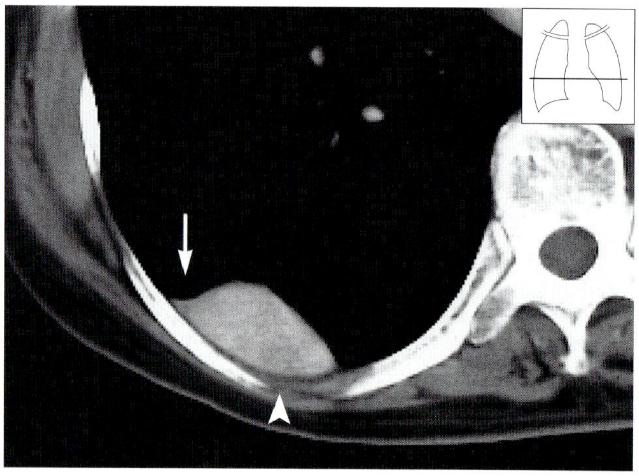

Figure 23. **Chest CT**

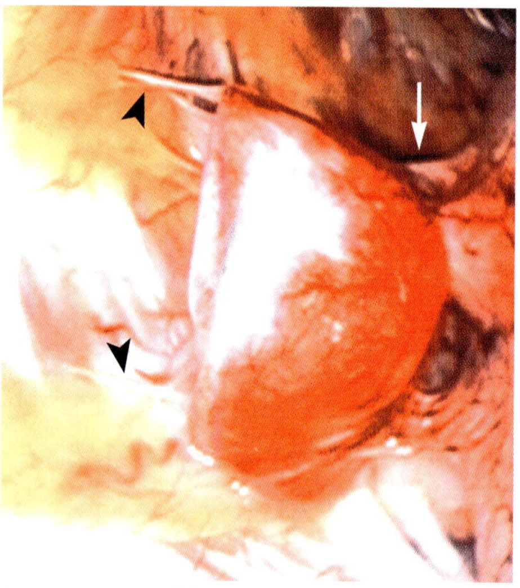

Figure 24. **View of the tumor at video assisted thoracoscopic surgery**

An abnormal shadow was detected on chest radiograph at mass screening.

Chest radiograph (frontal view) (*Fig. 22*) revealed faint round opacity in the right middle lung field (→).

Contrast-enhanced CT (*Fig. 23*) revealed a well-defined homogeneously enhanced flat triangular mass with tapering margin (→) along the right back. An extra pleural fat layer was apparent. Video assisted thoracoscopic surgery was conducted to remove the tumor. The tumor derived from visceral pleura and attached to the pleura through a narrow neck (→). There was some string-like adhesion (➤) between the tumor and parietal pleura (*Fig. 24*). The pathological diagnosis was solitary fibrous tumor.

Case 7 Solitary fibrous tumor
86-year-old male

An abnormal shadow was detected on chest radiograph at mass screening.

Chest radiograph (frontal view) (*Fig. 25*) revealed a well-defined solitary round opacity in the left middle lung field (→). Bilateral pleural thickening (➤) was present due to old tuberculous pleurisy.

Contrast-enhanced CT (*Fig. 26*) revealed a nonhomogeneously enhanced semicircular mass with smooth margin at the left anterior chest wall (→). The angle between the chest wall and the mass is sharp and an extra pleural fat layer is seen at the sternal side (➤).

Sagittal T2-weighted MRI (*Fig. 27*) revealed wedge shaped pleural fluid on the caudal side of the tumor, and the tumor was considered to have originated from the pleura. A solitary fibrous tumor derived from visceral pleura was removed by VATS.

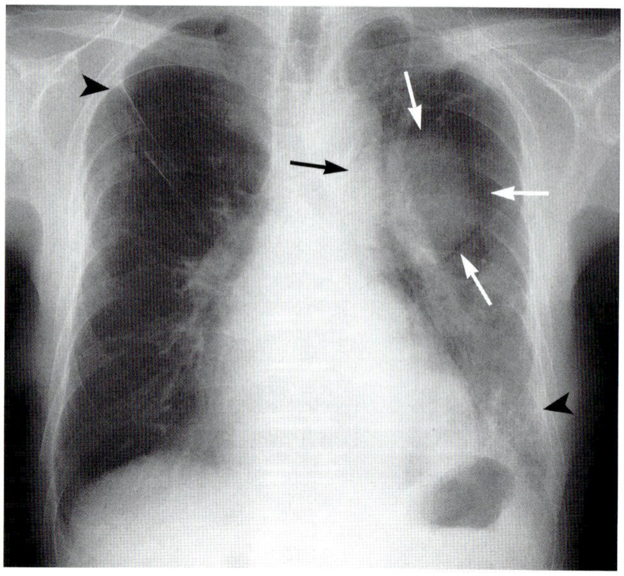

Figure 25. **Chest radiograph**

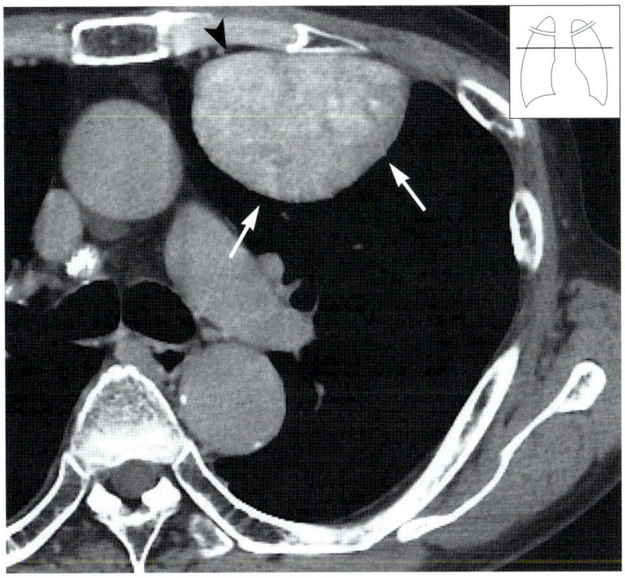

Figure 26. **Chest CT at the level of left pulmonary artery**

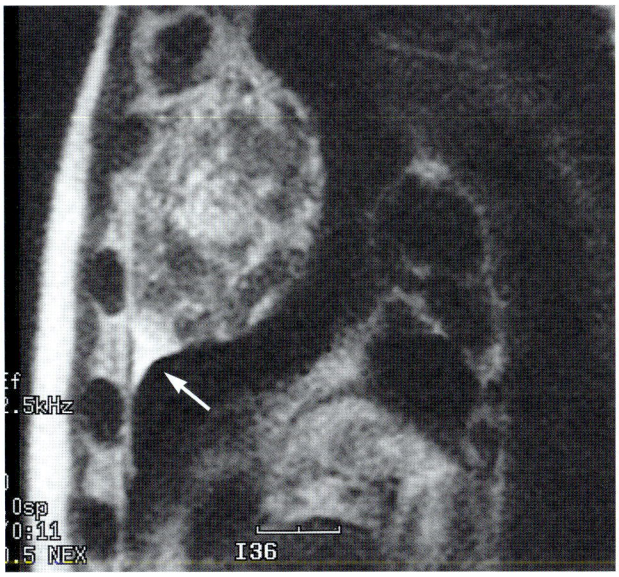

Figure 27. **Sagittal T2-weighted MRI**

Case 8 Loculated tuberculous empyema

22-year-old female

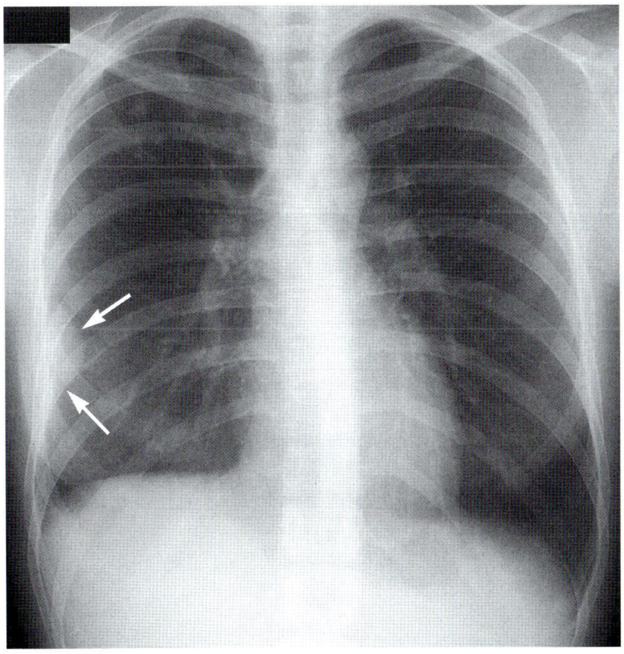

Figure 28. **Chest radiograph**

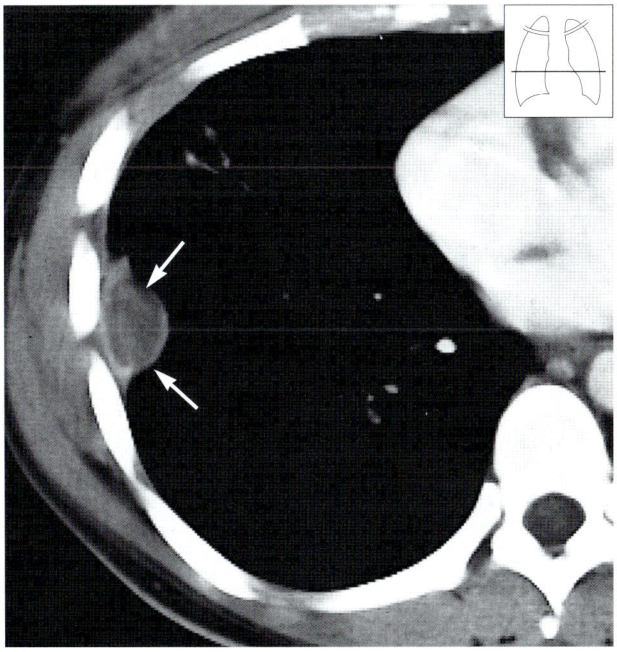

Figure 29. **Chest CT**

Although the patient had been treated with antituberculous drugs for one year, the pleural lesion had not improved. *Mycobacterium tuberculosis* was detected by aspiration from the mass.

Chest radiograph (frontal view) (*Fig. 28*) revealed a homogeneous mass shadow with an obtuse angle with the chest wall in the right middle and lower lung fields (→).

Contrast-enhanced CT (*Fig. 29*) revealed a well-defined mass with a smooth surface in the lateral chest. The angle between the chest wall and the mass is obtuse. Although there was no enhancement inside the mass, circumferential enhancement was observed (→). Decortication was performed.

Case 9 Tuberculous empyema with a bronchopleural fistula

31-year-old male

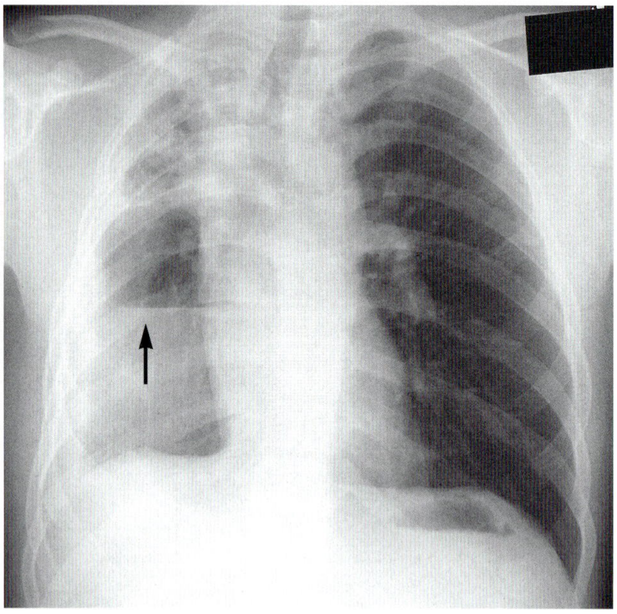

Figure 30. **Chest radiograph**

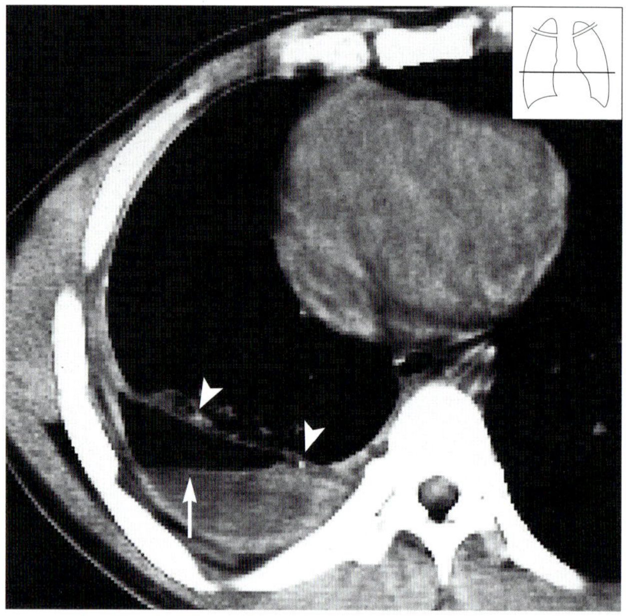

Figure 31. **Chest CT**

The patient complained of yellow sputum. He had been treated with antituberculous drugs for two years due to pulmonary tuberculosis.

Chest radiograph (frontal view) (*Fig. 30*) revealed shrunken right thorax and trachea and mediastinum displaced to the right side. Right chest opacity was increased by consolidation in the upper lung field and there was thickening of the pleura. A bronchopleural fistula was apparent because of air-fluid level in the right middle lung field (→).

Chest CT (*Fig. 31*) revealed fluid accumulation with air-fluid level in the posterior right chest (→). There was fine calcification on the thickened visceral pleura (➤). Decortication was performed.

Case 10 Chronic expanding empyema

66-year-old male

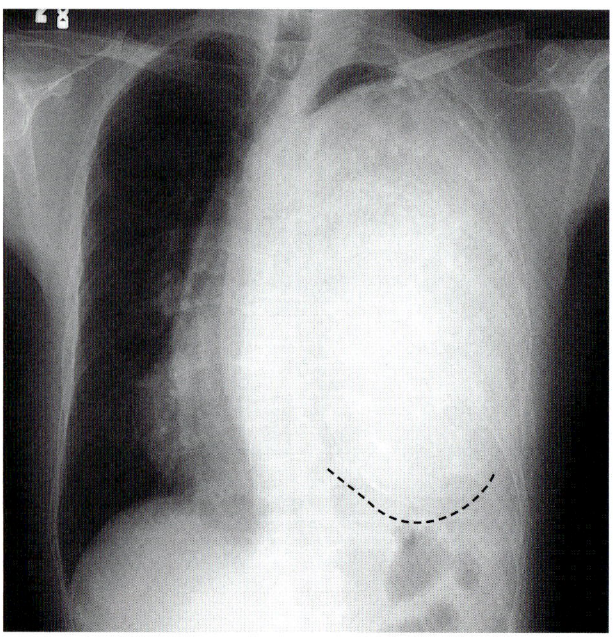

Figure 32. **Chest radiograph**

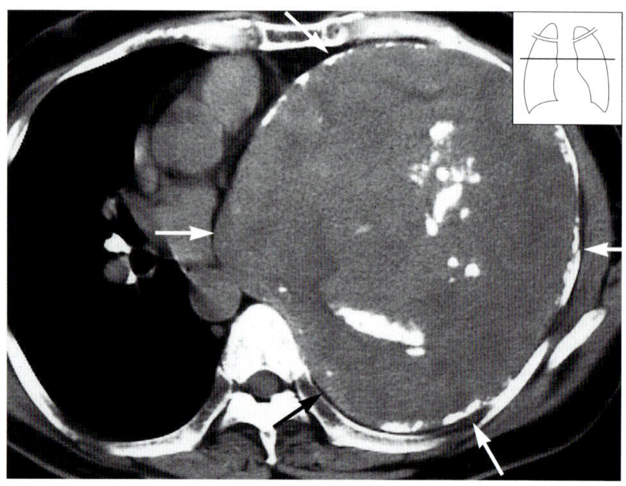

Figure 33. **Chest CT at the level of superior pulmonary vein**

The patient underwent therapeutic pneumothorax to treat pulmonary tuberculosis 45 years ago. He came to our respiratory disease center due to a mass in the left thorax that had been gradually expanding for several years.

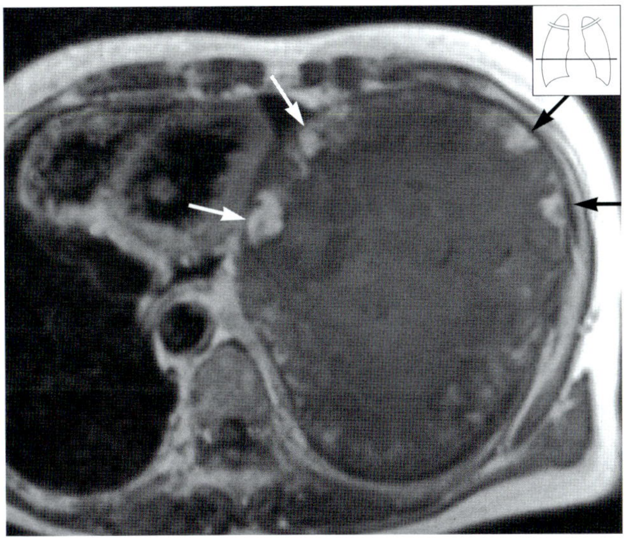

Figure 34. **Axial enhanced T1-weighted MRI**

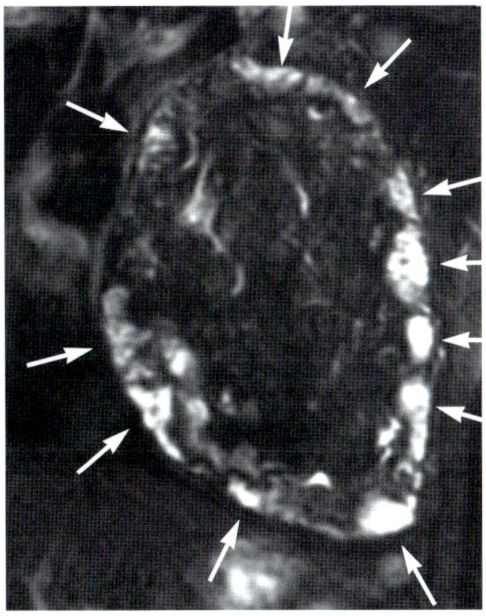

Figure 35. **Coronal T2-weighted MRI**

Chest radiograph (frontal view) (*Fig. 32*) revealed that a huge calcified opacity occupied the left thorax. The mediastinum, trachea, and heart were markedly shifted to the right side and the left hemidiaphragm had become inverted toward the abdominal side (broken line).

Chest CT (*Fig. 33*) showed a huge mass in the left thorax displacing the heart to the opposite side. There was some calcification around and inside the mass (→).

Axial enhanced T1-weighted MRI (*Fig. 34*) showed many islands enhanced by contrast medium at the periphery (→). Since coronal T2-weighted MRI (*Fig. 35*) showed islands with high or low intensity along the periphery (→), the mass seemed to be a hemangioma accompanied by both fresh bleeding and coagulated blood. We considered the mass to be a chronic expanding empyema and performed a pleuropneumonectomy.

A surgical specimen (*Fig. 36*) was cut in coronal section-like MRI (*d*). The mass size was 21 x 16 x 12 cm. There were many parts with comparatively fresh bleeding at the edge (→) and old thrombotic substance inside the mass. Flattened lung with the cut end of the left main bronchus and left pulmonary artery (➤) was observed on the left side of the mass.

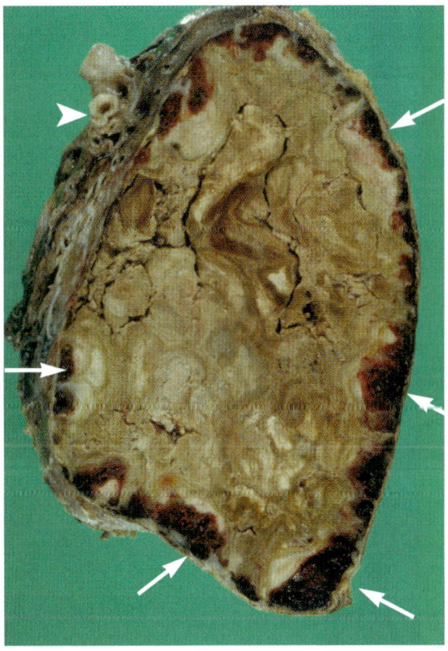

Figure 36. **Surgical specimen**

Conclusion

Diagnosis of pleural disease

Characteristics of pleural disease are pleural effusion, pleural thickening, and mass shadow. Plain chest radiographs are useful for observing the location and expanse of lesions and checking for any calcification. If effusion is not encapsulated, the decubitus position enables diagnosis by moving only a small amount of fluid. CT provides detailed observation of shield lung due to pleural effusion, lesions of the mediastinum, tumors in the thorax, pleural thickening, and fine calcification, while adding enhancement indicates blood inflow to the lesion. Tuberculous pleural disease, which we encounter most in daily work, is explained below and image diagnosis of pleural thickening and pleural effusion is demonstrated.

Tuberculous pleural disease

Tuberculous pleural disease includes tuberculous pleurisy (Case 4) and tuberculous empyema (Case 8, 9, 10). Tuberculous pleurisy is commonly caused by rupture of a subpleural caseous focus into the pleural space. Pleural fluid is a serous exudate that accumulates as a result of hypersensitivity and infrequently yields a positive culture. Tuberculous empyema is characterized by purulent pleural fluid which contains numerous tuberculous bacilli. In the past, tuberculous empyema used to be a common complication following therapeutic pneumothorax. These days tuberculous empyema generally results from incomplete therapy. Well-treated tuberculous pleurisy and empyema result in fibrothorax. Insufficiently treated tuberculous empyema changes to chronic empyema. Chronic empyema results in the reactivation of tuberculous bacilli that had remained dormant within the calcified space and suddenly develop into either a bronchopleural (Case 9) or pleurocutaneous fistula at a later date. Chronic empyema occasionally develops into chronic expanding empyema which bleeds repeatedly and slowly expands (Case 10). B-cell lymphoma sometimes arises from chronic empyema.

Imaging diagnosis of pleural effusion

Pleural effusion may originate from any number of disease processes and thoracentesis or pleural biopsy is required for accurate diagnosis. The effusion consists of transudative, exudative, purulent (pyothorax), bloody (hemothorax), or chylous (chylothorax) fluid. Classically, free fluid takes the shape of a meniscus, which appears as homogeneous increased density with a concave, upward sloping contour (Case 4). Blunting of the lateral costophrenic angle is a characteristic with a smaller amount of fluid, although detection requires approximately 200 mL of pleural fluid since the posterior costophrenic angle is lower than the lateral costophrenic angle. Much smaller quantities of fluid can be detected with a radiograph of the patient in the lateral decubitus position. Ultrasonography, CT, and MRI are more useful for detecting small amounts of fluid correction.

Pleural effusion sometimes accumulates underneath the lung and above the diaphragm and is called subpulmonic effusion. On a lateral radiograph, the pseudodiaphragmatic contour of subpulmonic fluid is typically a flat superior surface that slants sharply downward at the major fissure (Case 2). Loculated fluid in the fissure is called a fissural pseudotumor because it may simulate a mass on chest radiographs when adherence of the pleural layers in the peripheral portion of the fissure is present. These are most frequently seen in patients with congestive heart failure. Since the mass shadow easily disappears with appropriate treatment for congestive heart failure, it is called as a vanishing tumor (Case 3).

Pleural fluid freely moves around the thoracic cavity without adherence to the pleural layers, but encapsulated pleural effusion is a result of plural adhesion anywhere between the parietal and visceral pleura caused by pleural infection or hemothorax. Chronic empyema, which is a typical loculated effusion that is lenticular shaped in appearance, compresses pulmonary parenchyma displacing bronchi and vessels, and forms an obtuse angle with the chest wall. Visualization of intravenous contrast-enhancing thickened visceral and parietal pleura surrounding the fluid allows confident distinction of loculated empyema from a peripheral lung abscess (split pleura sign) (Case 8).

Imaging diagnosis of pleural thickening

Solitary small amounts of pleural thickening are called pleural plaque. A vast majority of the lesions are derived from asbestos exposure 20 or 40 years before. Characteristics of the plaque are solitary and sharply defined thickening up to 15 mm. Concerning the mechanism by which asbestos fibers produce plaques, it is thought that asbestos-fibers pierce the visceral pleura and then rub against and irritate the parietal pleura resulting in hyaline plaque which eventually calcifies. The calcification is seen as a dense white spot or line (Case 5).

Fibrothorax is the most common cause of diffuse pleural thickening. Fibrothorax is caused by tuberculosis, bacterial pleuritis, hemothorax, asbestosis, collagen disease, and so on. Fibrothorax is smooth pleural thickening ordinarily up to 1 cm occupying more than a quarter of the hemithorax but it occasionally develops until it is 2 cm thick. Although the costophrenic sinus disappears, the costophrenic angle in posteroanterior chest radiographs frequently remains sharp.

Pleural lesions are unilateral in patients with tuberculous pleurisy, hemothorax or bacterial pleuritis, while they are bilateral in patients with asbestos-related disease or collagen disease. Mediastinal extension is quite rare in these diseases, which differentiates them from diffuse mesothelioma. Parenchymal lesions and sheet-like calcification are characteristics of fibrothorax due to tuberculous pleurisy. Healed rib fracture and calcification are characteristics of fibrothorax due to traumatic hemothorax.

CT is quite useful for assessing diffuse pleural thickening. Signs suggesting mesothelioma are pleural thickening often with nearly rind-like encasement, irregular and often nodular thickening, parietal pleural thickening over 1 cm, mediastinal pleural thickening, or involvement of the chest wall or mediastinum.

References

- Fraser R. S., et al.: Diagnosis of diseases of the chest (4th ed.). Saunders, Philadelphia, 1999
- Light R. W.: Pleural disease (4th ed.). Lippincott Williams & Wilkins, Philadelphia, 2001
- Hood R. M., et al.: Surgical diseases of the pleura and chest wall. Saunders, Philadelphia, 1986
- Naidich D. P.: Computed tomography and magnetic resonance of the thorax (3rd ed.). Lippincottt-Raven, Philadelphia, 1999

Chapter 4

Radiographs of Intrapulmonary lesions with decreased radiolucency

1. Alveolar shadow: Consolidation [Pattern classification IV-A-1]

●Author — Shosaku Abe

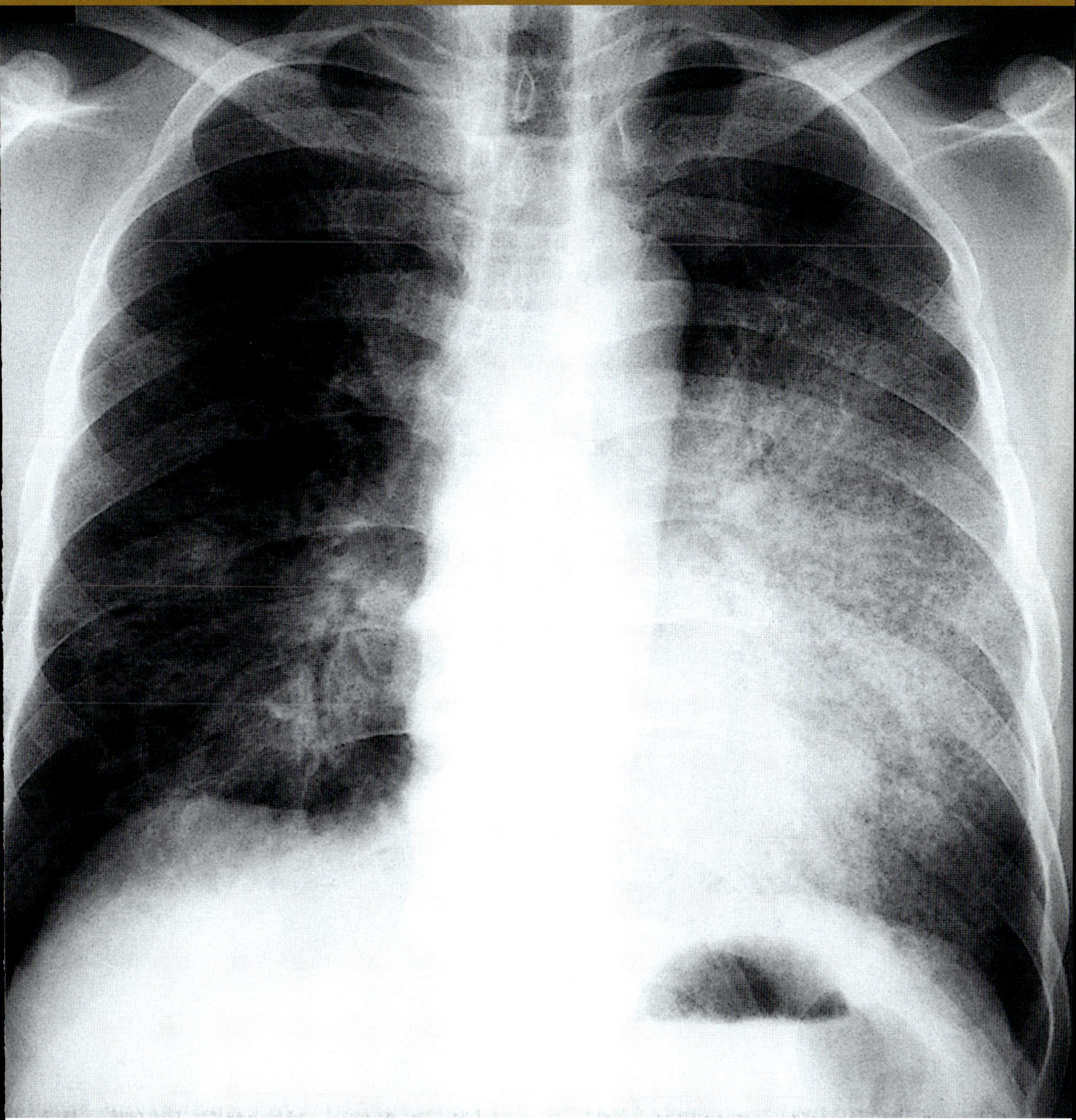

Keywords of this section

Consolidation
Air bronchogram
Pulmonary surfactant protein A (SP-A)
Pulmonary alveolar proteinosis
SP-D
Crazy-paving pattern
Pneumococcal pneumonia
Gram stain
Legionella pneumonia
Mycoplasma pneumonia
Bronchioloalveolar carcinoma
Pulmonary malignant lymphoma
Wegener's granulomatosis
Pulmonary hemorrhage
Pulmonary edema
Butterfly shadow

Consolidation
(filled intra-alveolar space)

Shosaku Abe
Honorary Director of Sapporo Minamisanjo Hospital, Hokkaido, Japan

Chest radiograph findings have been described as alveolar patterns, but in general the term currently used is consolidation. There is no appropriate Japanese equivalent and so an English term is used that has a meaning close to infiltrative shadow. Consolidation refers to pathology in which intra-alveolar spaces become filled with exudate or another substance. It is indicated by consolidation (increased attenuation areas) in images where intra-alveolar spaces are filled, and is accompanied by an air bronchogram of internal diameter 2 to 3 mm and no loss of pulmonary volume.

Case 1 49-year-old male

Chief complaint: Dyspnea on exertion
Medical history: Nothing notable
Family history: Nothing notable
Smoking history: 15/day for 19 years
Present illness:
Symptoms similar to the common cold were observed 6 months previously. Following this, a cough continued without recovery but as there was no sputum it was left untreated. From about 2 weeks previously, the patient felt short of breath during exertion. No wheeze was observed. A chest radiograph examination conducted at a local hospital indicated an abnormal diffuse shadow, and the patient visited this hospital for precise tests.
Physical findings:
No anemia, no jaundice, and no superficial lymph nodes apparent to the touch. No abnormal rales were heard with cardio-pulmonary auscultation. Laboratory findings showed LDH 765 IU/L, CEA 15 ng/mL, which were mildly elevated levels. Arterial blood gas analysis indicated mild hypoxemia with figures of PaO_2 72 torr, $PaCO_2$ 34 torr, and pH 7.41.

Chest radiograph findings (P. 33): From the hilum of both lungs to the central lower lung field a diffuse nodular shadow can be seen, with an air bronchogram. Distribution in the left lung is dense and widespread, with clear laterality. No enlargement of cardiac contour is seen, and the left heart borders are indistinct. No reduction in pulmonary capacity is seen, while there is also no indication of pleural thickening or pleural effusion retention.

Chest CT findings (*Fig. 1*): Consolidation is widespread, with the subpleural region maintained. An air bronchogram (→) can be seen in the increased attenuation area.

Diagnosis

Compared with the chest radiograph findings, subjective symptoms were comparatively mild. When bronchoalveolar lavage was performed, a milky-white, turbid liquid (*Fig. 2*) was recovered. PAS staining of a transbronchial lung biopsy sample indicated that alveolar spaces were filled with a PAS positive substance (*Fig. 3*), and that due

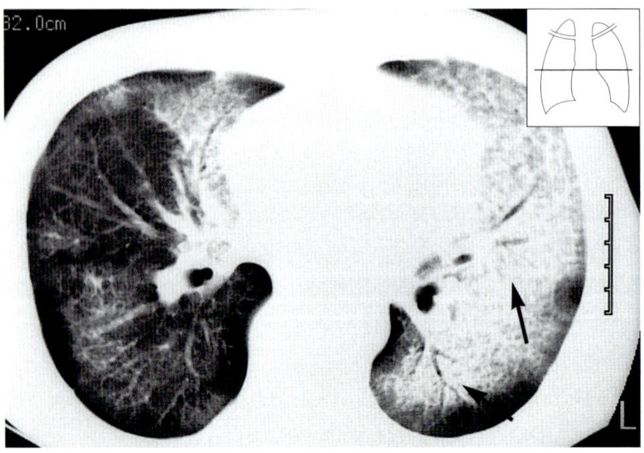

Figure 1. **Chest CT**

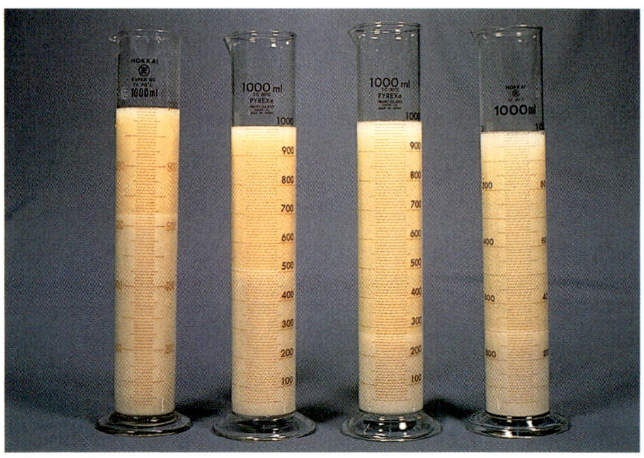

Figure 2. **BALF**

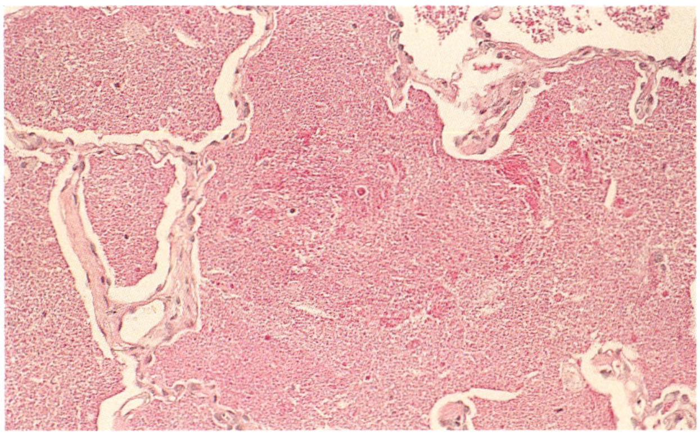

Figure 3. **Pathological findings: PAS stain**

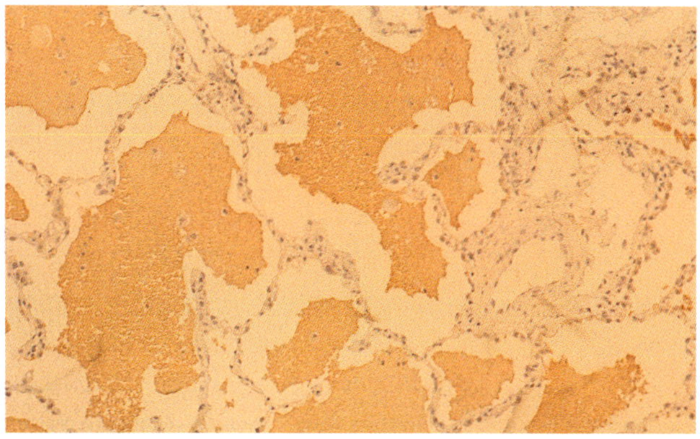

Figure 4. **Pathological findings: SP-A stain**

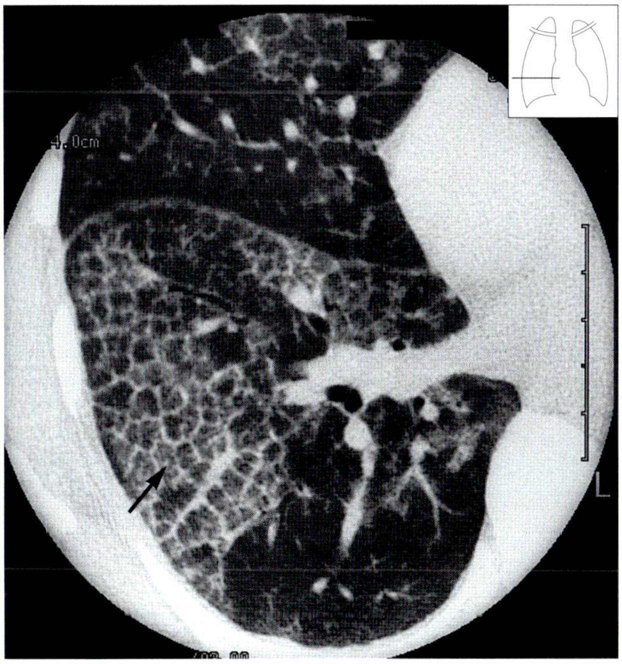

Figure 5. **Typical chest CT of PAP**

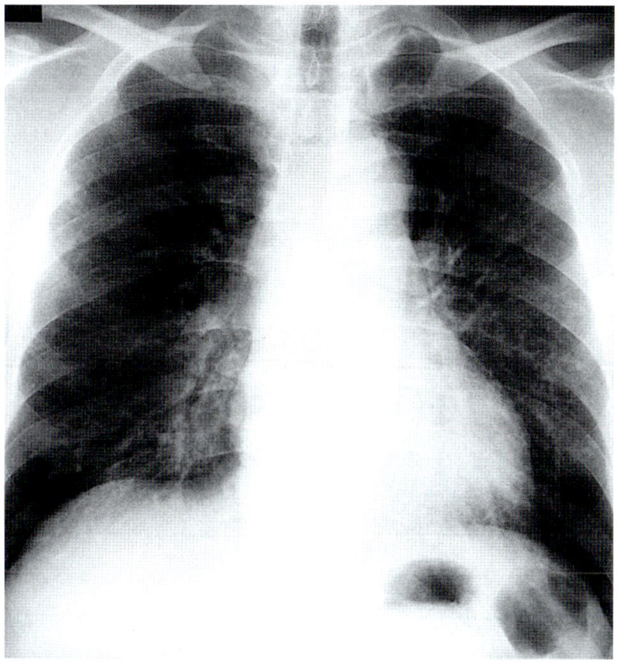

Figure 6. **Chest radiograph after BAL**

to pulmonary surfactant protein A (SP-A), the result of immunostaining of the substance in the alveolar spaces was strongly positive. For these reasons pulmonary alveolar proteinosis was diagnosed.

Conclusions of this case: Pulmonary alveolar proteinosis: PAP

PAP is a disease of unknown etiology characterized by the accumulation of amorphous, PAS-positive lipoproteinaceous material in the alveolar spaces. There is a congenital type of PAP which occurs due to the absence of GM-CSF function and a frame shift mutation in the SP-B gene, and acquired PAP due to alveolar macrophage function impairment leading to clearance function damage. Cases of acquired PAP may be of a primary type that is not induced by any specific factor, or of a secondary type associated with the inhalation of substances such as silicon and glass wool, or leukemia, malignant lymphoma and other diseases.

The substance filling the alveolar spaces is mainly composed of saturated phosphatidyl choline, and increased SP-A and SP-D are seen. Subjective symptoms in this case are mild. Laboratory findings indicate elevated LDH and mildly elevated CEA, and so there is a need to differentiate between PAP and bronchioloalveolar carcinoma. CT findings of PAP (*Fig. 5*) show a network of thickened interlobular septa superimposed on ground glass attenuation (decreased attenuation area). Networks of crazy-paving pattern or melon-skin appearance (→) are characteristic image findings.

Treatment is pulmonary lavage. It is performed either on one segmental bronchus at a time using a bronchoscope or one lobule ventilation is conducted under general anesthetic while the other lung is washed. *Figure 6* shows a chest radiograph of this case after lavage. Since coincidental pulmonary infections are often a problem, doses of steroids are not recommended.

Differentiation of consolidation

Diseases that present consolidation differ depending on the substance that fills the alveolar spaces. With substances such as exudate, mucus inflammatory cells and necrotic cells, the disease is pneumonia, with infusion it is pulmonary edema, with blood it is a pulmonary hemorrhage caused by SLE or Goodpasture syndrome, with malignant cells and mucus it is bronchioloalveolar carcinoma, and with lipoproteinaceous materials it is pulmonary alveolar proteinosis. It is difficult to judge what the substance is based on image findings alone. Consolidation must be discerned by the difference between images indicating atelectasis and images indicating ground glass attenuation.

The pathological characteristics of atelectasis are loss of air in the distal airspaces with no replacement by a substance, imaging findings that do not indicate air bronchogram, and reduced pulmonary volume seen as extensive consolidation.

With ground glass attenuation, existing air in the lungs is replaced by small amounts of a substance, imaging findings show ground glass attenuation, and air bronchogram and loss of pulmonary volume are not seen. As the pathology of ground glass attenuation progresses, there are cases in which consolidation leads to filling of intrabronchial spaces resulting in atelectasis-like shadows.

Case 2 Bacterial pneumonia (Pneumococcal pneumonia)

54-year-old male

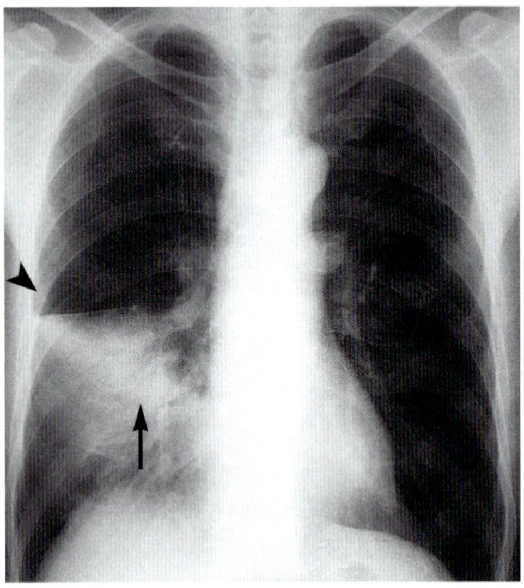

Figure 7. **Chest radiograph**

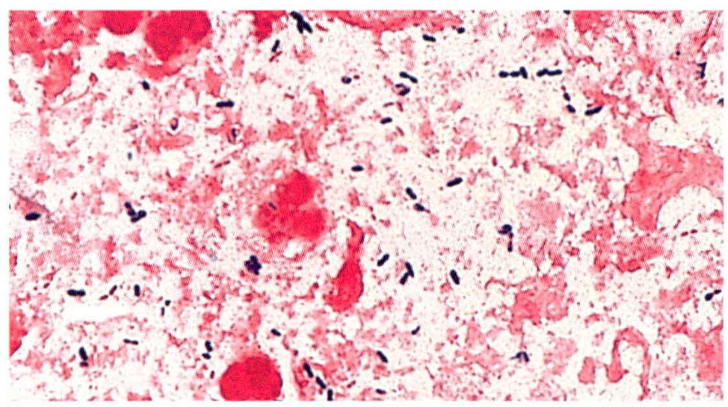

Figure 8. **Pathological findings: Sputum Gram stain**

The patient took nonprescription drugs 5 days after suffering from fever and cough, but there was no improvement. Yellow sputum was seen, and he received a medical examination.

A chest radiograph shows nonuniform consolidation, with pronounced air bronchogram (→) in the right middle lung field. The upper line clearly shows the boundary of minor fissure (➤). The right heart border is indistinct. No loss of pulmonary volume is seen. A Gram stain of sputum indicated a large number of Gram-positive diplococcus bacteria.

Case 3 *Legionella* pneumonia

55-year-old male

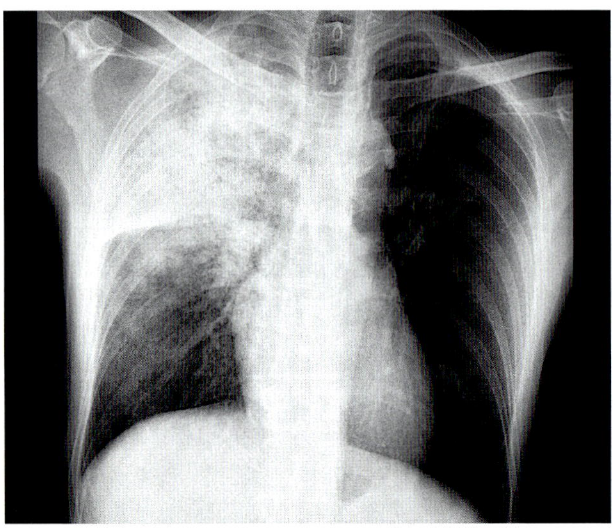

Figure 9. **Chest radiograph**

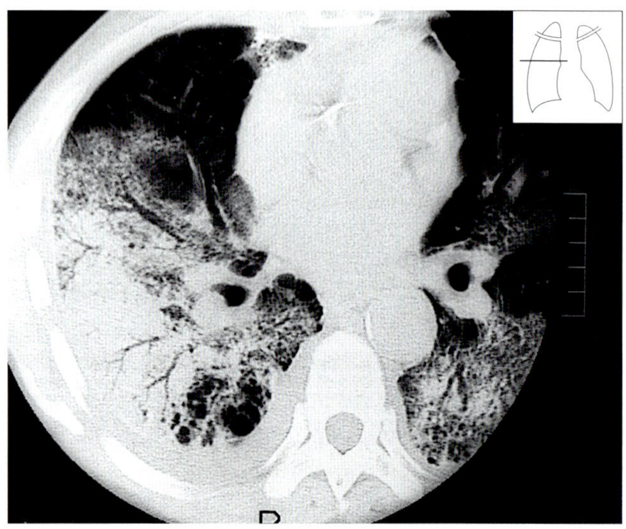

Figure 10. **Chest CT**

The patient received a medical examination for fever (40°C) and dyspnea by a local doctor.

A chest radiograph shows extensive consolidation from the right upper lung field to the middle lower lung field. No loss of pulmonary volume is seen.

A chest CT shows extensive consolidation with air bronchogram and retention of pleural effusion clearly visible.

Case 4 *Mycoplasma* pneumonia

28-year-old female

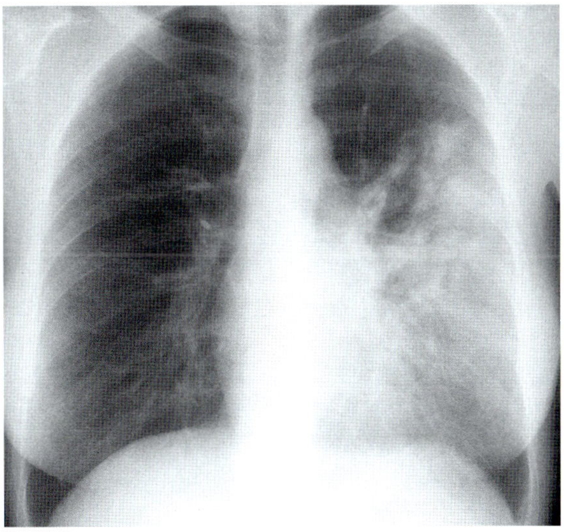

Figure 11. **Chest radiograph**

The patient received a medical examination for the major complaints of a 38°C fever and slightly yellow sputum accompanying a cough.

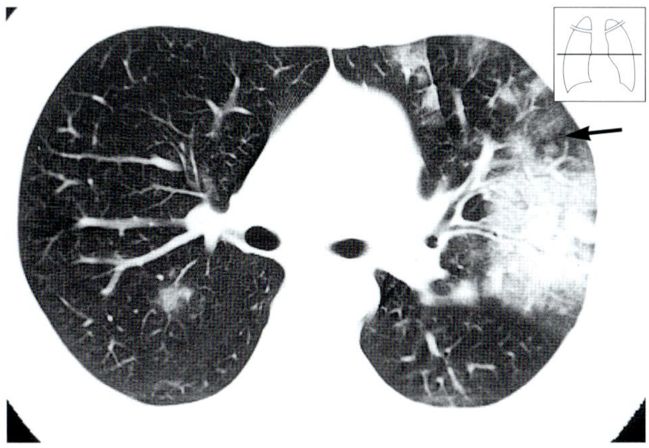

Figure 12. **Chest CT**

A chest radiograph shows nonuniform consolidation from the inside of the middle lung field to the lower lung field. Almost no loss of pulmonary volume is observed.

A chest CT shows the main focus of disease as extensive consolidation with an air bronchogram, but ground glass attenuation can be seen at the periphery (→). Thickening of the bronchial wall is clearly visible, possibly indicating bronchiolitis. No retention of pleural effusion is seen.

Case 5 Bronchioloalveolar carcinoma

52-year-old male

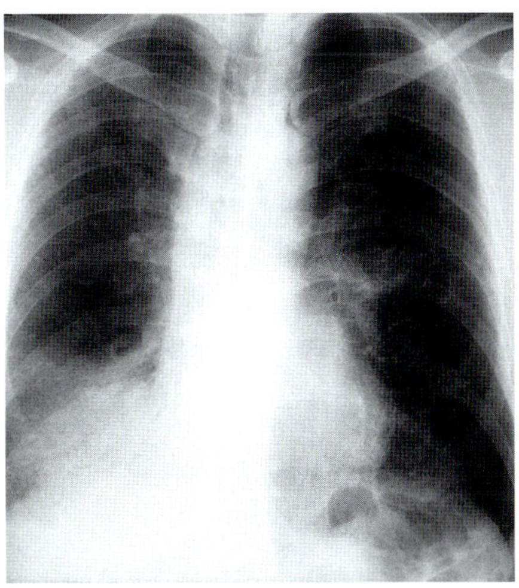

Figure 13. **Chest radiograph**

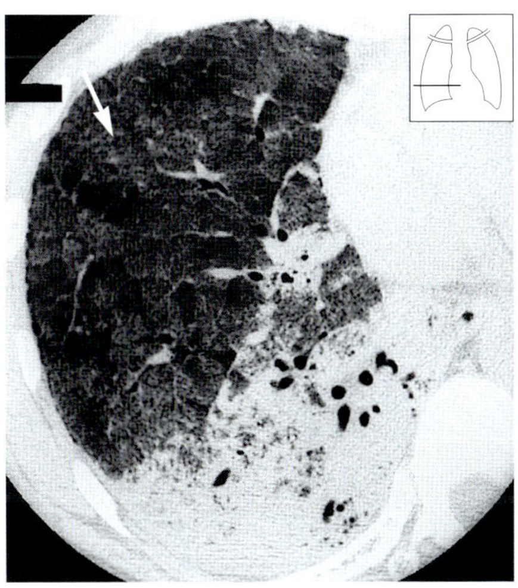

Figure 14. **Chest CT**

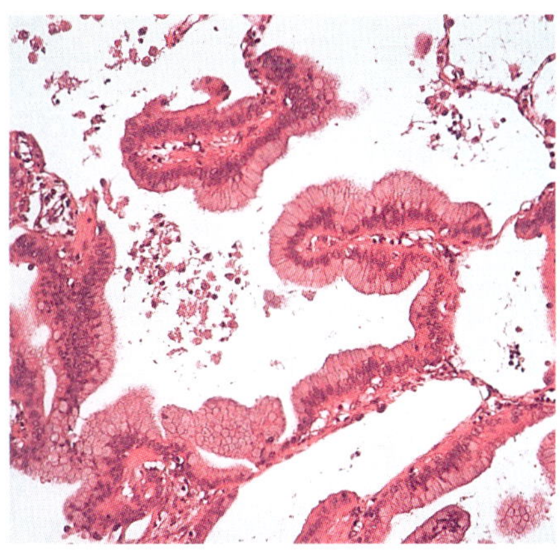

Figure 15. **Pathological findings by lung biopsy**

The patient received a medical examination for pain on the right side of the chest and a gradual increase in white colored sputum (20 to 30 mL/day).

A chest radiograph shows consolidation with indistinct border in the right lower lung field. The right heart border and diaphragm surface are indistinct, giving a positive silhouette sign. No loss of pulmonary volume is seen.

A chest CT shows extensive consolidation with an air bronchogram located dorsally, and ground glass attenuation (→) scattered in the anterior region. A transbronchial lung biopsy indicated mucus-secreting adenocarcinoma cells progressing along the alveolar wall.

Case 6 Pulmonary malignant lymphoma

67-year-old male

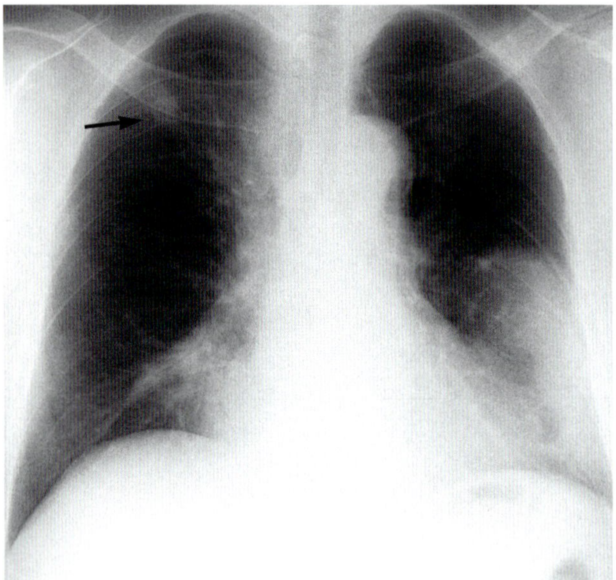

Figure 16. **Chest radiograph**

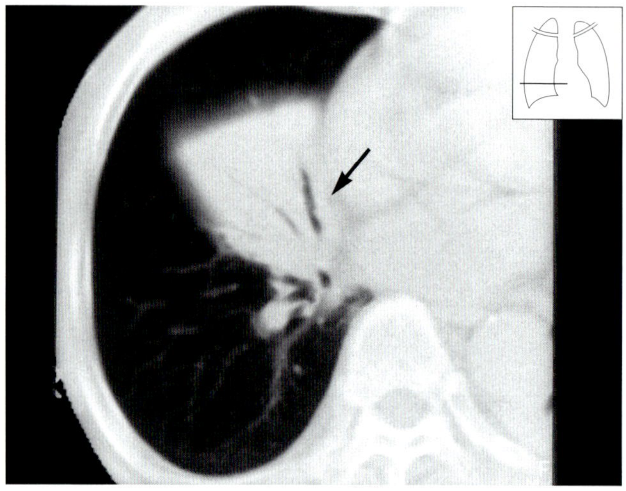

Figure 17. **Chest CT**

The patient received a medical examination for cough, fever and shortness of breath. Red rash was observed on anterior chest. Superficial lymph nodes were not palpable.

A chest radiograph shows consolidation in the outer zone of the left middle lung field and the mediastinal side of the right middle lower lung field. No loss of pulmonary volume is seen. A tumor-like shadow (→) with a diameter of 3 cm is also visible in the right upper lung field. The diaphragm surface is distinct on both sides, and no clear pleural effusion retention is observed.

A chest CT reveals findings of extensive consolidation with an air bronchogram (→). After a transbronchial lung biopsy and biopsy of the rash, malignant lymphoma was diagnosed.

Case 7 Wegener's granulomatosis

42-year-old female

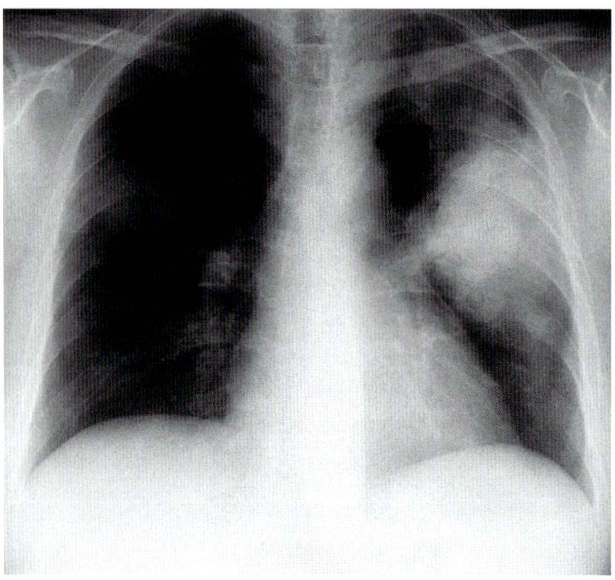

Figure 18. **Chest radiograph**

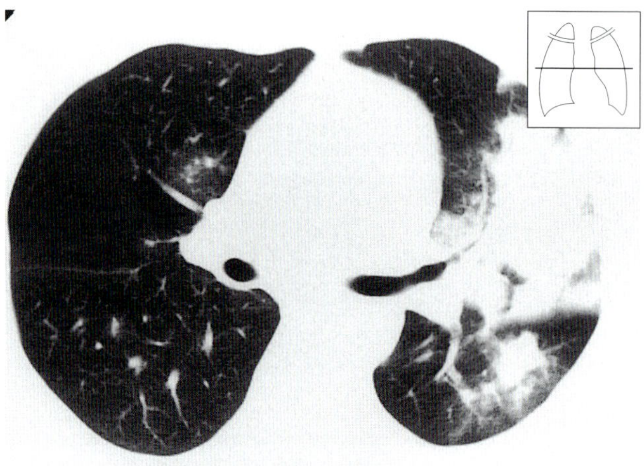

Figure 19. **Chest CT**

The patient received a medical examination for bloody sputum, cough and slight fever. Laboratory findings were RBC 3,710,000, Hb 11 g/dL, WBC 6,800, CRP 15 mm and ESR 117 mm/hr.

A chest radiograph shows consolidation in the center of the left middle lung field, with no loss of pulmonary volume. There is also an air bronchogram.

A chest CT also shows extensive consolidation with an air bronchogram. No clear change in the pleura can be seen. cANCA level was a high 150 IU.

Case 8 Pulmonary hemorrhage

46-year-old male

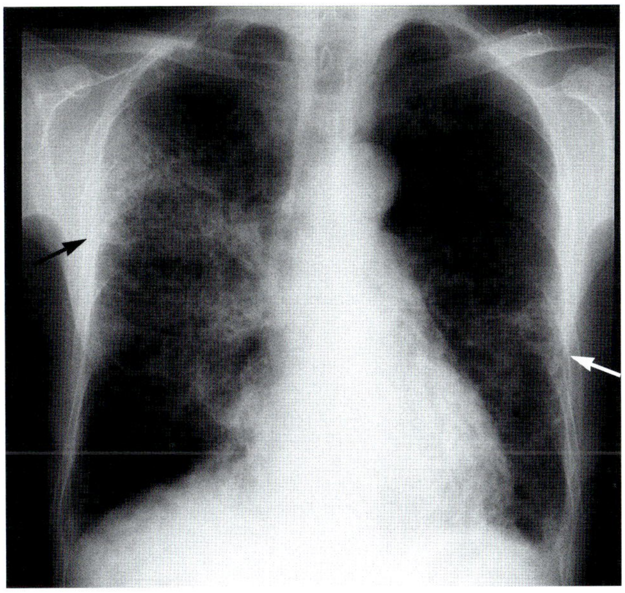

Figure 20. **Chest radiograph**

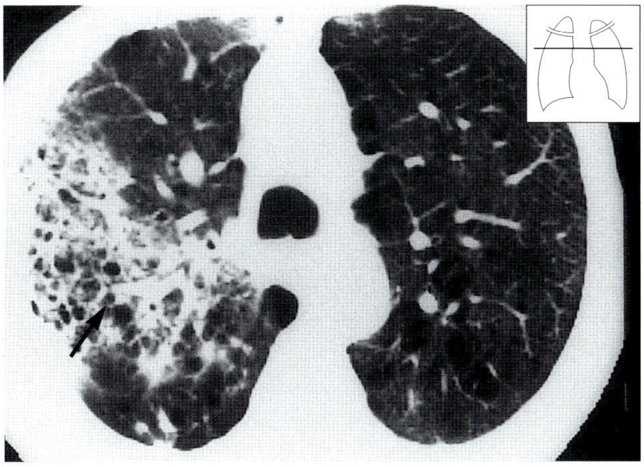

Figure 21. **Chest**

The patient received a medical examination for fever with dyspnea, and hemoptysis while under observation after discontinuation of steroid treatment for SLE.

A chest radiograph shows marginal indistinct consolidation (→) in both lungs, The right lung shadow is extensive and there is air bronchogram.

A chest CT shows extensive consolidation with a clear air bronchogram (→).

Case 9 Pulmonary edema

77-year-old male

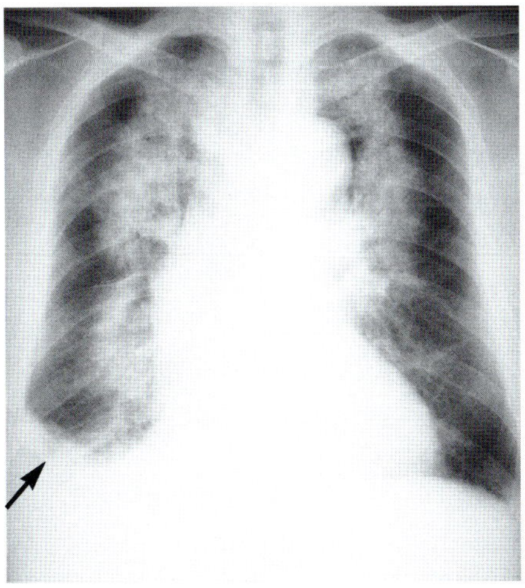

Figure 22. **Chest radiograph**

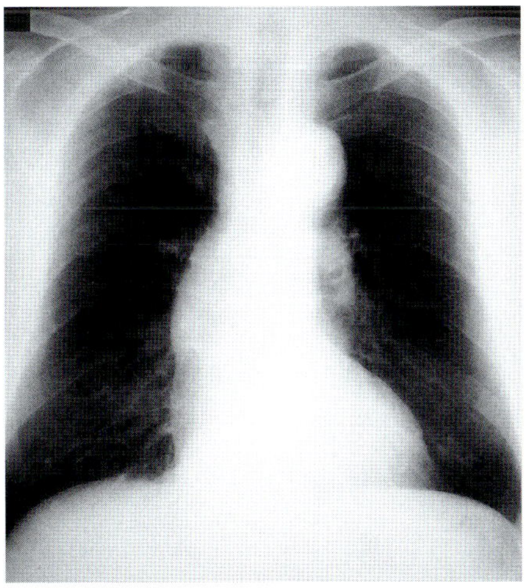

Figure 23. **Chest radiograph**: after improvement with treatment

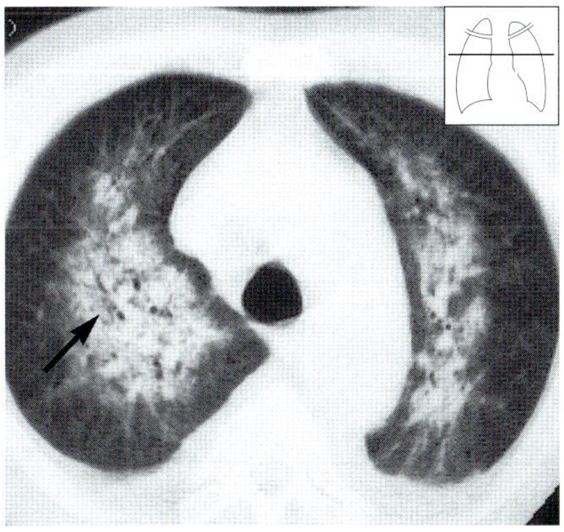

Figure 24. **Chest CT**

While receiving medical treatment for hypertension and diabetes, the patient developed common cold-like symptoms with fever and general fatigue for which he was treated with intravenous drip injection by a local doctor. After 2 days he exhibited shortness of breath and began coughing up foamy sputum. A chest radiograph indicated an abnormal shadow, and the patient received a consultation.

A chest radiograph shows consolidation with bilateral hilar lesions seen as a butterfly shadow. The diaphragm is elevated, with the costophrenic angle appearing as a half moon shape (→), indicating retention of pleural effusion. Extensive cardiac contour can be seen.

A chest CT reveals a typical butterfly shadow (→). The patient's condition improved with oxygen therapy and diuretics.

The principal pathology of consolidation is intra-alveolar lesions. Heitzman reported the characteristics of image findings (alveolar shadows) of intra-alveolar changes as being 1) lobular or segmental distribution, 2) poor margination of the process, 3) tendency of the process to coalesce, 4) air bronchogram and air alveologram, and 5) butterfly or batwing distribution of the process. As mentioned above, consolidation is characterized by increased attenuation areas, with an air bronchogram and no reduction of pulmonary volume. An air bronchogram is a bronchial shadow caused by filling of alveolar spaces due to intra-alveolar lesions at the bronchial periphery, which in turn results in air remaining in intrabronchial spaces.

It goes without saying that diseases showing consolidation should not be diagnosed using image findings alone. The patient's subjective symptoms, physical findings and laboratory findings are important for diagnosis. The following is an outline of typical diseases showing consolidation.

Bacterial pneumonia

With the increase in the number of elderly people, diabetics, administration of steroids and other factors, the incidence rate and mortality rate of community-acquired pneumonia is increasing. Diagnosis of community-acquired pneumonia and treatment are indicated in guidelines related to respiratory infections. The importance of a simple Gram stain for diagnosing bacterial pneumonia has been reported. Most cases of community-acquired bacterial pneumonia are pneumococcal pneumonia.

***Mycoplasma* pneumonia**

This is an atypical type of community-acquired pneumonia. The incidence in young people is comparatively high, and it is characterized by a persistent, dry cough and a markedly increased white blood cell count. Diagnosis is by an elevated serum mycoplasma antibody level, but usually, a nested PCR method is used. A typical image finding is ground glass attenuation, but consolidation is shown in many cases. A characteristic finding in CT is thickening of the bronchial walls and interstitial thickening in the areas surrounding the pulmonary artery, which is rarely seen with bacterial pneumonia. As yellow sputum is also seen in some cases, it could be a double infection with bacterial pneumonia.

Bronchioloalveolar carcinoma

This develops along alveolar walls, with cancer cells proliferating until they appear to fill alveolar spaces. A type that progresses diffusely is strongly mucus-secreting, with expectoration of a large volume (100 to 200 mL/day) of saliva-like, watery sputum in some cases. Diagnosis is by sputum cytology and transbronchial lung biopsy.

Pulmonary malignant lymphoma

Primary pulmonary malignant lymphoma is extremely rare, and accounts for just 0.3% of all cases of malignant lymphoma. Almost all are cases of indolent lymphoma, with most of these being B-cell lymphoma of mucosa-associated lymphoid tissue (MALT). Aggressive lymphomas account for 10% or less of cases, for which the prognosis is poor. Primary pulmonary malignant lymphoma forms lesions in intrabronchial spaces, and in some cases atelectatic shadow is indicated due to bronchial obstruction, but consolidation is indicated due to infiltration of tumor cells into the alveolar spaces.

***Legionella* pneumonia**

Genus Legionella bacteria exist in water and moist soil, and multiply most readily at body temperature. The source of infection is often bathing facilities such as hot springs. Diagnosis is by elevated Legionella antibody level, and by using a PCR method. Treatment with macrolides, fluoroquinolone and rifampicin is effective.

Wegener's granulomatosis

Lesions are multiple and there is involvement with a cavity, but in many cases pulmonary hemorrhage or exudation due to angitis results in consolidation being indicated. Refer to elevated cANCA levels for diagnosis.

Pulmonary hemorrhage

This is also called alveolar hemorrhage syndrome. Major pathogenic diseases include Goodpasture syndrome, general angitis, SLE and other collagen diseases, and pulmonary hemorrhage due to drugs. Ferruginous cells in alveoli and hemosiderin deposits on alveolar walls are seen. Diagnosis is by confirmation of iron stain of BALF cells and a positive macrophage image.

Cardiogenic pulmonary edema

Pulmonary edema is a pathological condition caused by the retention of large volumes of water in the extravascular areas of the lungs. In other words, it occurs when there is an imbalance between the discharge of water from microcirculation in the lungs and its elimination by the lymph ducts. Butterfly shadow is bilaterally symmetrical but in some cases it appears stronger on the right side. The mechanism of onset is unclear but it is thought that in the outer zone of the lung field, lymph duct development is good and thoracic movement is good so that elimination capability is high, resulting in little retention.

Radiographs of intrapulmonary lesions with decreased radiolucency

2. Alveolar shadow:

Atelectasis

[Pattern classification IV-A-2]

●Author — Tsuyoshi Okazaki

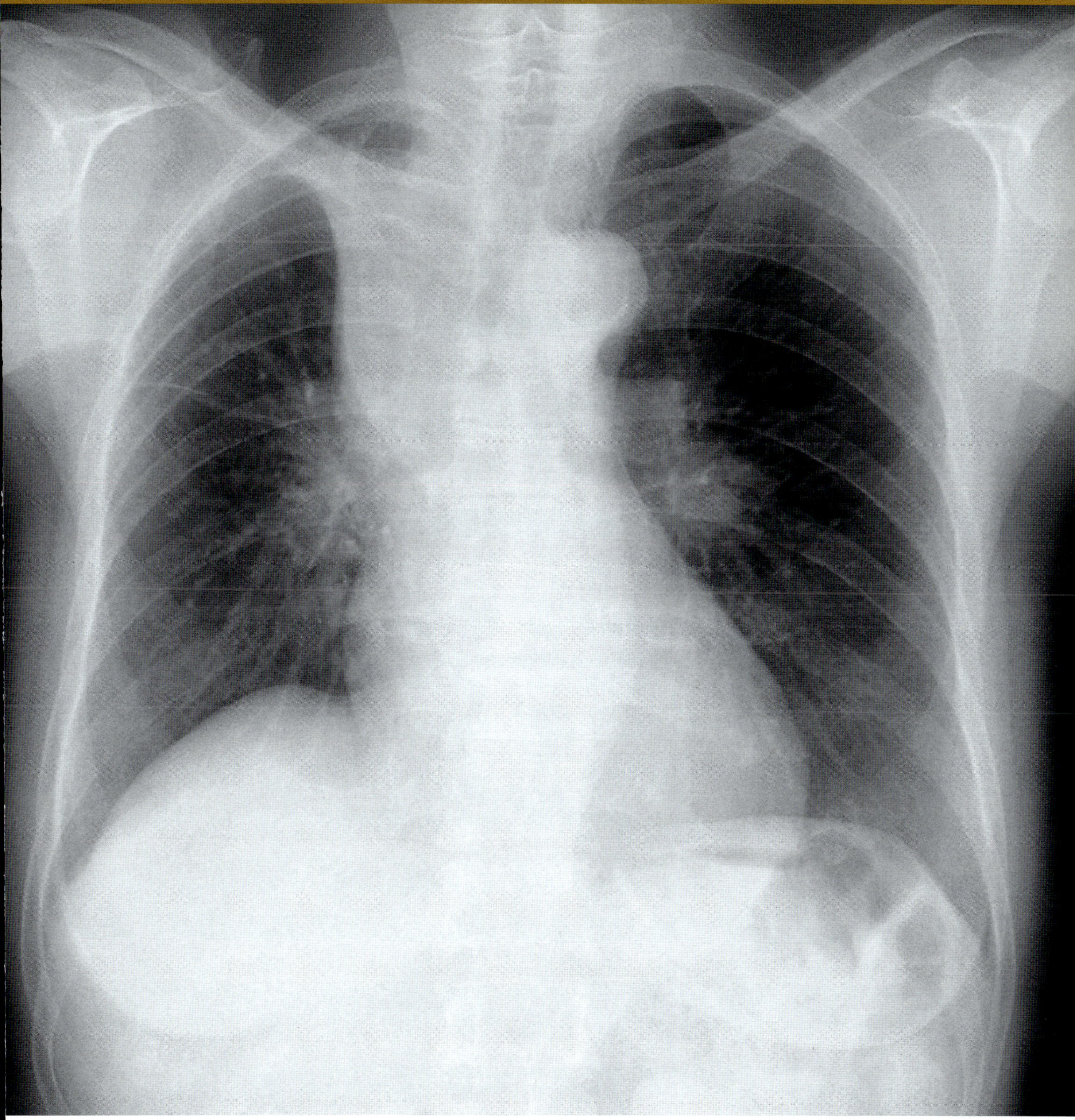

Keywords of this section

Atelectasis
Mediastinal lesions
Cicatricial contraction
Endotracheal foreign body
Atelectatic shadow
Mediastinal displacement
Compensatory overinflation
Air bronchogram
Pulmonary markings
Increased radiolucency
Overinflation
Pulmonary volume

Atelectasis

Tsuyoshi Okazaki
The Lung Cancer and Chest Diseases Center, Kusatsu General Hospital, Shiga, Japan

Atelectasis refers to a decrease in the volume of intrapulmonary air and lung volume. Its appearance in chest radiographs differs widely depending on its range and degree. Atelectasis is caused by various agents of disease and by lesions that obstruct segmental bronchi and lobar bronchi. This section focuses on atelectatic shadows resulting from obstruction of the lobar bronchi. Case 1 is a case in which the course over time of atelectasis was observed.

Case 1 73-year-old female

Chief complaints:
Cough, chest pain, blood-stained sputum
Medical history:
Anemia (under observation at another hospital)
Family history: Nothing notable
Present illness:
The patient was referred to this department after a chest radiograph taken one month ago indicated an abnormality in the right part of the hilum.

A chest radiograph (*Fig. 1*) showed an enlarged right hilar shadow (➤).

A bronchoscopy was conducted at the time, but no diagnosis was obtained. With a cough, chest pain and blood-stained sputum, the patient received a medical examination at this department.

A chest radiograph showed an enlarged abnormal shadow (P. 41, *Fig. 2*), and the patient was admitted. A silhouette-positive linear shadow in the right upper lung field (→), reduced right lung volume and elevated diaphragm could be seen.

Laboratory data on admission:
Mild anemia was observed, and arterial blood gas analysis indicated a satisfactory PaO_2 of 87.8 mmHg.
Course after admission:
Changes in chest radiographs over a period of 8 days indicated possible respiratory tract obstruction, and so a second bronchoscopic examination was scheduled. In the evening of the seventh day after admission, however, the patient suddenly lost consciousness, her SpO_2 level fell, and breathing difficulties suddenly became worse.

A chest radiograph (*Fig. 3*) showed reduced right lung volume (→), highly elevated diaphragm (➤), and displacement of mediastinal lesions to the right (➔), with progressive atelectasis. An emergency bronchoscopic examination was conducted after performing endotracheal intubation.

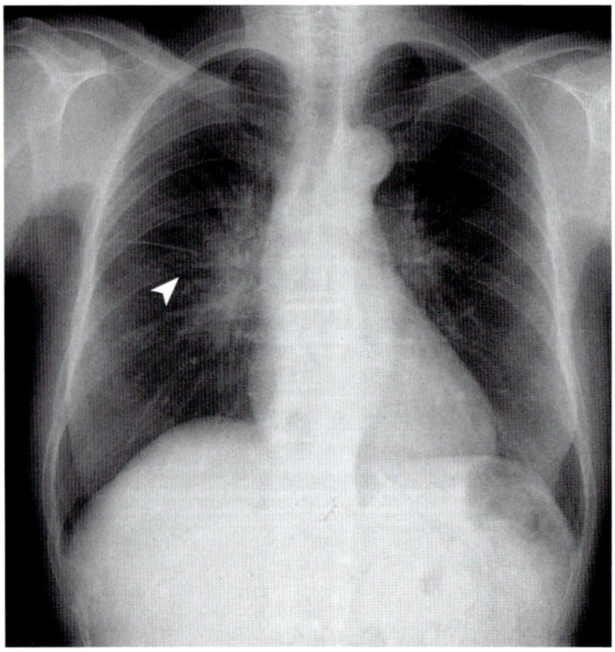

Figure 1. **Chest radiograph at first bronchoscopic examination**

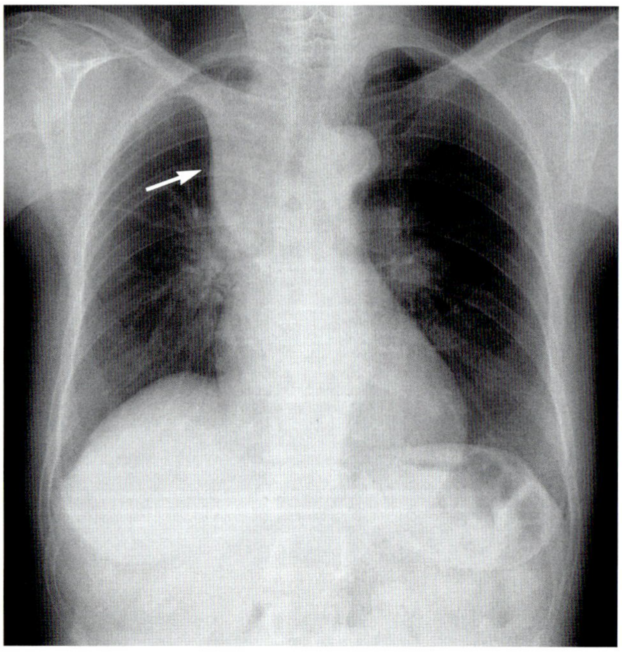

Figure 2. **Chest radiograph on admission**

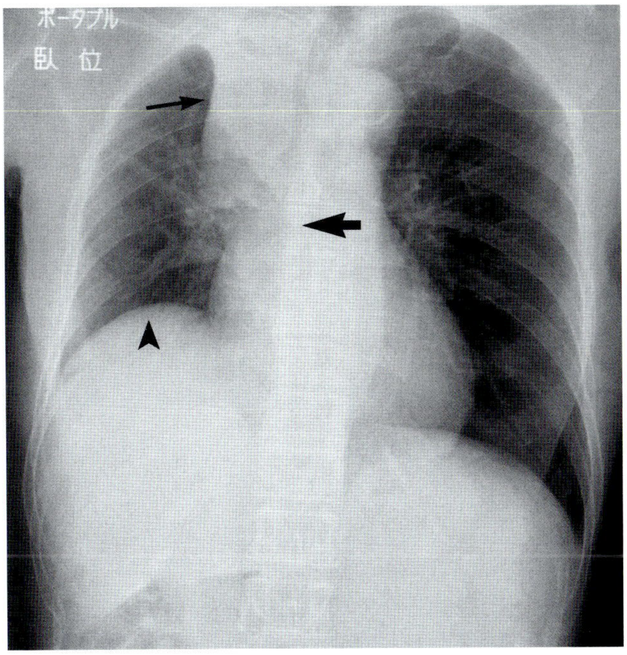

Figure 3. **Chest radiograph at the time of a sudden change**

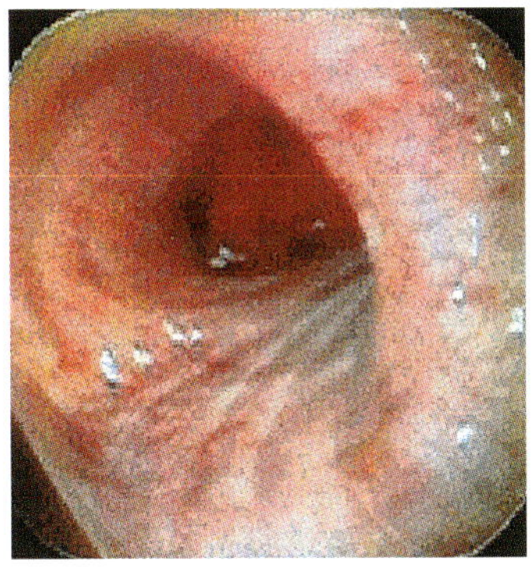

Figure 4. **Bronchoscopic findings:** right main bronchus

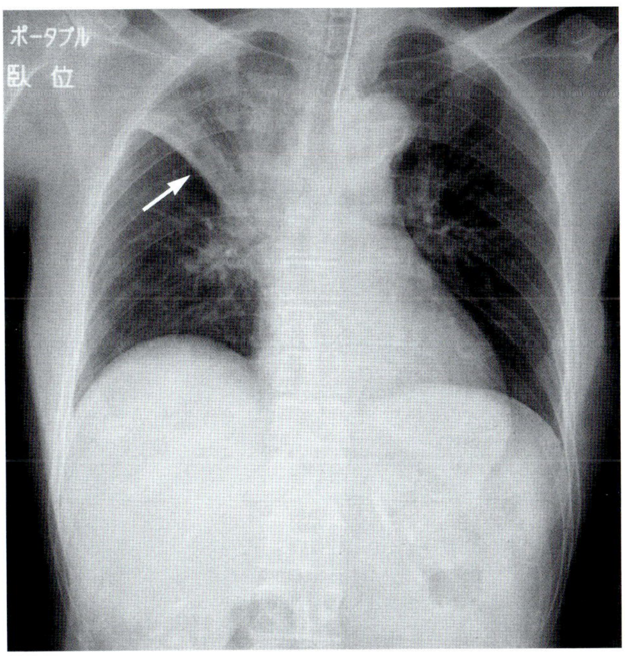

Figure 5. **Chest radiograph directly after blood clot removal**

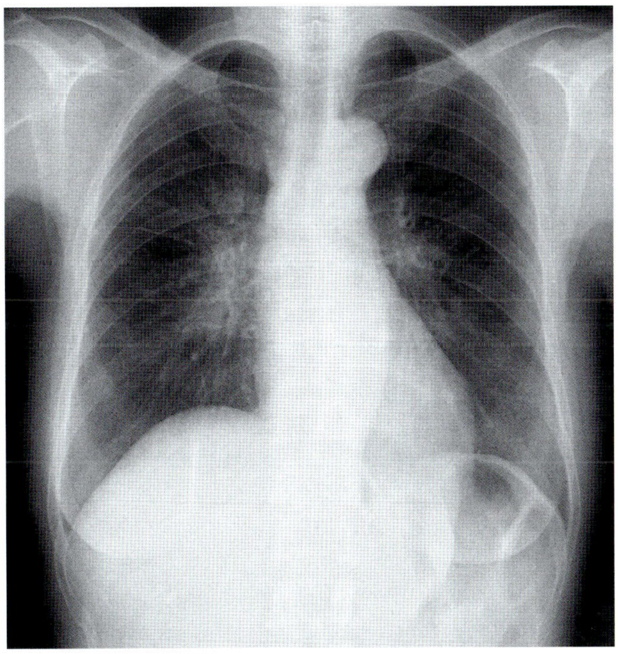

Figure 6. **Chest radiograph 3 days after blood clot removal**

The bronchoscopic examination revealed complete obstruction of the right main bronchus by a blood clot (*Fig. 4*), and it was decided at this department to remove the blood clot using a large pair of biopsy forceps inserted through the bronchoscope biopsy channel. After removal of the clot, the patient was immediately able to breathe, blood gas analysis showed improvement, and the intubation tube was removed.

Directly after removal of the blood clot, a chest radiograph (*Fig. 5*) showed air in the right upper lung field (→), and recovered pulmonary volume.

Following this, no blood-stained sputum was seen, no atelectasis was observed in a chest radiograph (*Fig. 6*), and the radiograph was almost the same as the one taken at the first medical examination.

For a definite diagnosis, a mediastinoscopy and lung biopsy were considered, but since there was a reduced tendency of hemorrhage and reduced blood platelet count, outpatient observation was conducted.

Course after being discharged

Since there was no particular change in course up to now, this was thought to be a case of idiopathic respiratory tract hemorrhage.

Atelectasis

Atelectasis is caused by tumors or foreign bodies directly obstructing the respiratory tract, and obstruction of the respiratory tract by external pressure due to tumors, inflammation, spontaneous pneumothorax, pleural effusion retention and other factors. In some cases obstruction is also caused by wall thickening. In other words, atelectasis is a disease condition that can be commonly observed.

Chest radiographs of complete atelectasis are often seen but by chance, Case 1 provided images of the process involved in the completion of atelectasis. Furthermore, because respiratory tract obstruction occurred over a short period of time, extreme respiratory symptoms were also observed. In cases where the course up to atelectasis is comparatively long, subjective symptoms are not clear, and some cases may be asymptomatic.

Classification of atelectasis

1. Respiratory tract obstruction
   - Inside the respiratory tract
   - Pressure from outside the respiratory tract
   - Inflammation or thickening of respiratory tract walls
2. Cicatricial contraction
3. Spontaneous pneumothorax
4. Tumor or inflammation in the pulmonary parenchyma
5. Surfactant disorder (radiation pneumonitis)

Causative diseases

I. Diseases causing obstruction inside the respiratory tract
   1. Foreign body in bronchus
   2. Obstruction due to bronchial mucus (sputum)
   3. Intrabronchial tumor (lung cancer, bronchial adenoma, etc.)

II. Diseases causing obstruction due to extrabronchial pressure
   1. Lymphadenopathy (lung cancer, pulmonary tuberculosis, malignant lymphoma, etc.)
   2. Vascular system disease (aortic aneurism, left atrial enlargement, etc.)
   3. Mediastinal tumor
   4. Pulmonary parenchyma disease (malignant tumor, cystic diseases, etc.)

III. Bronchial diseases (bronchial tuberculosis, traumatic bronchial disruption, broncholith, etc.)

IV. Nonobstructive atelectasis (bronchiectasis, pulmonary tuberculosis, radiation pneumonitis, etc.)

Interpretation points of chest radiograph

When an atelectatic shadow indicates an abnormality, the shape of a typical segment/lobe atelectatic shadow (direct change) should be ascertained. At the same time it is important to bear in mind the indirect changes that occur due to atelectasis, namely decreased lung volume and changes in intrapulmonary pressure.

Direct changes

Atelectatic shadows in different pulmonary lobes (*Fig. 7*)

Indirect changes

1. Elevated diaphragm shadow
2. Mediastinum displacement towards the atelectasis side
3. Compensatory overinflation of the normal lung
4. Narrowing of intercostal space on the atelectasis side
5. No air bronchogram
6. Fewer pulmonary markings on the affected lung

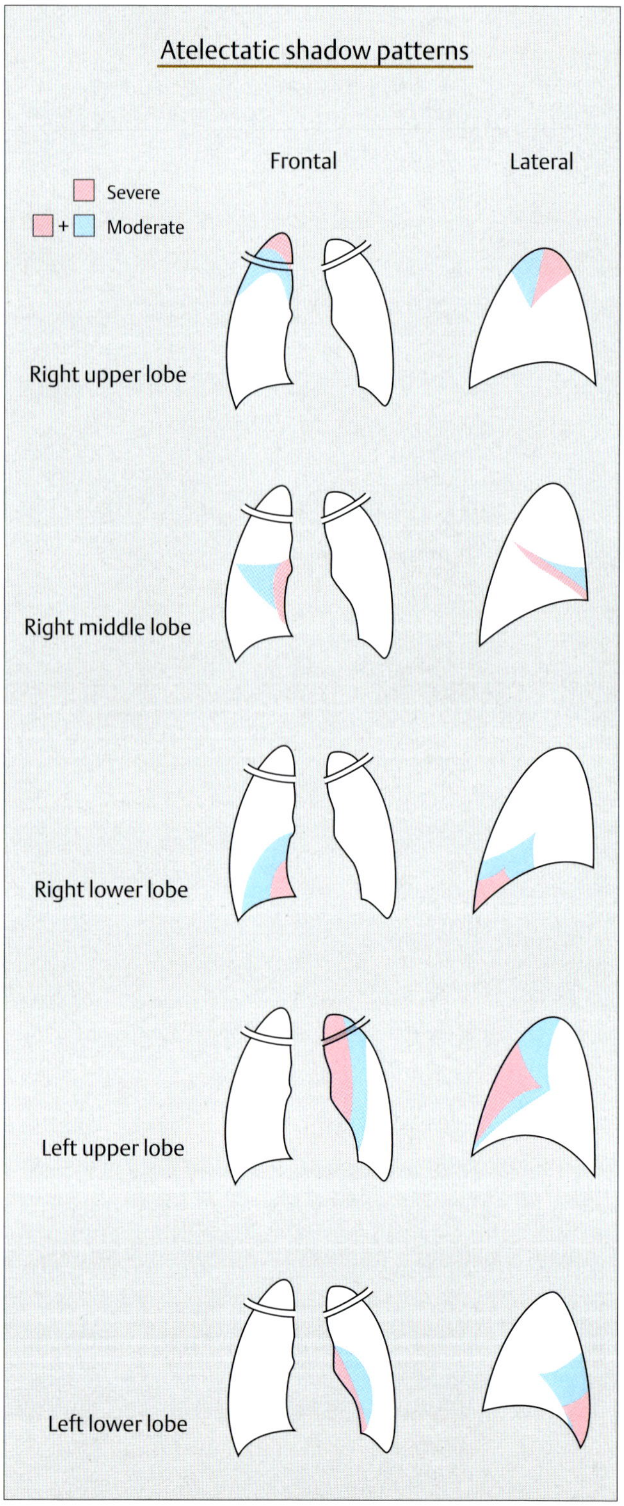

Figure 7. **Atelectatic shadows in different pulmonary lobes**

Case 2 Middle lobe syndrome
56-year-old male

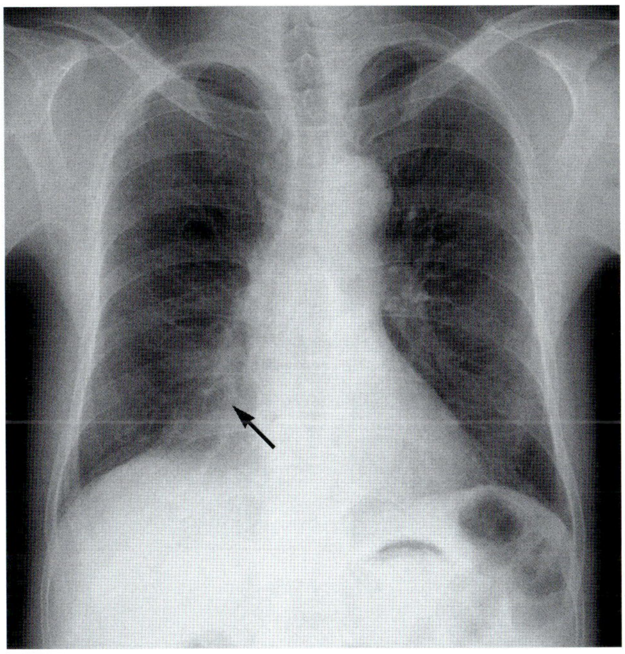

Figure 8. **Chest radiograph**

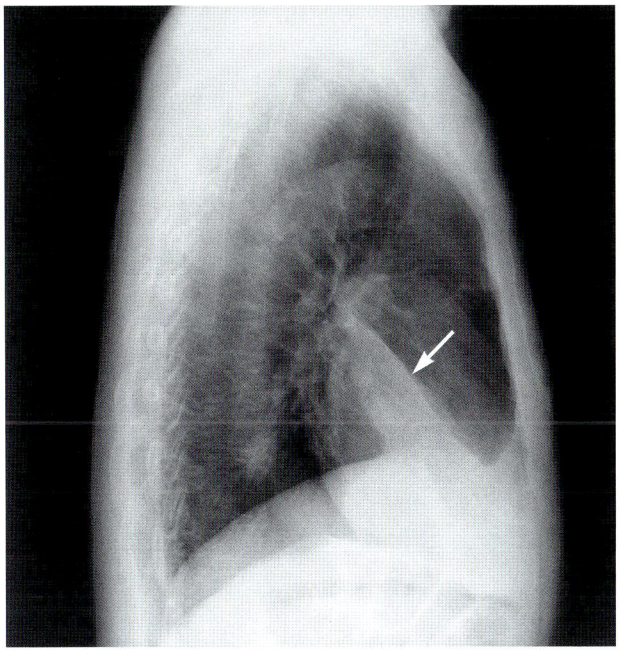

Figure 9. **Chest radiograph**

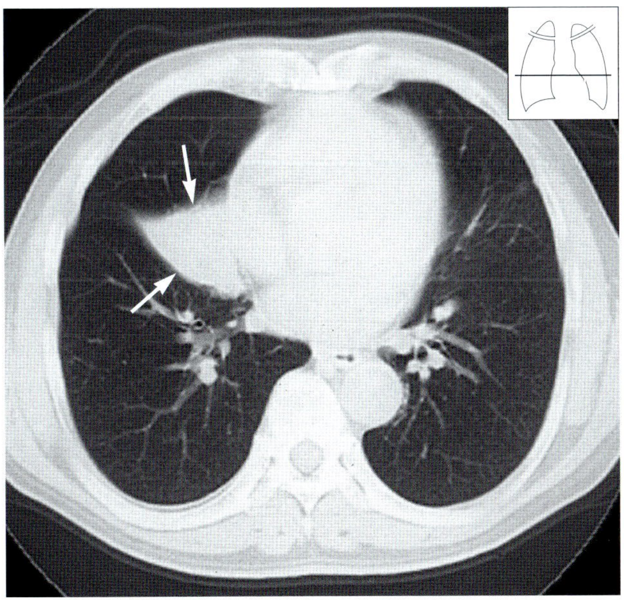

Figure 10. **Chest CT**

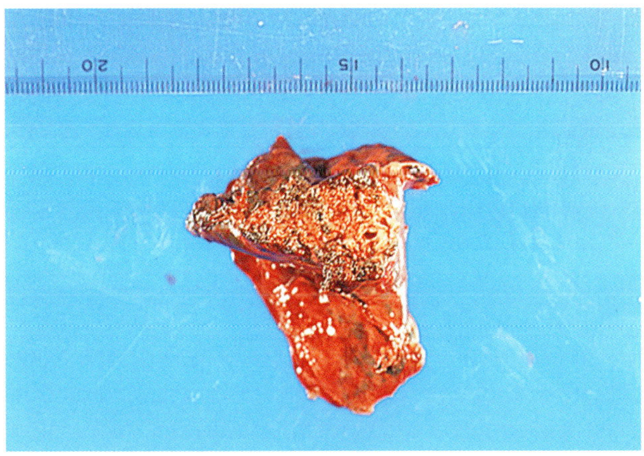

Figure 11. **Excised specimen**

A frontal chest radiograph (*Fig. 8*) shows a faint shadow in the right lower lung field, with the right ventricular segment (second border of the heart) indicating a silhouette-positive shape (→).

A lateral chest radiograph (*Fig. 9*) shows normal air spaces in the right upper and lower lobes but severe atelectasis is indicated in the middle lobe (→).

In a chest CT, the completely atelectatic middle lobe is seen as a triangular shape on the outside of the heart border (→).

In this case, excision of the middle lobe was conducted due to recurrent pneumonia.

The specimen is a middle lobe that has become completely atelectatic. Since there is no air in it and it has changed organically, the diagnosis was bronchiolitis obliterans with organizing pneumonia (BOOP).

Case 3 Lung cancer

53-year-old male

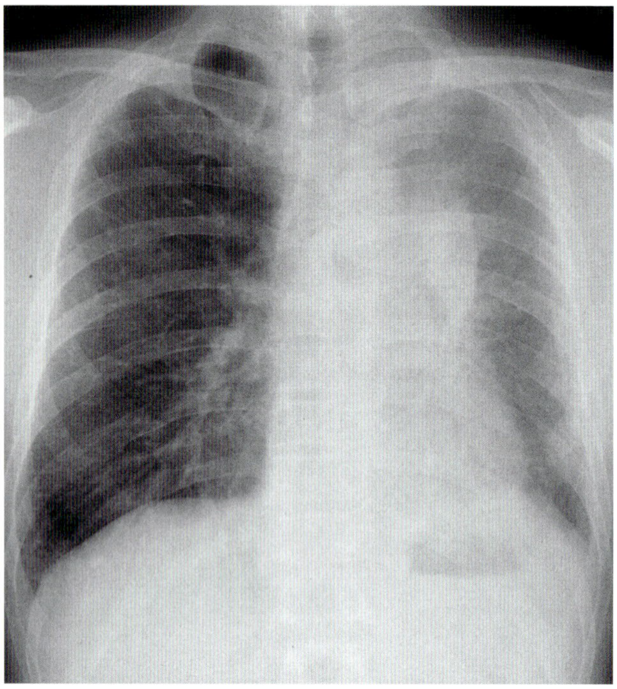

Figure 12. **Chest radiograph**

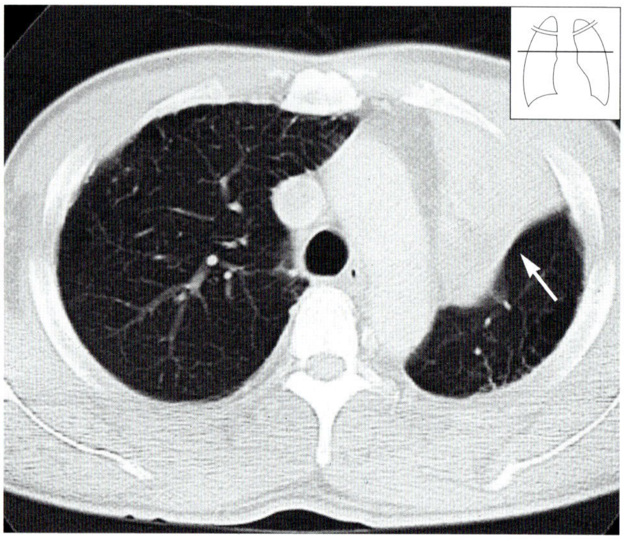

Figure 13. **Chest CT**

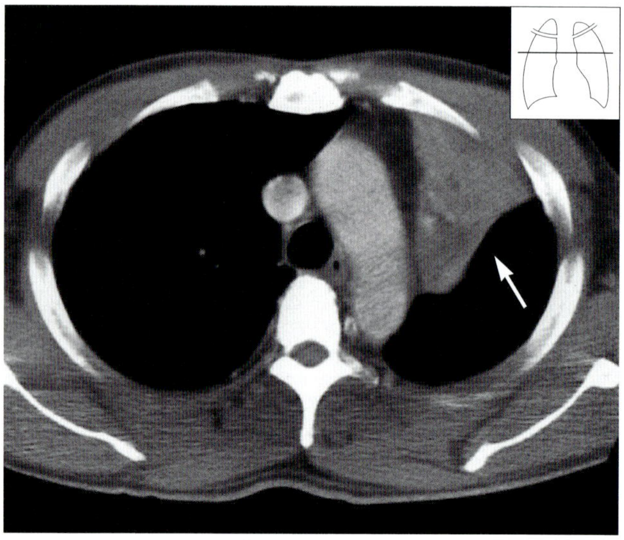

Figure 14. **Chest CT: Mediastinal window setting**

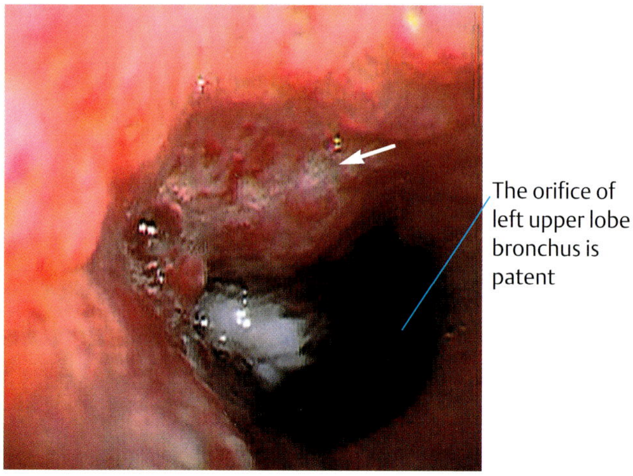

Figure 15. **Bronchoscopic findings**

A chest radiograph (*Fig. 12*) shows decreased radiolucency in the entire left lung, decreased left lung volume (direct change), mediastinal lesion displacement to the left, increased radiolucency and overinflation (indirect change) in the right lung.

In chest CT (*Figs. 13, 14*), left upper lobe opacity and occupation of the upper chest by the left lower lobe (S^6) (→) are seen, pointing to a diagnosis of complete atelectasis.

In this case, the patient received a medical examination at this hospital for the chief complaints of cough and dizziness. Left upper lobe atelectasis was observed in chest radiographs and chest CT. To ascertain the cause, a bronchoscopic examination was conducted (*Fig. 15*), during which a tumor (→) obstructing the left upper lobe bronchus was observed, and a cytological examination led to a diagnosis of lung cancer (adenocarcinoma). However, due to poor general physical condition, it was thought that chemotherapy using anticancer agents would be difficult. Rapid improvement of the atelectasis was desired, and so bronchial artery infusion with anticancer agents was conducted, resulting in atelectasis improvement. In addition, whole brain irradiation was conducted, and the patient was discharged.

Case 4 Lung cancer

69-year-old female

A chest radiograph (*Fig. 16*) indicates reduced left lung volume and the line of the descending aorta becoming opaque (➞) (direct changes). In addition, mediastinal lesions have in general been displaced to the left (indirect changes).

In chest CT (*Figs. 17, 18*), peripheral atelectasis from the left lower lobe branch is observed (➞), with obstruction of the left lower lobe bronchus by a tumor (➤).

Bronchoscopic findings (*Figs. 19, 20*) show obstruction of the left lower lobe bronchus by a tumor.

After sputum examination, this case was diagnosed as lung cancer (small cell lung cancer), and chemotherapy was conducted resulting in the tumor shrinking and improved atelectasis. Following this, chemotherapy was repeated and radiation therapy of the chest was conducted.

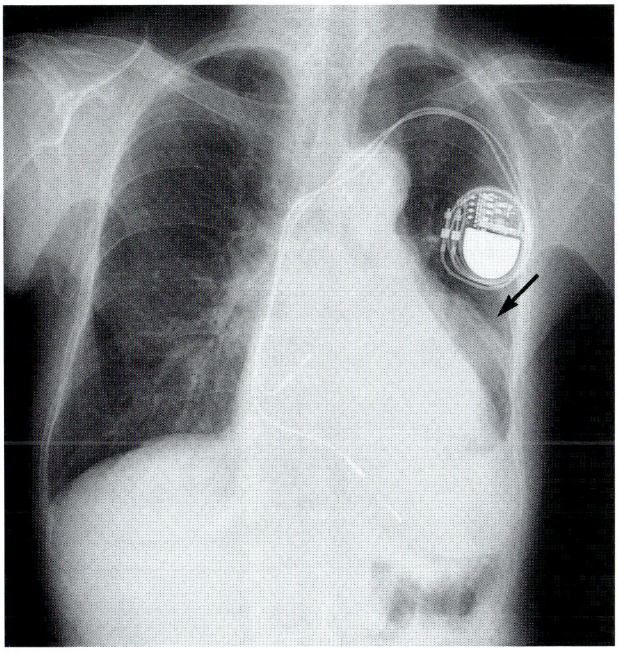

Figure 16. **Chest radiograph**

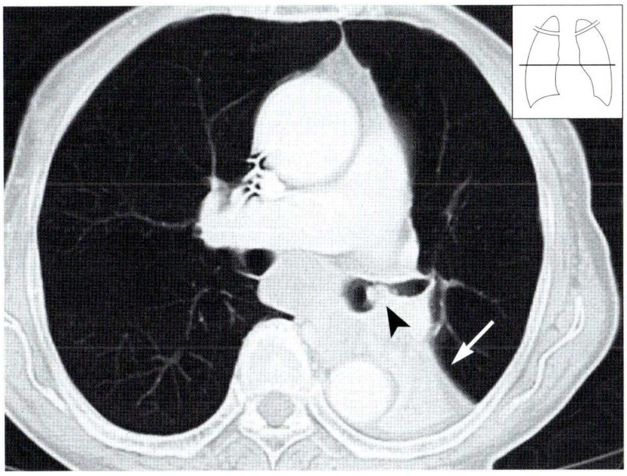

Figure 17. **Chest CT**

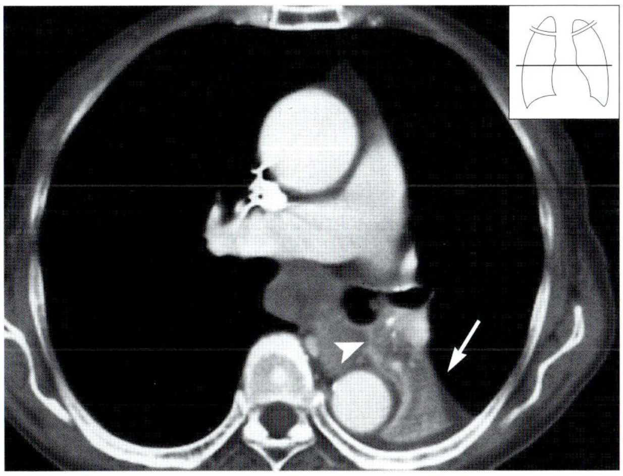

Figure 18. **Chest CT: Mediastinal window setting**

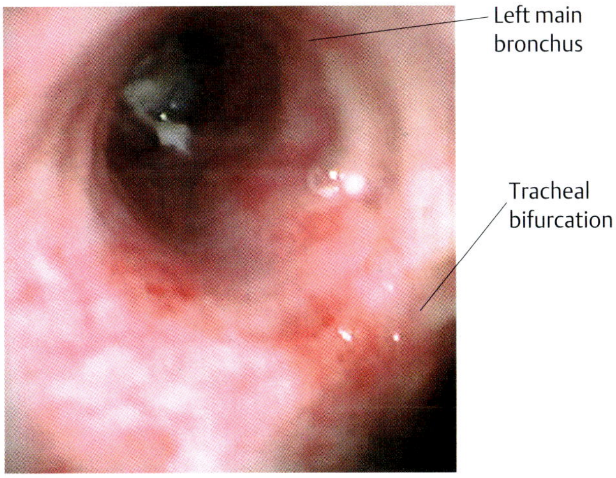

Figure 19. **Bronchoscopic findings**

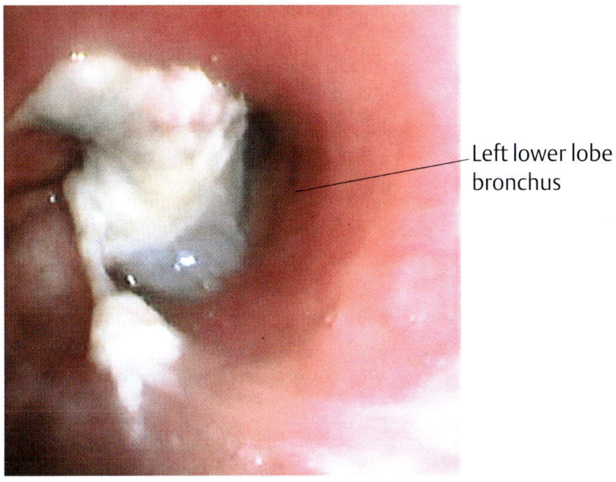

Figure 20. **Bronchoscopic findings: close-up view**

Atelectasis is a disease condition frequently observed in respiratory disease. In addition to the major cause of respiratory tract obstruction (foreign object, mucoid impaction, tumor), atelectasis is due to a wide range of causative factors such as external pressure on the bronchus (lymphadenopathy, aortic aneurism, mediastinal tumor), bronchial diseases (bronchial tuberculosis, traumatic bronchial disruption), and nonobstructive diseases (bronchiectasis, calcification of old tuberculous lesion). Atelectasis can be diagnosed using 1) direct findings and 2) indirect findings indicated by chest radiographs but a clearer diagnosis is possible with chest CT.

Points for interpreting chest CT include the internal structure of a shadow (absence of air), bronchopulmonary and lobar narrowing and obstruction, adjacent pulmonary lobes and their borders, mediastinal displacement, bronchial and vascular displacement, pleural effusion retention and elevated diaphragm, and in many cases these points enable easy diagnosis of atelectasis. However, with a regular diagnosis, after examining chest radiographs it is important to bear in mind the main cause of the abnormal shadow and what exactly is occurring.

To diagnose atelectatic shadows, it is important to first ascertain the atelectatic shadow shape and pattern in different pulmonary lobes. Rather than focusing on just direct findings, it is vital not to overlook indirect findings, that is, secondary changes. These secondary changes include elevated diaphragm, mediastinal displacement towards the atelectatic side, compensatory overinflation of the normal lung, narrowing of intracostal space on the atelectatic side and lack of air bronchogram.

When atelectasis develops, there is increased intrapleural negative pressure on the affected side which is compensated for by an elevation of the diaphragm. Normally, left/right intrapleural negative pressure is equal, and the mediastinum is located in the center. When a difference in intrapleural negative pressure occurs, however, the mediastinum is displaced towards the side of lower pressure. Due to the relationship with anatomical position, strong displacement of the bronchus is seen with upper lobe atelectasis, while there is little bronchial displacement with lower lobe atelectasis and cardiac contour displacement is observed. Another change seen with upper lobe atelectasis is hilar vascular shadow elevation on the affected lung side. Conversely, with lower lobe atelectasis, the hilar shadow is displaced downward. Due to the same principle, increased intrapleural negative pressure causes intracostal space narrowing on the affected side but this change is not observed in all cases and is also difficult to ascertain with a frontal chest radiograph. Furthermore, if air is absorbed as atelectasis progresses, the air bronchogram inside the shadow disappears. The remaining lung on the affected side also overinflates to compensate, resulting in reduced pulmonary markings.

For pathologies requiring differentiation of atelectatic shadows, factors to note include pleural effusion retention, lobar pneumonia and giant pulmonary cyst. However, working from the primary and secondary changes mentioned above, diagnosing atelectatic shadow is not so difficult. Nevertheless, when a large volume of pleural effusion is retained, there are many cases where this, together with external pressure, causes atelectasis. It is also necessary to differentiate between lower lobe atelectasis and pleural effusion. In the case of the right lower lobe, the costophrenic angle disappears, while with the left lower lobe there are many cases in which an opaque shadow is observed from the cardiac contour to the central part of the diaphragm. In many cases, decreased pulmonary markings are another important consideration. With lobar pneumonia, the presence or absence of an air bronchogram is a differentiating point, while for giant pulmonary cysts a differentiating point is that in many cases no decrease in pulmonary volume is observed.

To assure that nothing is overlooked in an atelectatic shadow, it is important to interpret radiographs in detail applying the information provided in this section.

Chapter 4

Radiographs of intrapulmonary lesions with decreased radiolucency

3. Interstitial shadow:

Granulomatous sign

[Pattern classification IV-B-1]

●Authors — Koichiro Yoshida, Nobuyuki Hara

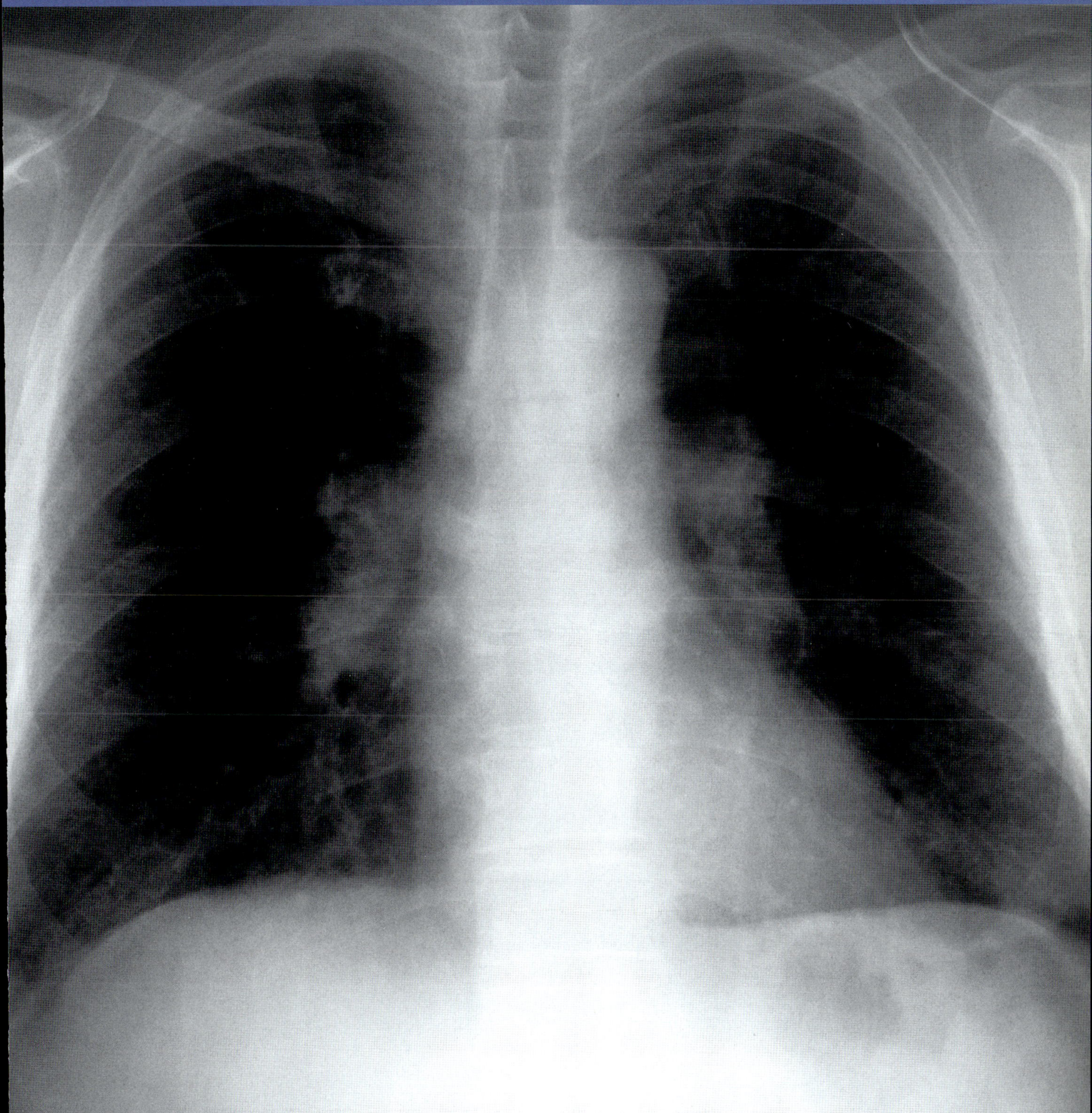

ywords of
s section

Granulomatous sign
BHL
Noncaseating granuloma
Pulmonary sarcoidosis
Trichosporon asahii
Pulmonary tuberculosis
Satellite lesions
Langhans' giant cell
Pulmonary atypical mycobacteriosis
M. avium
Pulmonary eosinophilic granuloma
Birbeck granule
Pulmonary cryptococcosis
Wegener's granulomatosis
Multiple nodules accompanying cavities
Centrilobular nodules
Peripheral lobular nodules
Necrotizing granulomatous inflammation

Granulomatous sign

Koichiro Yoshida,[1)] **Nobuyuki Hara**[2)]
1) Faculty of Medicine, Kyushu University, Fukuoka, Japan
2) Fukuoka Cancer Society, Fukuoka, Japan

Pulmonary granulomatous disease is characterized mainly by nodular patterns on chest radiographs caused by epithelial cells and multinucleated giant cells. Imaging diagnosis is important for diagnosis of the disease, with morphological analysis on the secondary lobule level using high-resolution CT (HRCT) in particular being used to ascertain the primary site of the lesion.

Case 1 65-year-old male

Chief complaint: Cough
Past history: Psoriasis from the age of 50
Medical history: Mother with hypertension, elder sister with hepatitis
Smoking history: 30/day for 50 years
Present illness:
The patient exhibited a cough from around September 1999 and received a medical examination at a local hospital. Chest radiographs indicated an abnormality and he was referred to this department as an outpatient. In October he received a medical examination as an outpatient and chest radiographs indicated bilateral hilar lymphadenopathy and diffuse granular shadow. Sarcoidosis was suspected and the patient was admitted.
Physical findings on admission:
Height 153 cm, weight 65 kg, normal breath sounds, no other findings of note.
Laboratory data on admission:
Positive tuberculin skin reaction, and elevated ESR of 9 mm/hour, 23 mm/2 hours, ACE of 29 U/L, and lysozyme of 25 μg/mL. Other serologic tests, blood gas and pulmonary function tests indicated no abnormalities. A Ga scintigram showed bilateral mediastinal abnormalities.

Chest radiograph (P. 49): A diffuse granular shadow is observed throughout bilateral lung fields. Nodules are faint, 2 to 3 mm in diameter. Findings show accompanying bilateral hilar lymph node swelling indicating bilateral hilar lymphadenopathy (BHL).

Chest CT: A lung window setting image shows multiple diffuse granular shadows throughout the lung fields. Distribution is almost uniform but it is slightly more concentrated on the posterior side. Nodules are about 2 to 3 mm in diameter, with most of them being centrilobular. Thickening of the interlobular septal wall touching the pleura is observed in places, as well as nodal thickening along the interlobar pleura, central bronchus and blood vessels (→) (*Figs. 1, 2*). Hilar lymph node swelling is also observed in the mediastinum (→) (*Figs. 3, 4*).

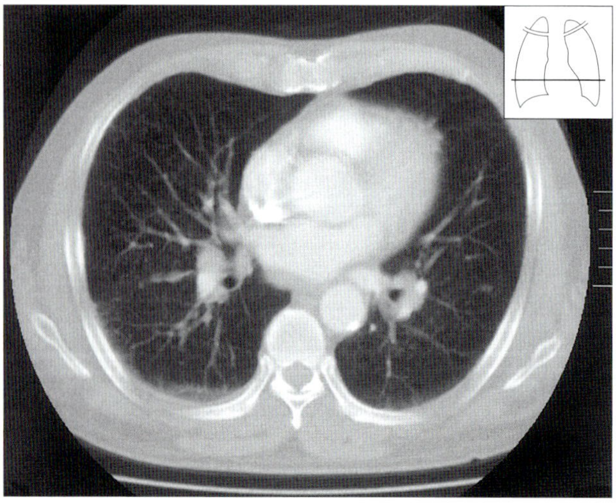

Figure 1. **Chest CT: Lung window setting**

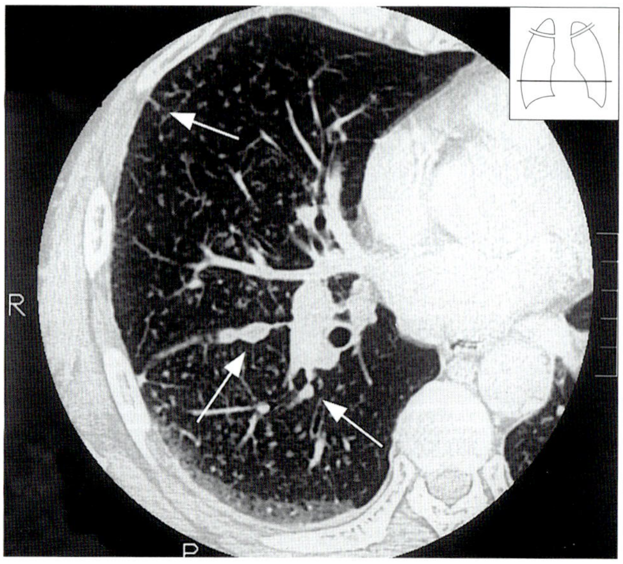

Figure 2. **High-resolution CT: Lung window setting**

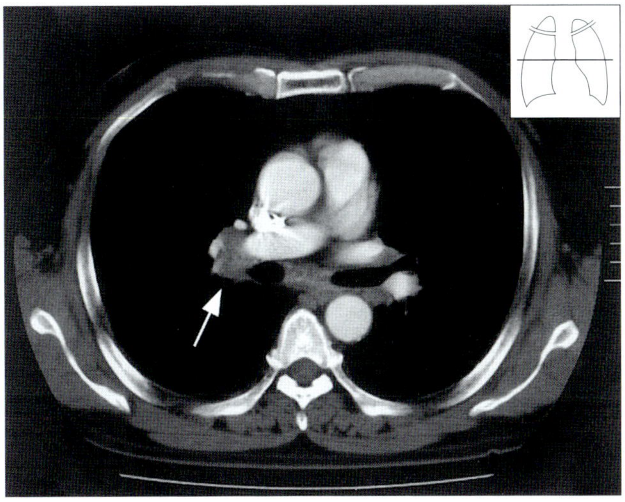

Figure 3. **Chest CT: Mediastinal window setting**

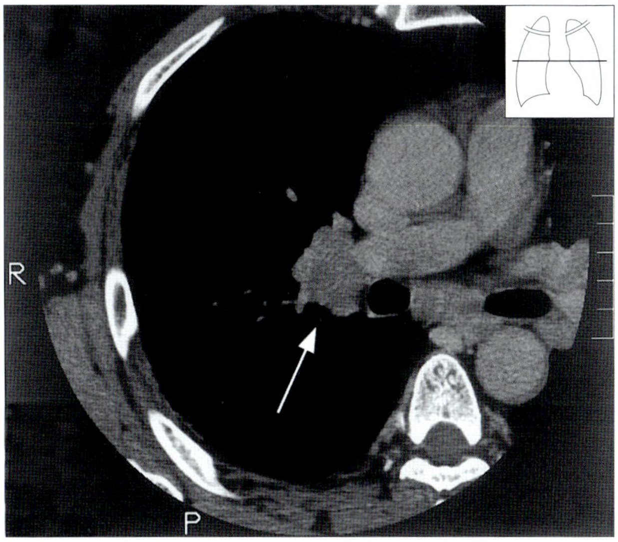

Figure 4. **High-resolution CT: Mediastinal window setting**

Diagnosis

From imaging findings such as nodules in both centrilobular and perilobular tissues, and accompanying multiple mediastinal and hilar lymph nodule swelling, sarcoidosis was first considered as the differential diagnosis. The tuberculin skin test was positive but serological test and Ga scintigram results did not contradict the diagnosis of sarcoidosis. For a histological diagnosis, bronchoscopy was conducted.

Bronchoalveolar lavage (BAL): Cell count was elevated at 4.48 x 10^5/mL, cell fractionation showed a macrophage count of 50% and elevated lymphocyte count of 50%. CD4/CD8 ratio was mildly elevated at 5.49.

Transbronchial lung biopsy (TBLB) (*Figs. 5, 6*): Non-caseating granuloma including histiocytes and multinuclear giant cells are observed. Due to this and other test results, the diagnosis was sarcoidosis.

Conclusions of this case: Pulmonary sarcoidosis

Sarcoidosis is a systemic disease of unclear cause that forms non-caseating epithelial cell granulomas. With spontaneous remission occurring in 70 to 80% of cases, it is a disease with a favorable prognosis but some cases are difficult to treat, leading to progressive fibrosis and organ dysfunction.

Chest radiograph findings classify three stages of the disease. In Stage I the findings are hilar and mediastinal lymphadenopathy, otherwise known as BHL. Stage II is the stage when the lung parenchyma becomes diseased as indicated by bilateral diffuse granular, reticular shadow. In Stage III, fibrosis progresses and BHL disappears.

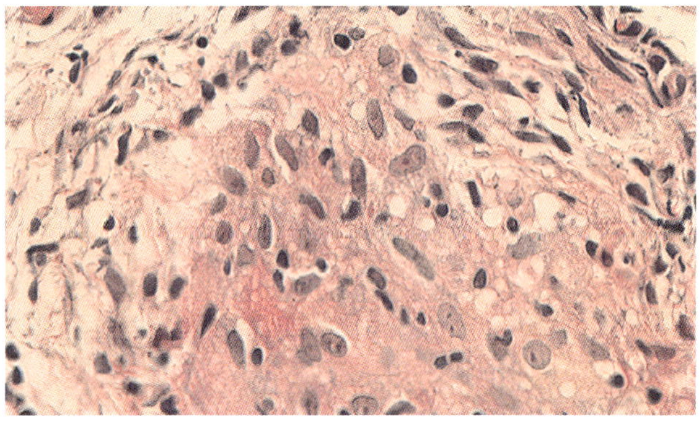

Figure 5. **Pathological findings by transbronchial lung biopsy (x 200)**

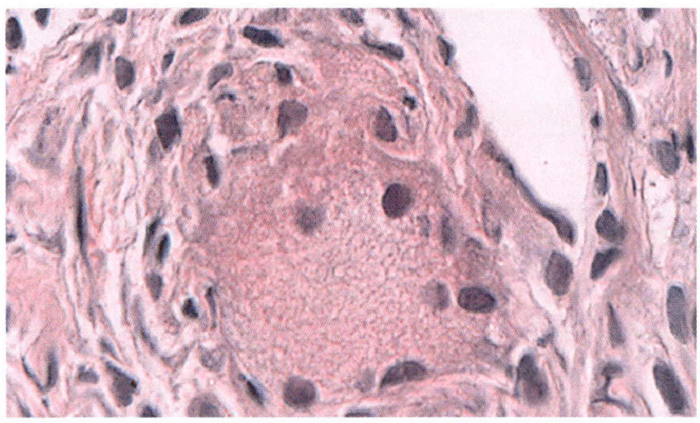

Figure 6. **Pathological findings by transbronchial lung biopsy**

High-resolution CT shows that lung field lesions are characterized by the formation of granulomas predominantly in centrilobular and perilobular tissue including lymphatics. Typical findings show uniform or nodular-like thickening of bronchial arteries and pulmonary vein. In addition, when small granulomas are diffusely formed in the surrounding tissue of the lower bronchioles and alveolar septum, ground glass opacity is sometimes exhibited. When granulomas clump together, nodular shadows may also have irregular borders.

In cases that progress to fibrosis, findings include reduced capacity predominantly in the upper lung field, fibrotic shadow and honeycomb lung.

Granulomatous sign and its differentiation

A granuloma is caused by the accumulation and proliferation of mainly mononuclear leukocytes resulting from a chronic inflammatory reaction. The disease occurs in foci that show as nodular shadows. Since diseases that cause the formation of these granulomas have widely differing pathologies (*Table 1*), the definition of granulomatous pulmonary disease is at present still vague.

In many cases, imagings of granulomatous pulmonary disease show nodular shadows of varying size, while in chest radiographs findings include diffuse granular shadow, nodular shadow and granular reticular shadow. As a result, it is necessary to differentiate between other diseases that exhibit diffuse granular and nodular shadows (*Table 2*).

Currently, CT clearly shows the relationship between the disease and the spread from the primary site, localization, and vascular and bronchial factors, and differential imaging diagnosis of granulomas is now easy. In particular, high-resolution CT enables analysis on the secondary lobule level, and has in many cases become a conclusive method for the imaging diagnosis of noninfectious granuloma.

Infection	Pulmonary tuberculosis Atypical (nontubercular) mycobacteriosis Fungal infection
Chemical substances	Beryllium lung disease, silicosis
Extrinsic allergies	Hypersensitivity pneumonitis
Cause unclear	Sarcoidosis Pulmonary eosinophilic granuloma Wegener's granulomatosis Allergic granulomatosis angitis Lymphomatoid granulomatosis

Table 1. **Classification of granulomatous pulmonary disease**
(From reference literature 1)

	Common	Rare
Acute	Viral pneumonia Miliary tuberculosis, pulmonary edema ARDS	Metastatic lung cancer Pulmonary mycosis Septic emboli
Chronic	Metastatic lung cancer Sarcoidosis Pulmonary tuberculosis Pneumoconiosis (especially silicosis) Diffuse panbronchiolitis (DPB)	Malignant lymphoma Pulmonary eosinophilic granuloma Hypersensitivity pneumonitis Alveolar carcinoma Pulmonary mycosis Alveolar hemorrhage Chronic beryllium lung Other bronchiolitic disease

Table 2. **Diseases exhibiting diffuse granular shadow (Heitzman)**
(Changed from reference literature 2 and 3)

Case 2 **Hypersensitivity pneumonitis**
49-year-old female

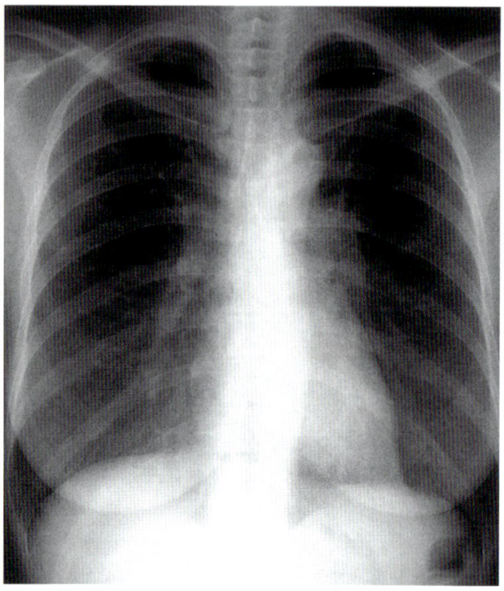

Figure 7. **Chest radiograph**

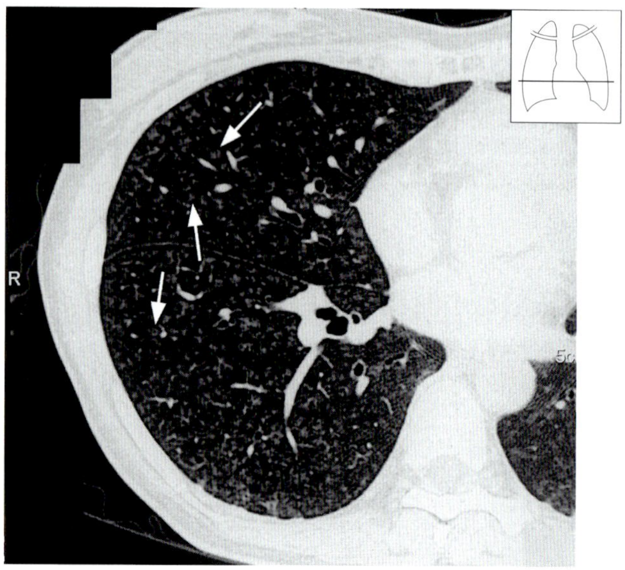

Figure 8. **Chest CT**

Chief complaint: Dyspnea on exertion
This case received a medical examination at this department with the chief complaint of dyspnea. A bronchoalveolar lavage indicated an elevated lymphocyte count and a reduced CD4/CD8 ratio, and elevated antibody titer for *Trichosporon asahii*. These findings, together with image findings, resulted in a diagnosis of hypersensitivity pneumonitis.

Chest radiograph: Increased density of faint ground glass opacity in both lower lung fields is observed.

Chest CT: Diffuse small nodular shadows are observed throughout bilateral lung fields. Nodules (→) are centrilobular and faint, with comparatively indistinct borders.

Case 3 Pulmonary tuberculosis

22-year-old male

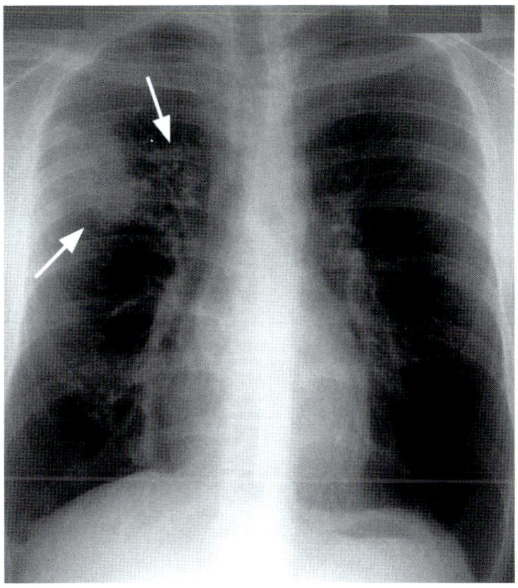

Figure 9. **Chest radiograph**

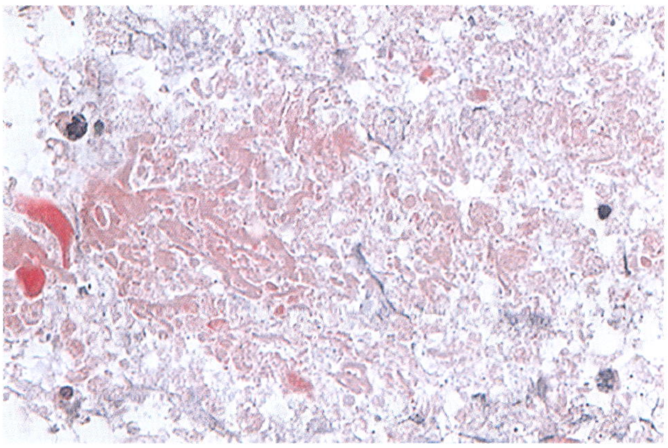

Figure 11. **Pathological findings by transbronchial lung biopsy (x 100)**

Chief complaint: None

Chest radiographs during examination indicated abnormalities, and the case was referred to this department. A transbronchial lung biopsy showed nodules with *Mycobacterium* spp. in the center and accompanying necrosis, from which evidence pulmonary tuberculosis was diagnosed.

Chest radiograph: Nodular-like, approximately 5 cm diameter shadows with comparatively distinct borders are observed in the outer areas of the right upper lung

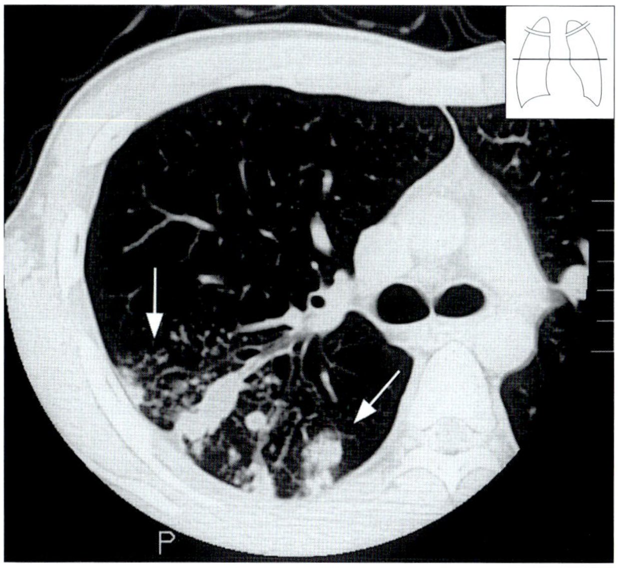

Figure 10. **Chest CT**

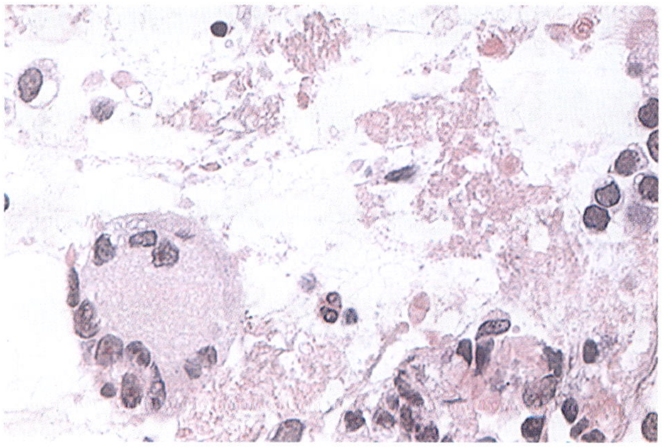

Figure 12. **Pathological findings by transbronchial lung biopsy (x 200)**

field. A number of small nodular shadows are observed in the area surrounding the bronchus in the center, which could be satellite lesions (→).

Chest CT: Multiple nodular shadows 1 cm or more in diameter are observed throughout the right lung S^2. Numerous centrilobular nodules and intralobular branch-like shadows (→) are also observed. The hilar side of the shadow joins with the bronchus connecting to the hilum.

Transbronchial lung biopsy: Necrotic tissue sparsely infiltrated with neutrophiles is observed. Langhans' giant cells can also be seen.

Case 4 Pulmonary atypical mycobacteriosis

44-year-old female

Chief complaint: Hemoptysis

The patient has a medical history of hemoptysis 8 years ago. From 6 years ago, chest radiographs pointed to abnormalities but they were left untreated. This time, with the recurrence of hemoptysis, the patient received a medical examination at a local hospital. As tuberculosis was suspected, a sputum examination was conducted. *Mycobacterium* (*M.*) *avium* was detected in culture and the patient was referred to this department. *M. avium* was detected in repeated sputum cultures, and since *M. avium* was detected with bronchoalveolar lavage PCR analysis, pulmonary atypical mycobacteriosis was diagnosed.

Chest radiograph: There are multiple nodular shadows with irregular borders in the left lower lung field, with a

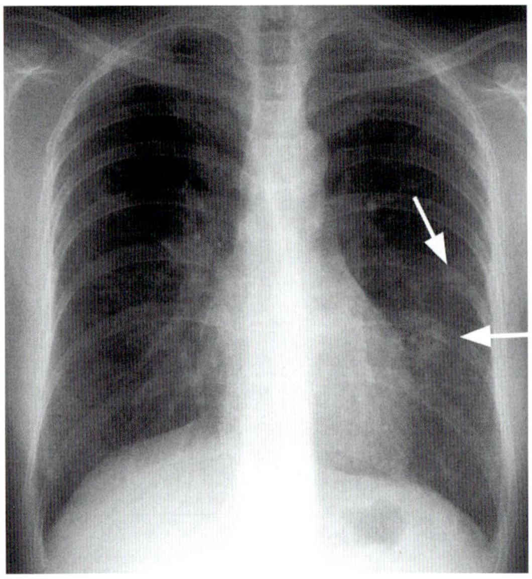

Figure 13. **Chest radiograph**

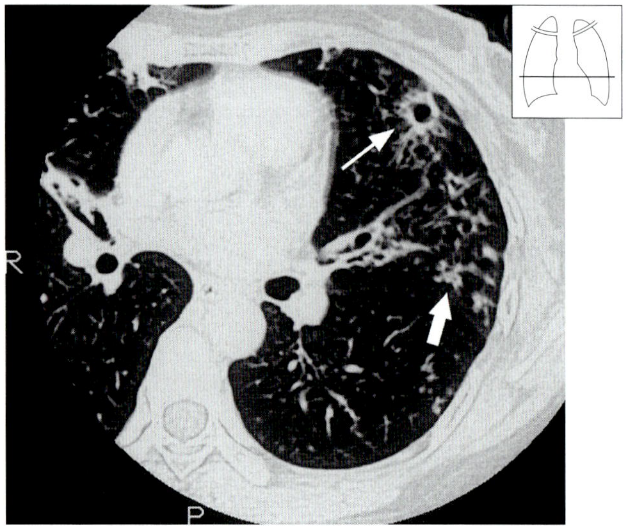

Figure 14. **Chest CT**

number of spot-like small nodular shadows (→) visible below.

Chest CT: In the center of the lingular segment multiple nodular shadows can be seen, with cavities (→) also visible in places. There are also a number of nodules in the central lower interlobar pleura (→), and under them numerous nodular shadows that could be satellite lesions.

Case 5 Pulmonary eosinophilic granuloma

17-year-old male

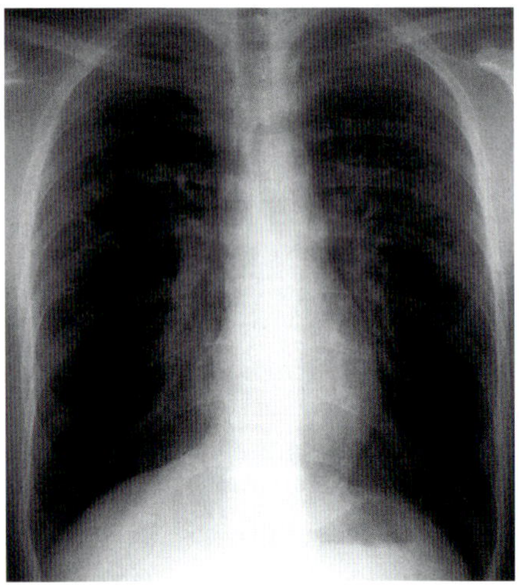

Figure 15. **Chest radiograph**

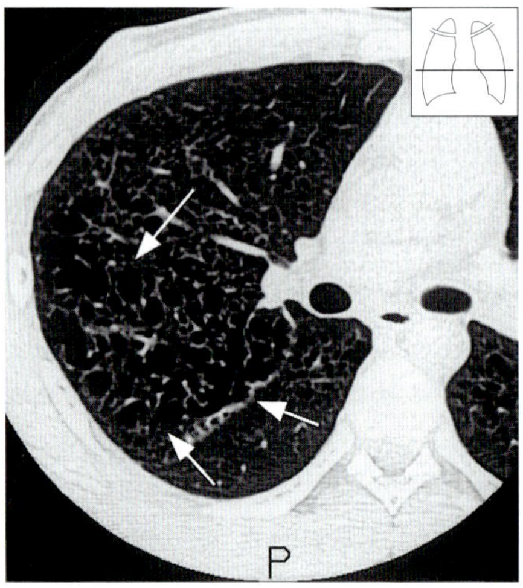

Figure 16. **Chest CT**

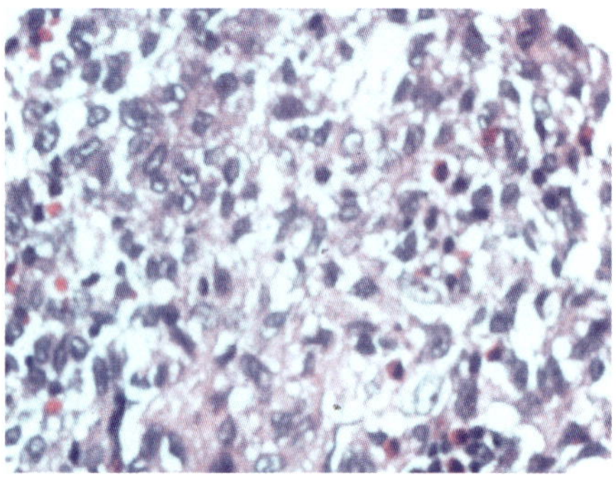

Figure 17. **Pathological findings by open lung biopsy**

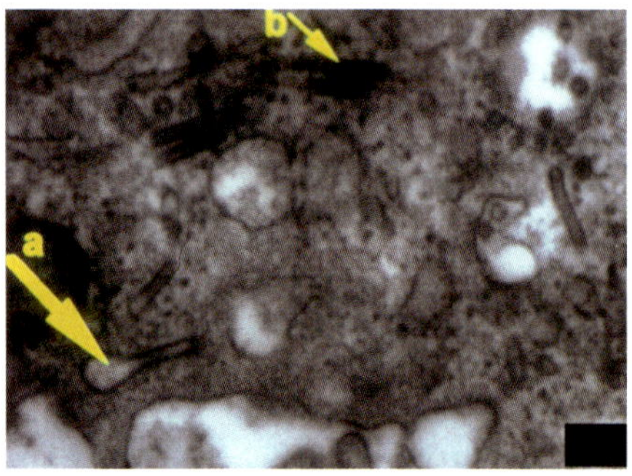

Figure 18. **Pathological findings by open lung biopsy** (electron microscopic finding)

Chief complaints: Fever, sputum, dyspnea on exertion The patient has a history of spontaneous pneumothorax on two occasions. When pulmonary eosinophilic granuloma was suspected after hospitalization for pneumonia, he was referred to this department. An open lung biopsy was conducted, and from image findings and pathological findings a diagnosis of pulmonary eosinophilic granuloma was reached.

Chest radiograph: Bilateral, diffuse, faint reticular shadow observed.

Chest CT: Multiple diffuse cysts observed throughout bilateral lung fields. The walls are comparatively thick particularly in the upper lung field, and numerous large, oval cysts (→) can be seen.

Pathological findings: Numerous eosinophils can be seen scattered in the center of histiocytes.

Electron microscope findings showed typical Birbeck granules (*a*, *b*⇨), and the diagnosis was pulmonary eosinophilic granuloma.

Case 6 Pneumoconiosis

60-year-old male

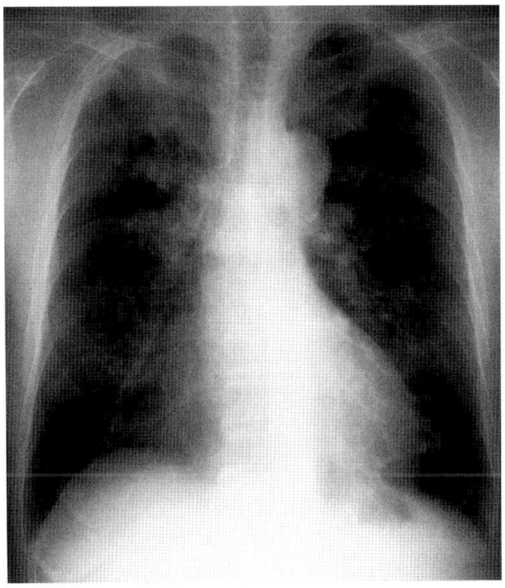

Figure 19. **Chest radiograph**

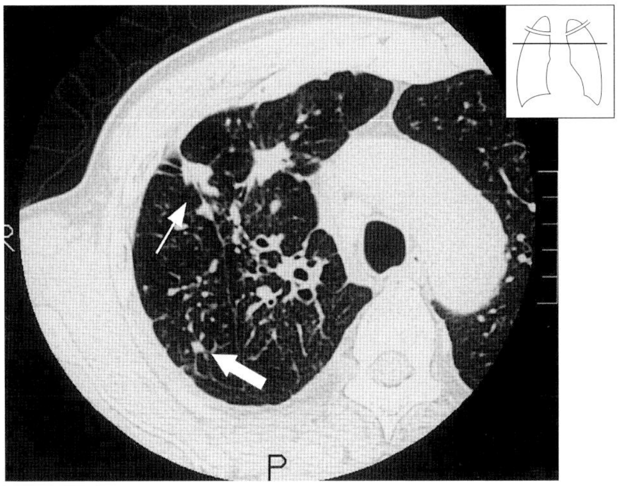

Figure 20. **Chest CT**

Chief complaint: None

The patient has a history of having worked in a mason's shop for 4 years.

Chest radiograph: Numerous nodular shadows can be seen in the right upper lung field, with nodular shadows in the apex of the lung appearing as hard shadows that could be due to calcification. Egg shell calcification is also seen in bilateral hilar lymphoducts, with diffuse, linear, reticular shadows and small granular shadows seen throughout bilateral lung fields.

Chest CT: In the right upper lobe, two 1 to 2 cm diameter hard nodular shadows can be seen that could be calcification (→). Surrounding scattered small nodular shadows can be seen, together with thickening of the interlobular septal wall and a linear shadow (➡). There are also findings of bronchodilation.

Case 7 Pulmonary cryptococcosis

69-year-old male

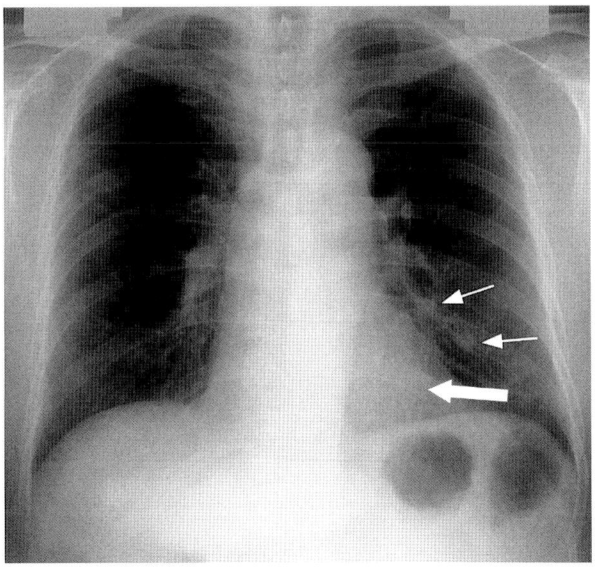

Figure 21. **Chest radiograph**

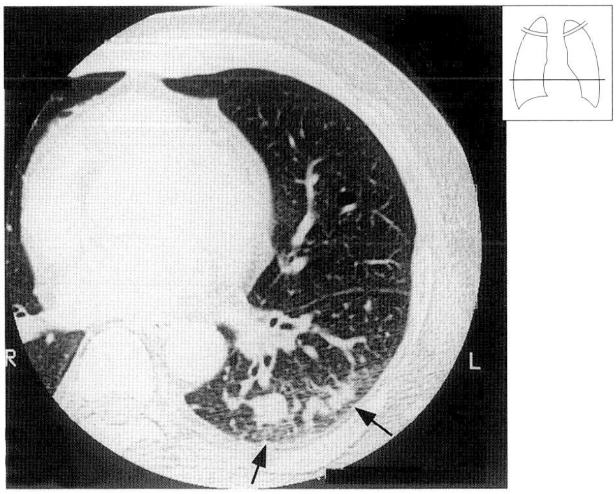

Figure 22. **Chest CT**

Chief complaint: Cough

This is a case of smoldering adult T cell leukemia (ATL) who while being treated with an external preparation of steroids by a dermatologist developed a cough. A chest radiograph indicated infiltrative shadow and he was referred to this department. An elevated level of blood Cryptococcus antigen (x 16) was observed, and pulmonary cryptococcosis was diagnosed.

Chest radiograph: two nodular shadows lying along the left lower lung field cardiac contour (→), and faint infiltrative shadow (➡) behind the cardiac contour can be seen.

Chest CT: two nodular shadows with comparatively distinct borders can be seen in the subpleura of the left lower lobe (→), with surrounding shaded infiltrative shadow.

Pathological findings

A granuloma is defined as a nodular lesion caused by the accumulation of mononuclear leukocytes resulting from a chronic inflammatory reaction. The cause of chronic inflammation varies widely, ranging from mycobacterial, fungal and other infections, silicon and other dusts to extrinsic allergies and unknown causes. If these causative agents are not removed from the lungs and the inflammation becomes protracted, a granuloma formation reaction frequently occurs.

Chest radiograph findings

There are a wide range of image findings indicating pulmonary granulomatous disease, such as diffuse granular shadows, nodular shadows and reticular shadows. Typical examples of pulmonary granulomatous disease that show diffuse granular shadows are sarcoidosis, miliary tuberculosis, and fungal and viral infections. There are also other less frequently occurring diseases that show the same shadows such as pulmonary eosinophilic granuloma, pneumoconiosis and chronic beryllium lung.

Diseases indicated by nodular shadows include Wegener's granulomatosis, pneumoconiosis and tuberculosis. A typical finding with Wegener's granulomatosis is multiple nodular shadows accompanied by cavities. A typical finding in the early stage of pneumoconiosis is diffuse granular shadows, but as the disease progresses large and small nodular shadows are shown. Nodular shadows are also seen with tuberculosis, but cavities frequently form, and in many cases satellite lesions are observed surrounding the primary lesion.

With sarcoidosis, since lesions are formed in lobular and bronchiole areas, granular shadows and linear reticular shadows become mixed. For this reason the shadows shown are called reticular granular shadows.

High-resolution CT findings

Since high-resolution CT enables morphological analysis up to the pulmonary secondary lobule level, it plays an important role in the differential diagnosis of diffuse pulmonary diseases. Differentiation of pulmonary granulomatous diseases using high-resolution CT depends on the ability to ascertain the sites of principal lesions on the secondary lobule level, the ability to ascertain intrapulmonary distribution and other points. Intrapulmonary distribution provides useful information for differential diagnosis such as upper/lower distribution and inner/outer layer distribution trends.

Lesions caused by pulmonary granulomatous diseases on the secondary lobule level include centrilobular nodules, peripheral lobular nodules and primary lesions not related to lobular construction.

A characteristic of centrilobular nodules is that the nodules are contiguous with the broncho-pulmonary artery bundles, with a small amount of normal lung field existing between the nodules and perilobular tissue. The disease includes the early stage lesion of infectious diseases such as mycobacterial, fungal and other infections, hypersensitivity pneumonitis, pneumoconiosis and pulmonary eosinophilic granuloma. Nodules in perilobular tissue accompany uniform or nodule-like thickening of interlobular septum and bronchial vascular bundles, indicating such diseases as sarcoidosis and pneumoconiosis. A typical disease not related to lobular construction is miliary tuberculosis in which there is hematogenous dissemination. Other diseases include Wegener's granulomatosis in which necrotizing granulomatous inflammation is seen.

References

1) Masashi Takahashi et al.: Granulomatous Pulmonary Diseases and Hematogenous Pulmonary Diseases, Japan Medical Radiology Society Magazine, 59 (Supplement 13) : 9-12, 1999
2) Takahide Izumi: Diagnosis and Treatment of Diffuse Pulmonary Diseases, Kinpodo Inc., 1995
3) Heitzman, E.R.: The lung: Radiologic-pathologic correlations. 2nd ed. Mosby, St. Louis, 1984

- Japan Medical Radiology Society Chest X-Ray Research Association: Imaging Diagnosis Guidelines for Diffuse Pulmonary Diseases, Igaku-Shoin, 1998
- Roland, M., et al.: Granulomatous Processes Chapter 7.5.1, 1925-1938 (edited by R. G. Crystal et al.: The Lung: Scientific Foundations). Raven Press Ltd., New York, 1991

4. Interstitial shadow:

Fibrotic shadow

[Pattern classification IV-B-2]

●Author — Kingo Chida

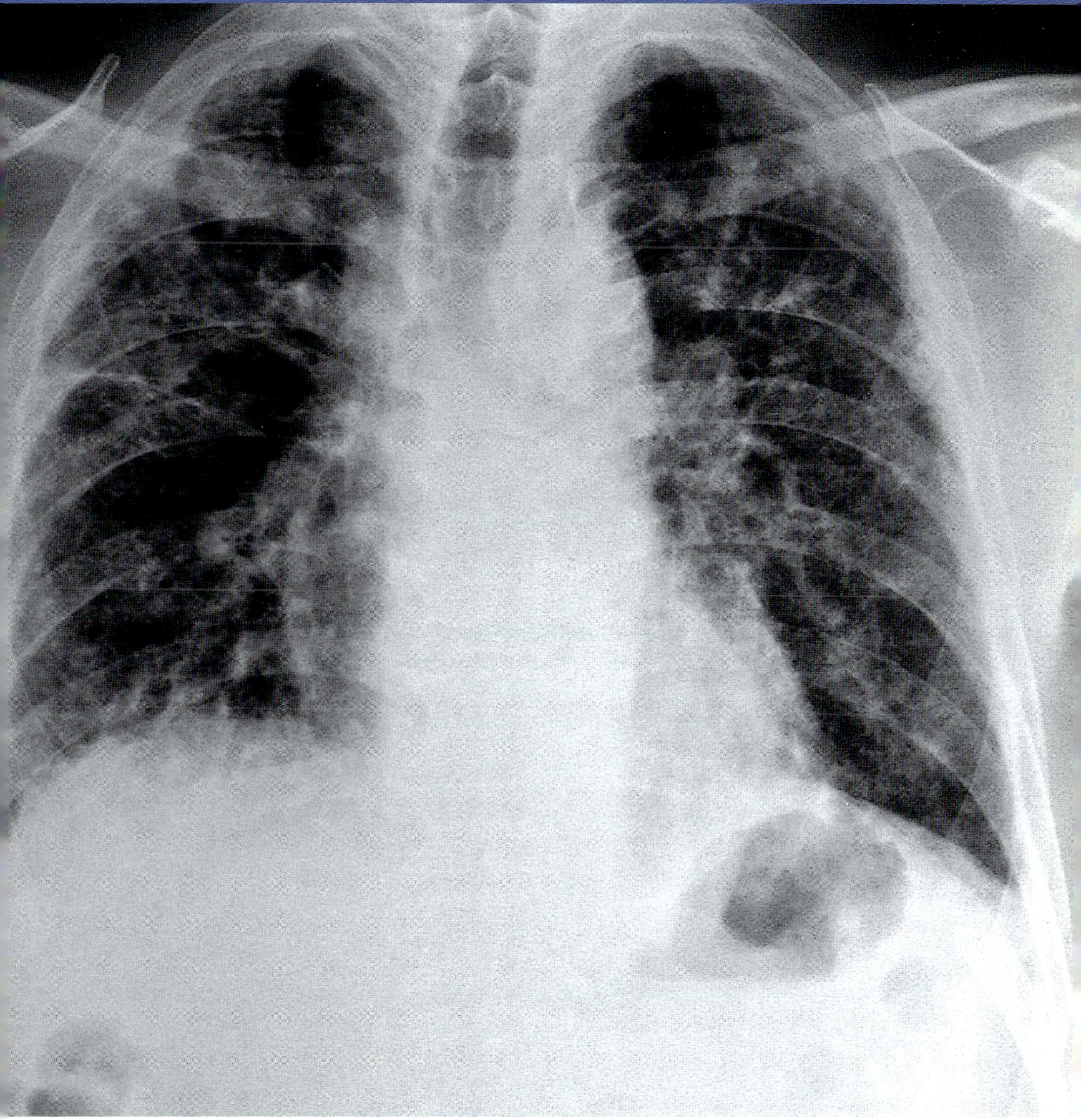

Keywords of this section

Ground glass opacity (GGO)
Traction bronchiectasis
Microscopic honeycomb lung
Idiopathic interstitial pneumonia
Silicosis
Dermatomyositis
Drug-induced pneumonia
Chronic hypersensitivity pneumonia
Sarcoidosis
Desquamative interstitial pneumonia
Alveolar macrophage pneumonia
Desquamative interstitial pneumonia-like reaction
Respiratory bronchiolitis
Obstructive bronchiolitis
Bronchiolitis obliterans organizing pneumonia
Eosinophilic pneumonia
Nonspecific interstitial pneumonia
Antineutrophil cytoplasmic antibody
Pneumocystis pneumonia (PCP)
Video-assisted thoracoscopic surgery (VATS)

Fibrotic shadow

Kingo Chida
Second Division, Department of Internal Medicine, Hamamatsu University School of Medicine, Hamamatsu, Shizuoka, Japan

For the early diagnosis of fibrosing lesions, look for the presence of ground glass opacity (hazy increased attenuation), fine nodular shadows, linear shadows and reticular shadows (small or large). Detailed analysis of these findings is possible with CT. Traction bronchiectasis, air space enlargement and intralobular reticular opacity (small reticular shadow) on CT often point to the early stage of the contraction mechanism of alveolar septa. The significance of ground glass opacity (GGO) and microscopic honeycombing in terms of CT-pathologic correlation must await further study.

Case 1 64-year-old male

Chief complaints: Dry cough, dyspnea on exertion
Medical/family history: Nothing of note
Occupational history: No history of dust inhalation
Smoking history: 10/day for 35 years
Present illness:
For 6 months the patient had symptoms of gradually worsening dry cough. Since dyspnea on exertion was also observed, he received a medical examination at the hospital and was admitted for detailed examination. There were no findings suggesting collagen vascular diseases.
Physical findings on admission:
Weight loss of 3 kg in 6 months. Fine crackles heard on inspiration, no heart murmur or irregular pulse. No abnormal abdominal or neurological findings. Positive mild finger clubbing. No skin lesions.
Laboratory data on admission:
Increased erythrocyte sedimentation rate of 45 mm/hour and mildly positive CRP of 0.6 mg/dL, but leukocyte count and Hb level both normal. Electrolytes, liver function and renal function were all within normal limits. Elevated KL-6 level of 1,116 U/mL while pulmonary function tests showed reduced VC of 2,083 mL (%VC 58%). $FEV_{1.0}$ was 1,920 (86%). Arterial blood gas analysis showed pH of 7.394, $PaCO_2$ level of 37 mmHg and PaO_2 level of 68 mmHg indicating the presence of hypoxia.

A chest radiograph at the time of admission (P. 57) shows reduced lung volume (right diaphragm is at the level of the ninth posterior rib instead of at the normal level of the tenth posterior intercostal space), with a fusion of reticulonodular shadows throughout the entire lung field that are prominently seen in the lower lung fields and subpleural regions. Tracheal displacement, thickening of hair line and fluffing of the contour of the diaphragm are also seen.

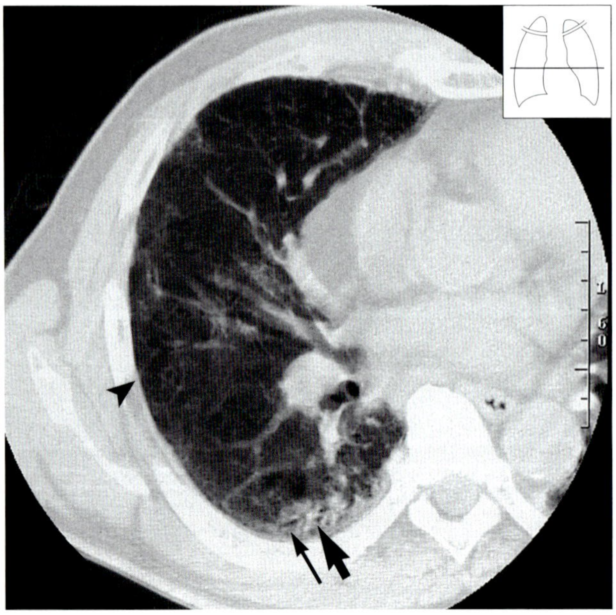

Figure 1. **Chest CT**

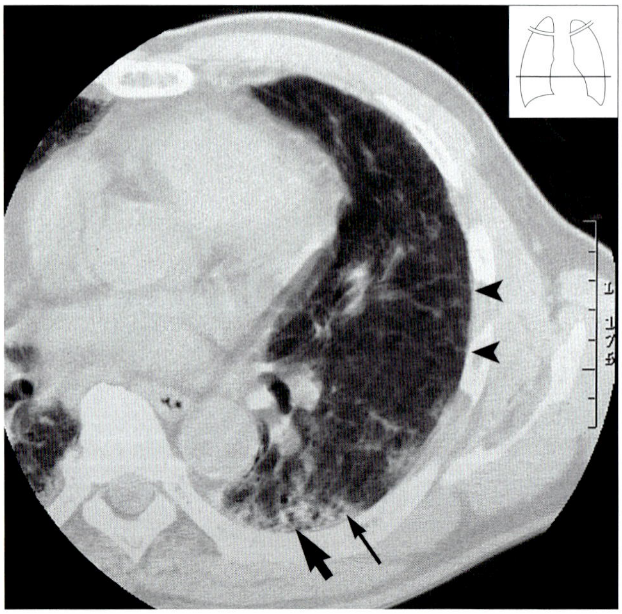

Figure 2. **Chest CT**

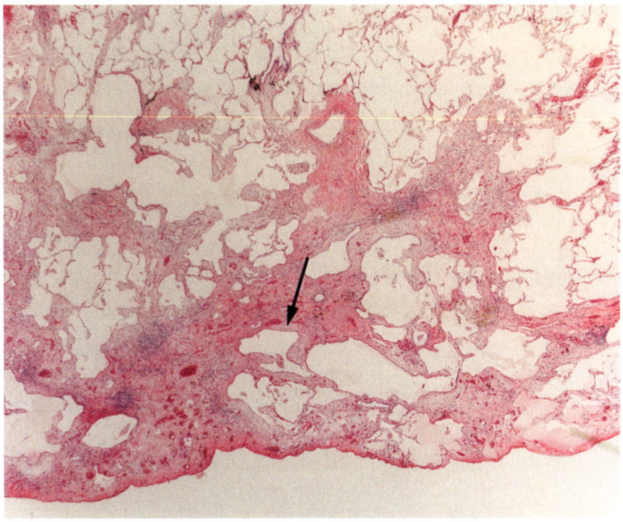

Figure 3. **Microscopic picture: HE stain**

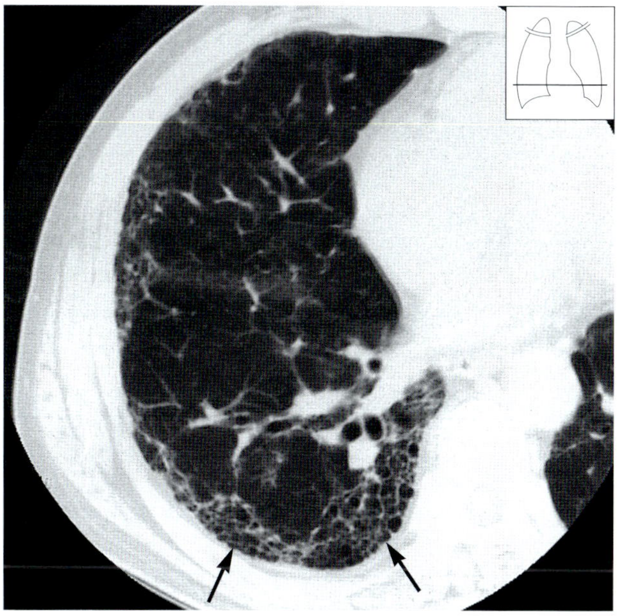

Figure 4. **Chest CT of a case other than Case 1: honeycomb lung**

Chest CT (*Figs. 1, 2*) shows shadows having nonsegmental distribution predominantly in the subpleura and posterior zone. The characteristics of these shadows are ground glass opacity (GGO) accompanied by reticular shadows (in the entire lung field in *Figure 2*). Slight bronchial dilatation (traction bronchiectasis) (→ in *Figures 1 and 2*), enlarged air spaces (➡ in *Figures 1 and 2*) and interlobular septal thickening (➤ in *Figures 1 and 2*) are evident. No typical findings of honeycomb lung are indicated.

Diagnosis

To reach a definite diagnosis, video-assisted thoracoscopic surgery (VATS) was conducted. In the microscopic picture (low magnification, HE stain) (*Fig. 3*), fibrotic thickening and honeycomb lung can be seen particularly in subpleural regions. With the low magnification, microscopic findings are distinctly varied, reflecting the characteristic nonuniform distribution of abnormalities ranging from normal alveoli to prominent collagen deposition with honeycombing. The air spaces in the honeycomb were 0.5 mm or less in diameter, which corresponds to the definition of microscopic honeycomb lung. Fibroblastic foci are typically scattered at the edges of dense scars (→ *in Figure 3*). Even if there was alveolar wall inflammation and macrophage accumulation in the alveolar spaces, it stayed at insignificant levels. Since clinically no underlying disease could be identified, the patient was given a diagnosis of a type of idiopathic interstitial pneumonia (IIP), specifically usual interstitial pneumonia (UIP).

Microscopic honeycomb lung

When a chest CT reveals no typical findings of honeycombing changes as in this case, examination of surgically-biopsied specimens is required for an accurate diagnosis of UIP. It is also important to note that early-stage honeycombing changes are thought to be microscopic. The findings that should be considered microscopic honeycombing on high-resolution CT (HRCT) include 1) air space consolidation accompanied by an air bronchiologram, 2) irregular borders between parenchyma and pleura, 3) GGO accompanied by fine reticular shadows and 4) intensified dense shadows with translucent areas along the subpleura.

In another case, a chest CT (*Fig. 4*) demonstrated honeycomb lung (→) predominantly in the lower lung field. In addition to the honeycombing change, if the cause cannot be specified, the possibility of UIP is quite high among the IIPs. However, an open-lung biopsy or VATS should be employed in the following situations: 1) patients aged 65 or less, 2) cases with progressive deterioration in 6 to 12 months, 3) involvement with upper lung predominance, 4) cases exhibiting nodular and patchy shadows, 5) cases with lymph node swelling or pleural effusion, 6) cases with bloody sputum, 7) cases with a history of recurrent pneumothorax, and 8) cases of inexplicable pulmonary hypertension.

Conclusion of this case: Idiopathic interstitial pneumonia

Although interstitial pneumonia is diagnosed without difficulty with HRCT, VATS or other measures are required to reach a definite diagnosis of subtypes. The flow chart in *Figure 5* indicates how to differentiate between subtypes based on the consensus statement of the joint committee of the American Thoracic Society (ATS) and the European Respiratory Society (ERS).

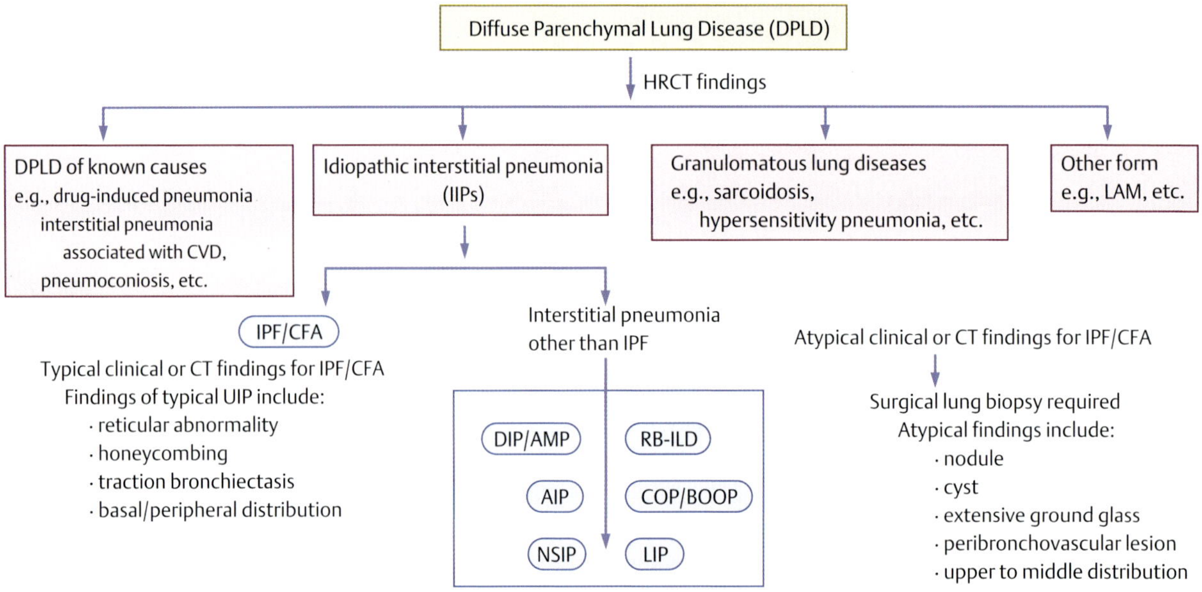

Abbreviations

AIP : acute interstitial pneumonia
AMP : alveolar macrophage pneumonia
BOOP : bronchiolitis obliterans organizing pneumonia
CFA : cryptogenic fibrosing alveolitis
COP : cryptogenic organizing pneumonia
CVD : collagen vascular disease
DIP : desquamative interstitial pneumonia
DPLD : diffuse parenchymal lung disease
IPF : idiopathic pulmonary fibrosis
LAM : lymphangiomyomatosis
LIP : lymphocytic interstitial pneumonia
NSIP : nonspecific interstitial pneumonia/fibrosis
RB-ILD : respiratory bronchiolitis associated with interstitial lung disease

Figure 5. **Differentiation flow chart (96th ATS Conference, Travis, Lynch, Bateman)**

Findings indicating fibrotic changes on chest radiographs and their differentiation

The existence of interstitial shadows and/or fibroblastic foci should be taken into consideration if chest radiographs show nodular shadows, reticular shadows, honeycomb, GGO (hazy increased attenuation) and dense consolidation in bilateral lungs. Since the lung is an organ in which reduced volume can easily occur if fibrosis is extensive, the displacement of tracheal or minor fissure (normally at the anterior third intercostal space) should be noted.

The location of fibrosing lesions is important for diagnosis, and if areas of subpleura, supradiaphragm or costophrenic angles are intact, IIP can be ruled out.

It is necessary to identify the causative agents to differentiate diffuse parenchymal lung diseases, which include inhalation factors (due to airborne particles, to include pneumoconiosis) (*Fig. 6*), pulmonary lesions associated with collagen vascular diseases (*Fig. 7*), drug-induced pulmonary diseases (*Fig. 8*), interstitial pneumonia forming granulomas (*Figs. 9–11*), and specific infectious diseases (virus or fungus).

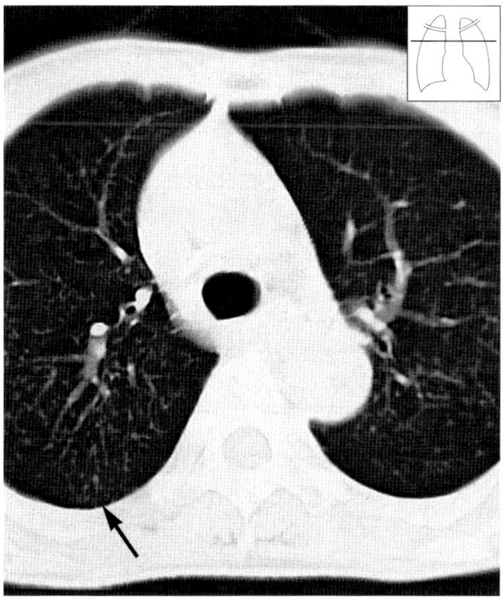

Figure 6. **Chest CT: Silicosis**
Scattered, distinct nodular shadows.

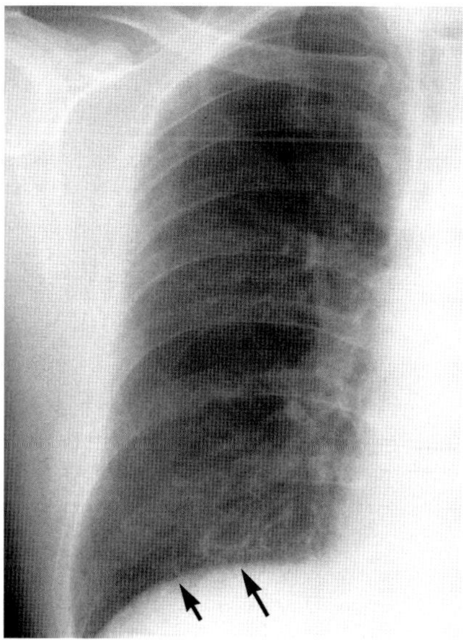

Figure 7. **Chest radiograph: UIP due to dermatomyositis**
Honeycombing formation can be seen in the lower lung fields just above the diaphragm.

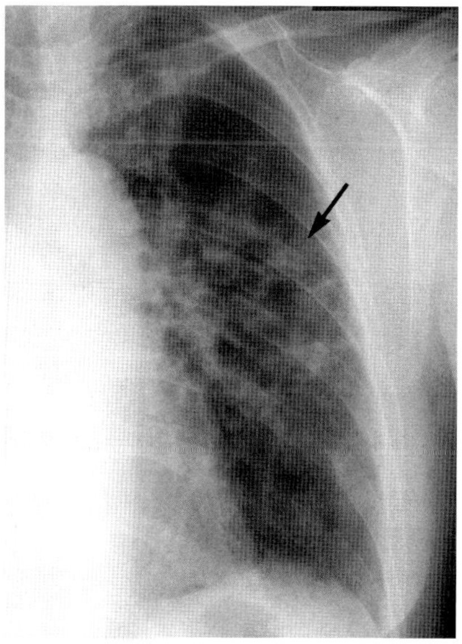

Figure 8. **Chest radiograph: Drug-induced (gold compounds) pneumonia**
Fine, patchy shadows can be seen in the middle lung fields, which correspond to alveolar pattern surrounding the bronchovascular bundles on CT (CT not shown).

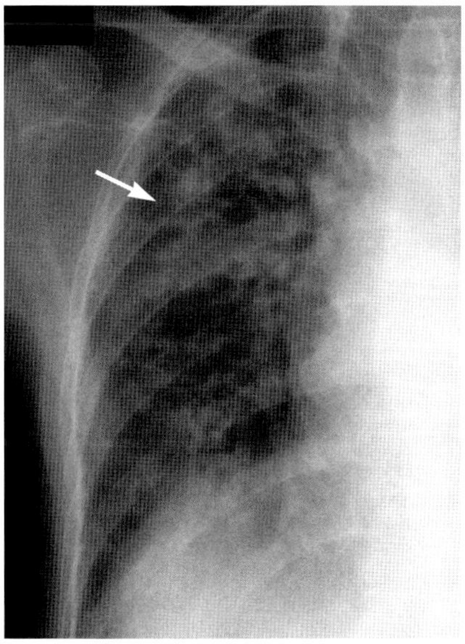

Figure 9. **Chest radiographic: Chronic hypersensitivity pneumonitis**
The shadow is more extensive in the upper lung field, decreased lung volume is conspicuous, and the shadow looks patchy due to emphysematous changes (confirmed with CT).

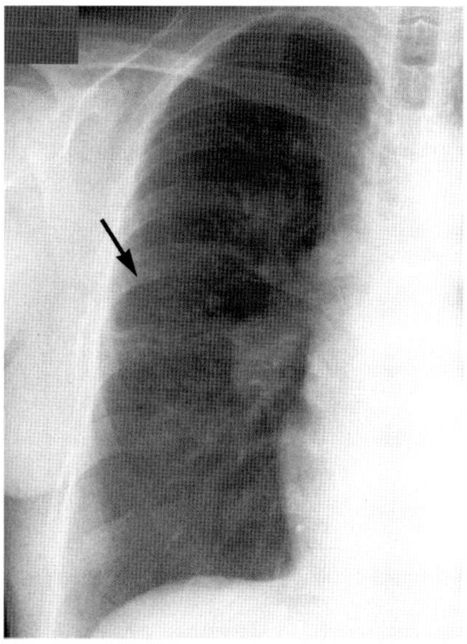

Figure 10. **Chest radiograph: Sarcoidosis**
There is enlargement of lymph nodes in the areas of the hilum and azygos, and scattered granular and nodular shadows together with reticular shadows can be seen mainly in the middle lung field.

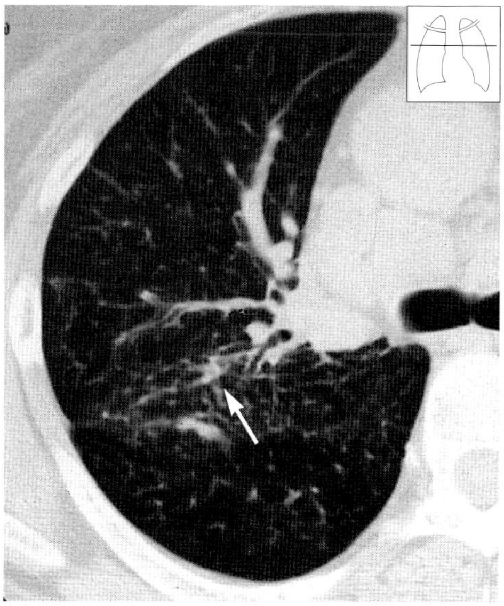

Figure 11. **Chest CT: Sarcoidosis**
Nodular reticular shadows, together with the enlargement and irregularity of bronchovascular bundles can be seen.

Case 2 Idiopathic interstitial pneumonia (DIP/AMP: Desquamative interstitial pneumonia/alveolar macrophage pneumonia)

57-year-old male

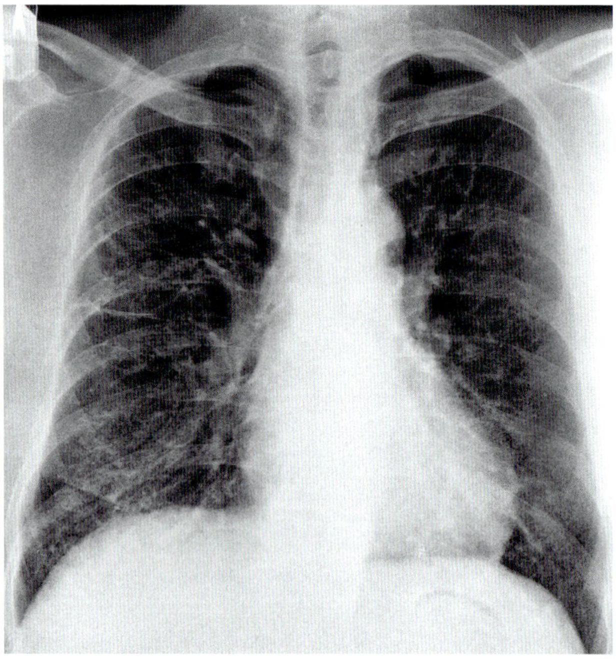

Figure 12. **Chest radiograph**

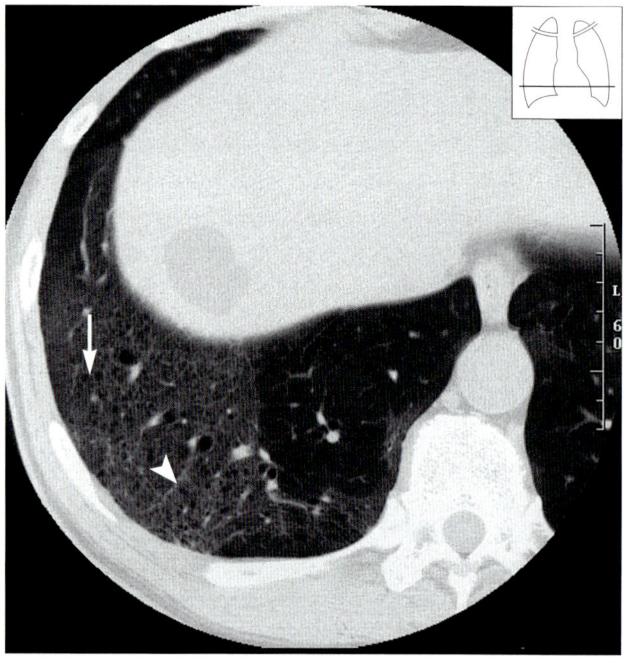

Figure 13. **Chest CT**

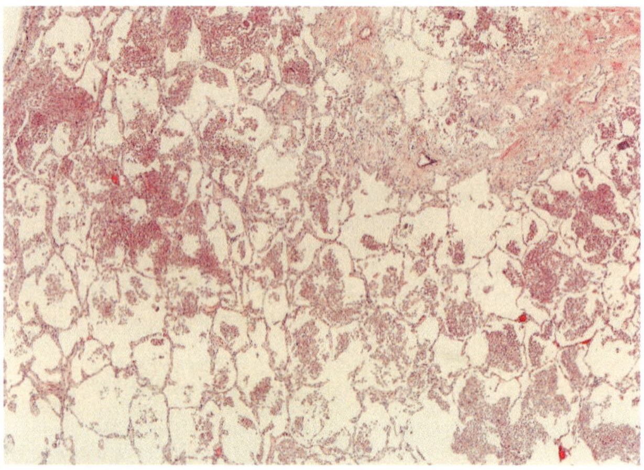

a. Low magnification showing moderate, fairly uniform disease

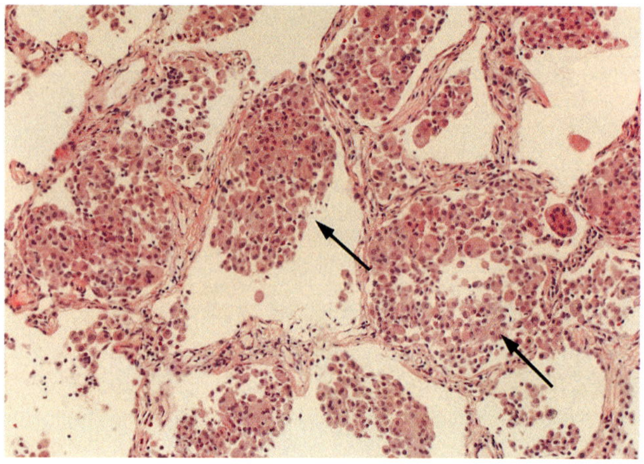

b. High magnification demonstrating interstitial thickening as well as the accumulation of numerous macrophages in adjacent air spaces

Figures 14 a–c. **Microscopic pictures: HE stain, low magnification**

This is a case with no symptoms in which the disease was suspected on regular health checkup. A smoking history of 20/day for 35 years.

Chest radiograph (*Fig. 12*) shows GGO mainly in subpleural regions of middle and lower lung fields. On the other hand, ring shadows can be seen in the upper lung fields, probably reflecting emphysematous change or cyst formation due to smoking.

Chest CT (*Fig. 13*) shows GGO. Since image changes are homogeneous, it is inferred that the lesion phase is also uniform. There is accompanying formation of small cysts (→) while there are no findings suggesting honeycombing change. Because vascular shadows are visible

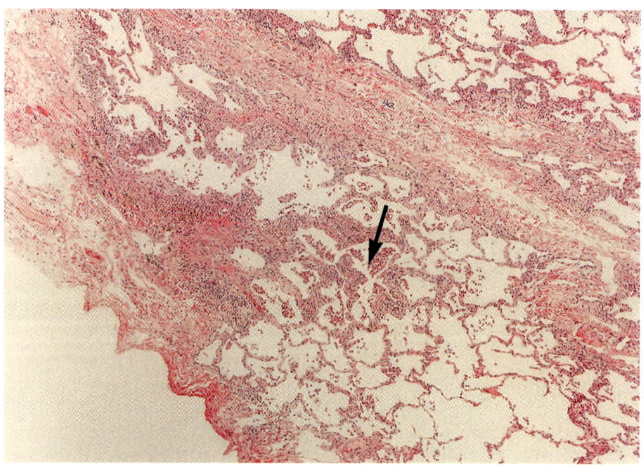

c. DIP-like reaction in the case of UIP

through GGO (➤), it can be ascertained that lobular structure was well preserved with a lack of parenchymal alteration.

The findings of specimens with VATS (*Figs. 14 a–c*) indicated a uniform inflammation of alveoli (*a*) that contrasts sharply with the heterogeneous distribution in UIP. The most striking finding is that a large number of macrophages (→) are seen in the air spaces (*b*). Fibroblastic foci are absent.

The disease was progressive in spite of cessation of smoking, and hence steroids were orally administered, resulting in mild improvement.

GGO

The GGO indicated in plain chest radiograph is equivalent to fine nodular shadows, and basically suggests early stage interstitial shadows (alveolar cell infiltration or slight fibrosing change). On the other hand, the GGO (hazy increased attenuation) in chest CT can imply not only interstitial lesions, but also alveolar lesions. So it is necessary to differentiate the two. An example of the latter is intra-alveolar lesions caused by exudate with the preservation of air in alveolar space (early stage pneumonia, pulmonary edema, pneumocystis pneumonia often showing geographic appearance). As mentioned before, GGO is exhibited even in cases of microscopic honeycomb lung.

DIP-like reaction

In diseases such as UIP *(Fig. 14 c)*, eosinophilic granuloma, asbestosis, malignancy and smoker's bronchiolitis, accumulation of macrophages in adjacent air spaces is often observed (→). Since this localized reaction is not rare, giving a diagnosis of DIP with transbronchial lung biopsy specimens is still problematic.

Case 3 Idiopathic interstitial pneumonia (RB-ILD: Respiratory bronchiolitis associated with interstitial lung disease)

48-year-old male

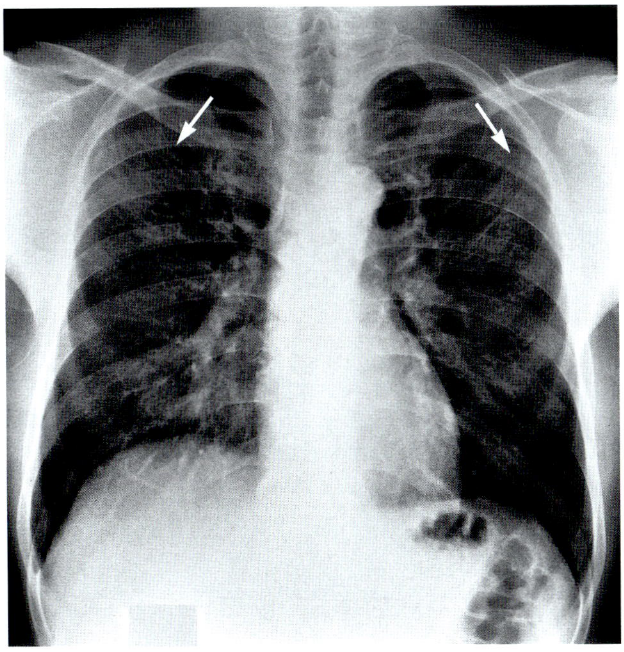

Figure 15. **Chest radiograph**

A smoking history of 20 to 40/day for 28 years. Admitted for further examination because dry cough was seen to worsen. The symptom improved on cessation of smoking.

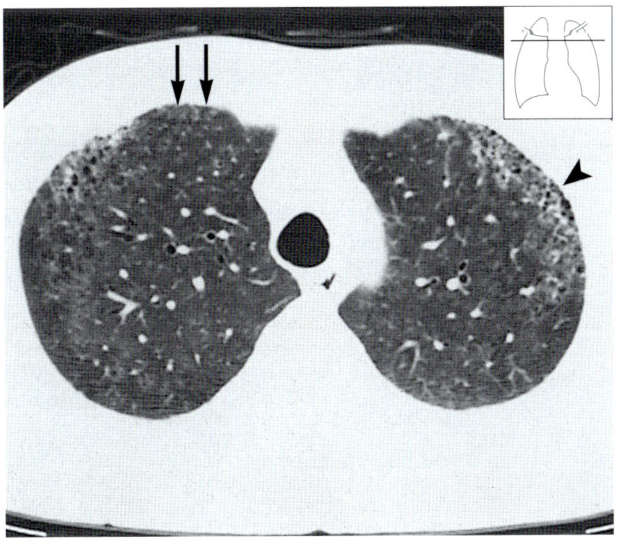

Figure 16. **Chest CT**

A chest radiograph shows bilateral, linear reticular shadows mainly on the outer sides of upper lung fields (→), but no decrease in lung volume can be seen.

A chest CT shows increased fine density in bilateral lungs. This is not homogeneous density resulting from the existence of centrilobular shadows (→). There are also areas of strongly increased density along the chest wall, inside which small cysts and reticular shadows can be seen (➤).

VATS to examine pulmonary tissue changes shows peribronchiolar distribution exhibiting bronchiolocentricity (→) with accumulation of macrophages only in air spaces that are adjacent to thickened interstitium.

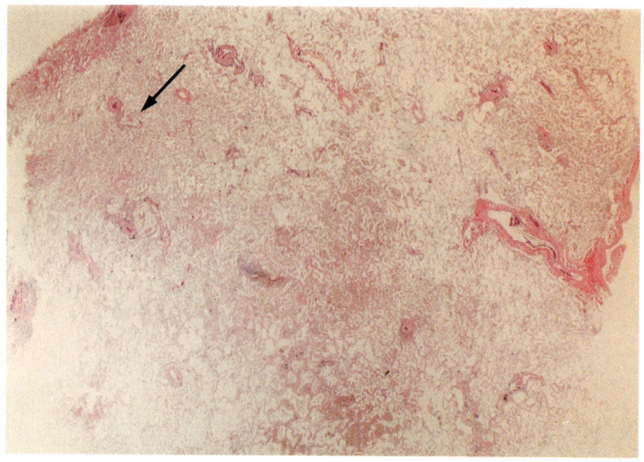

Figure 17. **Microscopic picture: HE stain**

Difference between RB-ILD and DIP

In both disease entities, the patients are males aged around 50 with a mild-to-severe smoking history. Points of difference include 1) the symptoms are more severe in DIP, and then many cases have hypoxia, 2) alveolitis in DIP is rather uniform but in RB-ILD there is bronchiolocentric distribution, and 3) the prognosis is worse for DIP.

Case 4 Idiopathic interstitial pneumonia (COP/BOOP: Cryptogenic organizing pneumonia/bronchiolitis obliterans organizing pneumonia)

76-year-old female

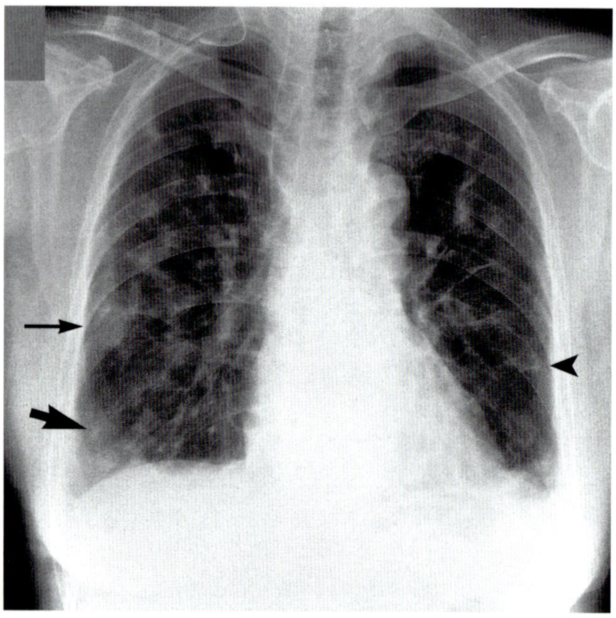

Figure 18. **Chest radiograph**

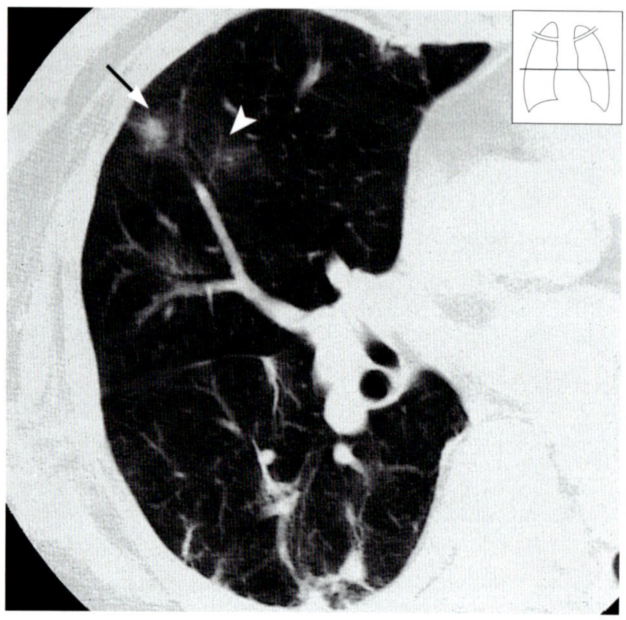

Figure 19. **Chest CT**

Received a detailed examination due to symptoms of slight fever, dry cough and dyspnea on exertion. Nothing of note in family or smoking history, and no clinical symptoms or physical examination findings suggesting collagen vascular diseases.

A chest radiograph shows bilateral multiple nonsegmental consolidation, which contains GGO, small patchy shadows (→), nodular shadows (➡) and linear shadows (➤). Despite the lack of clear fibrotic shadows, decreased lung volume is notable.

A chest CT shows bilateral shadows ranging from nodular to small patchy shadows in subpleural regions (→), with scattered GGO (➤). Another slice shows swollen contour of bronchovascular bundles (CT not shown).

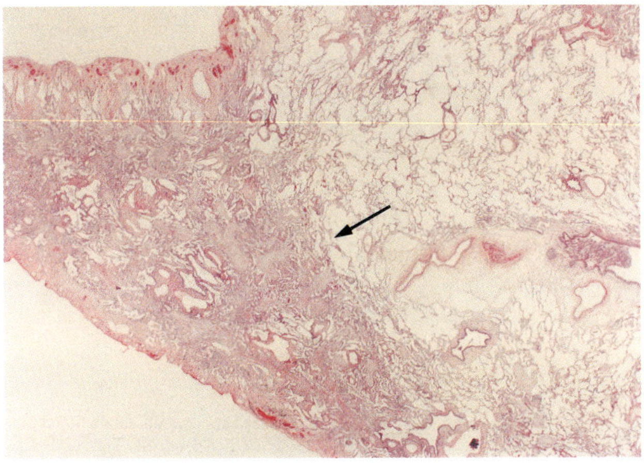

a. Low magnification

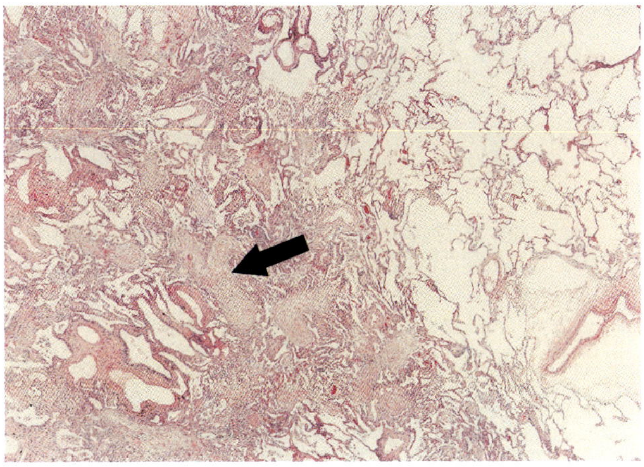

b. High magnification

Figure 20 a–b. **Microscopic picture: HE stain**

VATS to examine pulmonary tissue changes reveals dispersion of patchy lesion (→) in the microscopic findings (low magnification). The higher magnification image demonstrates the excessive proliferation of granulation tissue (polyp-shaped organization) in the alveolar spaces (➨) and surrounding interstitial lymphocyte infiltration.

The course of the disease was slow but progressive, and then oral doses of steroids were administered. Symptoms and shadows improved.

Differentiating diseases that cause BOOP pattern

With a chest CT, the findings of bilateral, nonsegmental GGO mixed with patchy or nodular shadows along the pleura are called "BOOP/eosinophilic pneumonia (EP) pattern". It is difficult for CT findings to differentiate BOOP from eosinophilic pneumonia. It is also necessary to exclude other diseases causing the BOOP/EP pattern, such as infectious diseases (bacterial, mycoplasmal, viral, fungal, etc.), vascular lesions (Wegener's granulomatosis, alveolar hemorrhage, etc.), and allergies (drug-induced pneumonia, radiation pneumonitis, etc.).

Case 5

Idiopathic interstitial pneumonia (Cellular NSIP: Nonspecific interstitial pneumonia)

49-year-old female

Received a medical examination at our hospital for dyspnea on exertion. Nothing of note in occupational or smoking histories, and no clinical symptoms or examination findings to suggest collagen vascular disease.

A chest radiograph shows a mild decrease in lung volume. Because there are linear and reticular shadows in bilateral lower lung fields (→), vascular structures in this area cannot be traced.

A chest CT shows bilateral lung field increased density, predominantly in the posterior region (→). Mild consolidation running along the bronchovascular bundles is also seen. There are no obvious findings indicating traction bronchiectasis or honeycombing formation.

VATS to examine pulmonary tissue changes shows infiltration of inflammatory cells of alveolar septa with little thickening of interstitium in the microscopic pic-

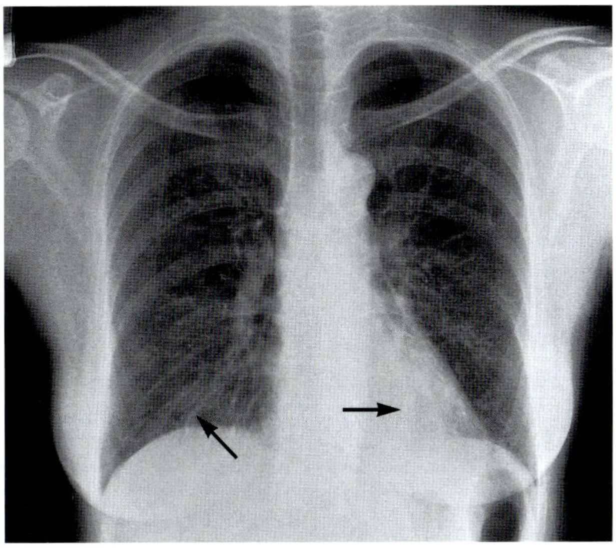

Figure 21. **Chest radiograph**

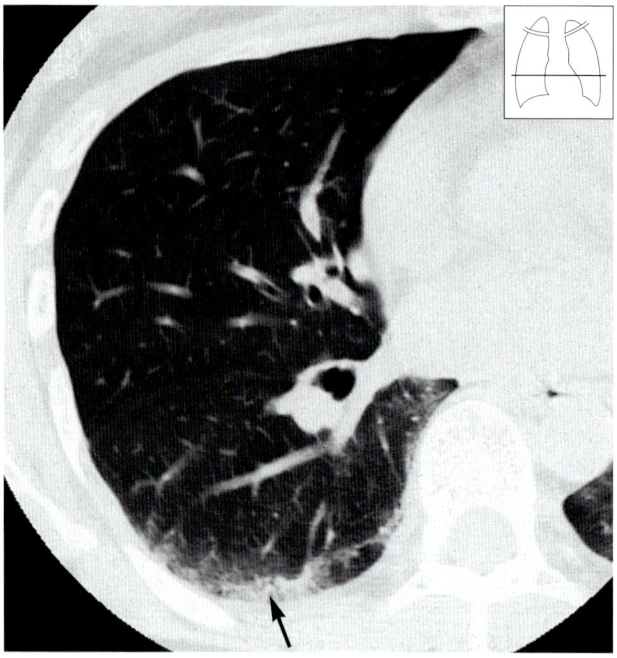

Figure 22. **Chest CT**

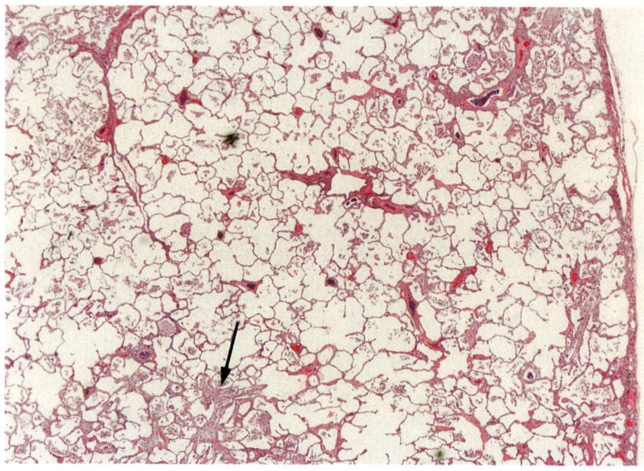

Figure 23. **Microscopic picture**

ture. These lesions are diffuse, the lesion phase is uniform, and tissue structure is maintained. Slight macrophage aggregation in spaces and inconsequential organization (→) can be seen.

There was a favorable response to treatment with steroids.

Case 6

Idiopathic interstitial pneumonia (fibrotic NSIP)

60-year-old male

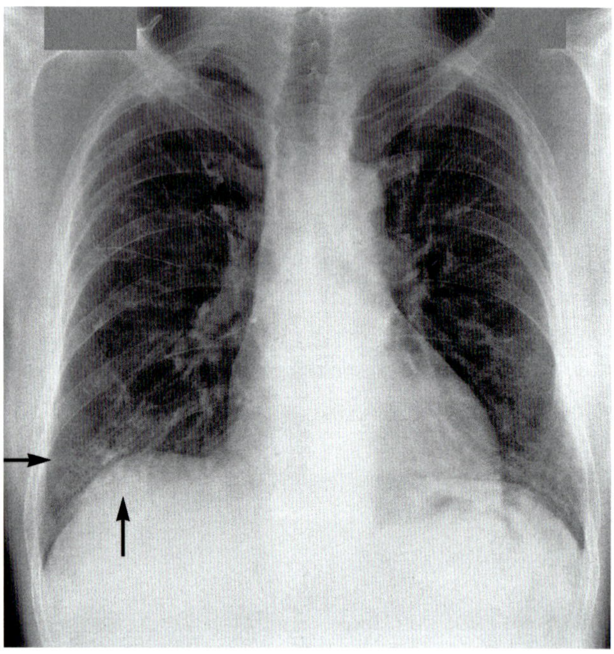

Figure 24. **Chest radiograph**

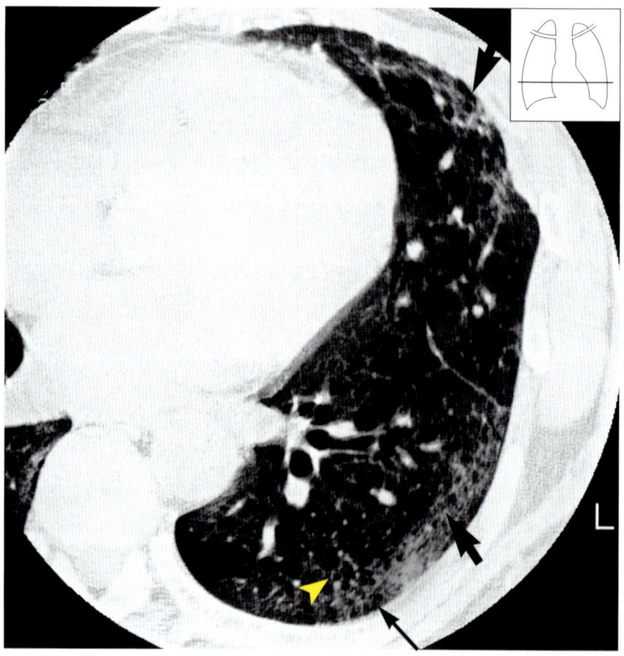

Figure 25. **Chest CT**

Received a medical examination at the hospital for dyspnea on exertion, and was admitted for detailed examination. There were no clinical symptoms or examination findings to suggest collagen vascular diseases. Past history was pulmonary tuberculosis in apex.

A chest radiograph shows a clear decrease in lung volume. There is bilateral GGO (→) mainly in the costophrenic angle extending to the outer areas of the middle lung field. Thickening of apical pleura (apical cap) and linear shadows extending to the hilum can be seen.

A chest CT shows increased lung field density mainly in the subpleural regions. The increased density includes dilation of air spaces (→) as well as interlobular and intralobular reticular opacity, resulting in inhomogeneous density (➨). Traction bronchiectasis can be identified (➤).

VATS to examine pulmonary tissue changes was performed. The microscopic picture shows a very small area of structural change accompanied by partial slight fibroblastic foci, but basically lesion distribution is diffuse with phase uniformity.

With regard to idiopathic NSIP subgrouping, it should be understood that at present it has not been conclusive. That is to say, Katzenstein[1)] published the classification of NSIP, namely Group I: Cellular interstitial pneumonia with little fibrosis, Group II: Infiltration of lymphocytes and plasma cells into the interstitium together with fibrotic lesions, and Group III: Diffuse fibrotic lesions or patchy shadows with more severe derangement of lung architecture. Nevertheless, there are many problems with this classification. Katzenstein herself reported later that 10% of cases in Group III are excluded from NSIP. Travis[2)] also reported that in Group I there are absolutely no cases of death, and the BAL lymphocyte fraction level is considerably higher, which is conspicuously different from the other two groups, and hence there are doubts as to whether it is included in NSIP. From this viewpoint, there is great significance in classifying NSIP as cellular NSIP and fibrotic NSIP for the time being.

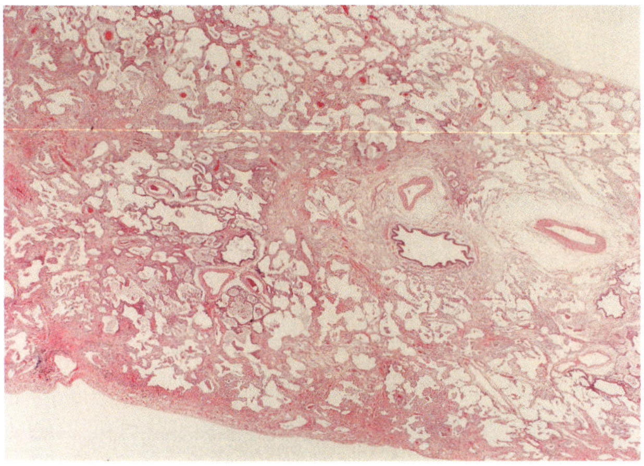

Figure 26. **Microscopic picture: HE stain**

Differentiating between fibrotic NSIP and UIP

Unlike UIP lesions, NSIP lesions are of uniform phase with diffuse distribution, but there is debate on how to deal with NSIP, and consequently, the ATS/ERS joint committee has adopted a provisional stance on NSIP. The reason for this is that there is no consensus of opinion among pathologists regarding the extent to which the presence of honeycombing and fibroblastic foci is permissible for NSIP.

Conclusion

Pulmonary fibrosis is a remodeling, resulting from two major mechanisms. First, persistent inflammation of alveoli progresses to fibrosis, a process sometimes seen in chronic hypersensitivity pneumonia. Secondly, aberrant wound healing response to repeated epithelial injuries, for example, UIP, results in fibrosis. Abnormal deposition of extracellular matrix is a common feature seen in prolonged injury regardless of the type of insults or causes. However, there is a relationship between the fibrotic pattern and the cause, which can be reflected in images. The following are typical examples.

Interstitial fibrosis related to inhalation factors

Chest radiographic findings of silicosis are multiple, well-circumscribed nodules throughout the entire lungs predominantly in the upper lung fields (*Fig.* 6). Massive fibrosis and emphysematous changes are seen in advanced cases. Eggshell calcification of hilar lymph nodes is a characteristic feature. Silicosis has a high incidence of complication of pulmonary tuberculosis, in which case the image is modified. In chest radiographs of asbestosis, linear and/or reticular shadows are observed mainly in the middle to lower lung fields because of more ventilation. Pleural plaque is a characteristic feature. It is necessary to pay attention to associated lung cancer and mesothelioma. In general the accumulation of dust and the tissue reaction by pneumoconiosis starts from the respiratory bronchiole and adjacent alveolar interstitium, producing bronchiolocentric opacities with HRCT (subpleural dot-like lesions).

Chest radiographs of acute hypersensitivity pneumonitis show scattered diffuse fine nodular shadows. CT shows ill-defined centrilobular nodules accompanied by GGO (fine increased density). In the chronic type, chest radiographs demonstrate irregular linear opacities and honeycombing involving mainly upper to middle lung zones (*Fig. 9*).

Interstitial fibrosis associated with systemic diseases

Each of the collagen vascular diseases (CVD) can involve the interstitium, resulting in the resemblance to one form of the idiopathic interstitial pneumonias (IIPs) (*Fig. 7*). However, interstitial fibrosis caused by CVD is often NSIP or BOOP. It should be noted that NSIP or BOOP tissue changes indicate lung disease associated with CVD. Pleural effusion can often be seen in CVD other than systemic sclerosis. With the pulmonary lesions accompanying rheumatoid arthritis, a characteristic feature is follicular bronchiolitis or obstructive bronchiolitis. The former appears as nodular shadows in a CT, but the latter appears as patchy low-attenuation areas. During treatment with immunosuppressive agents, the risk of drug-induced lung injuries or opportunistic infections should be kept in mind.

Chest radiographs of sarcoidosis show nodular and linear shadows extending from the middle to upper lung fields (*Fig. 10*), which are diagnostic if seen together with lymph node swelling in the hilum. GGO may also be seen. With CT, perilymphatic distribution along the perihilum, pleural surface, bronchovascular bundle and interlobular septum is important (*Fig. 11*).

Cases with positive myeloperoxidase-antineutrophil cytoplasmic antibodies (MPO-ANCA), depending on the degree of damage, have the corresponding findings to each of hemorrhage, diffuse alveolar damage (DAD) and BOOP lesions.

Drug-induced interstitial fibrosis

In recent years, reports on drug-induced lung injury by such agent as Chinese medicines, interferon, antibiotics, anticancer agents, G-CSF and methotrexate have been notable. Any of these agents can give rise to DAD, BOOP, NSIP, UIP, eosinophilic pneumonia, granulomatous inflammation and other changes. Risk is increased in older people, in smokers, in patients receiving combined cytotoxic agents, in irradiated patients and in patients with preexisting pulmonary fibrosis. Because amiodarone contains a large amount of iodine, a characteristic feature of CT findings is increased lung field density. (*Fig. 8*)

Interstitial fibrosis related to specific infections

Too strong an emphasis cannot be laid on the fact that chest radiographs of mycobacterial infections show a wide range of imaging patterns, including, needless to say, typical cavitary lesions. However, assessing findings suggesting endobronchial spread of lesions is useful for differentiation. That is to say, with CT, if tree-in-bud (TIB) appearance (the presence of dilated centrilobular bronchioles, their lumina impacted mucus, fluid, or pus, and peribronchiolar inflammation) is visible, tuberculosis should be listed for differential diagnosis even though TIB is not a pathognomonic finding for tuberculosis.

With pneumocystis pneumonia (PCP), chest radiographs of the early stage show fine reticular shadows extending from the hilum to the periphery. In most cases, because patients become aware only after the disease has progressed, extensive GGO can be seen. CT findings show geographical distribution of GGO with a tendency to become locally contracted and denser over a short period. Cystic formation is often seen in PCP with AIDS. Pneumothorax is a common complication.

Tree-in-bud appearance

This appearance corresponds to finger-in-glove findings in larger airways. It was first reported as a characteristic finding of endobronchial spread pulmonary tuberculosis, but it is also seen with other infectious diseases (viral infections, bronchopneumonia, etc.), immunologic disorders (hypersensitivity pneumonia, airway lesions of Sjögren's syndrome, etc.) and aspiration (pneumonia and bronchiolitis).

References

1) Katzenstein, A. L. A., Fiorelli, R. F.: Nonspecific interstitial pneumonia/fibrosis: Histologic features and clinical significance. Am. J. Surg. Pathol. 18: 136-147, 1994
2) Travis, W. D., et al.: Idiopathic nonspecific interstitial pneumonia: Prognostic significance of cellular and fibrosing patterns: Survival comparison with usual interstitial pneumonia and desquamative interstitial pneumonia. Am. J. Surg. Pathol. 24: 19-33, 2000

Further reading

- Naidich, D. P., et al.: Computed Tomography and Magnetic Resonance of the Thorax (2nd ed.). Raven Press, New York, 1991
- Webb, W. R., et al.: High-Resolution CT of the Lung. Raven Press, New York, 1992

Radiographs of intrapulmonary lesions with decreased radiolucency

Chapter 4

5. Alveolar-interstitial shadow

Pulmonary edema, reverse pulmonary edema shadow [Pattern classification IV-C]

●Author — Masamitsu Nakajima

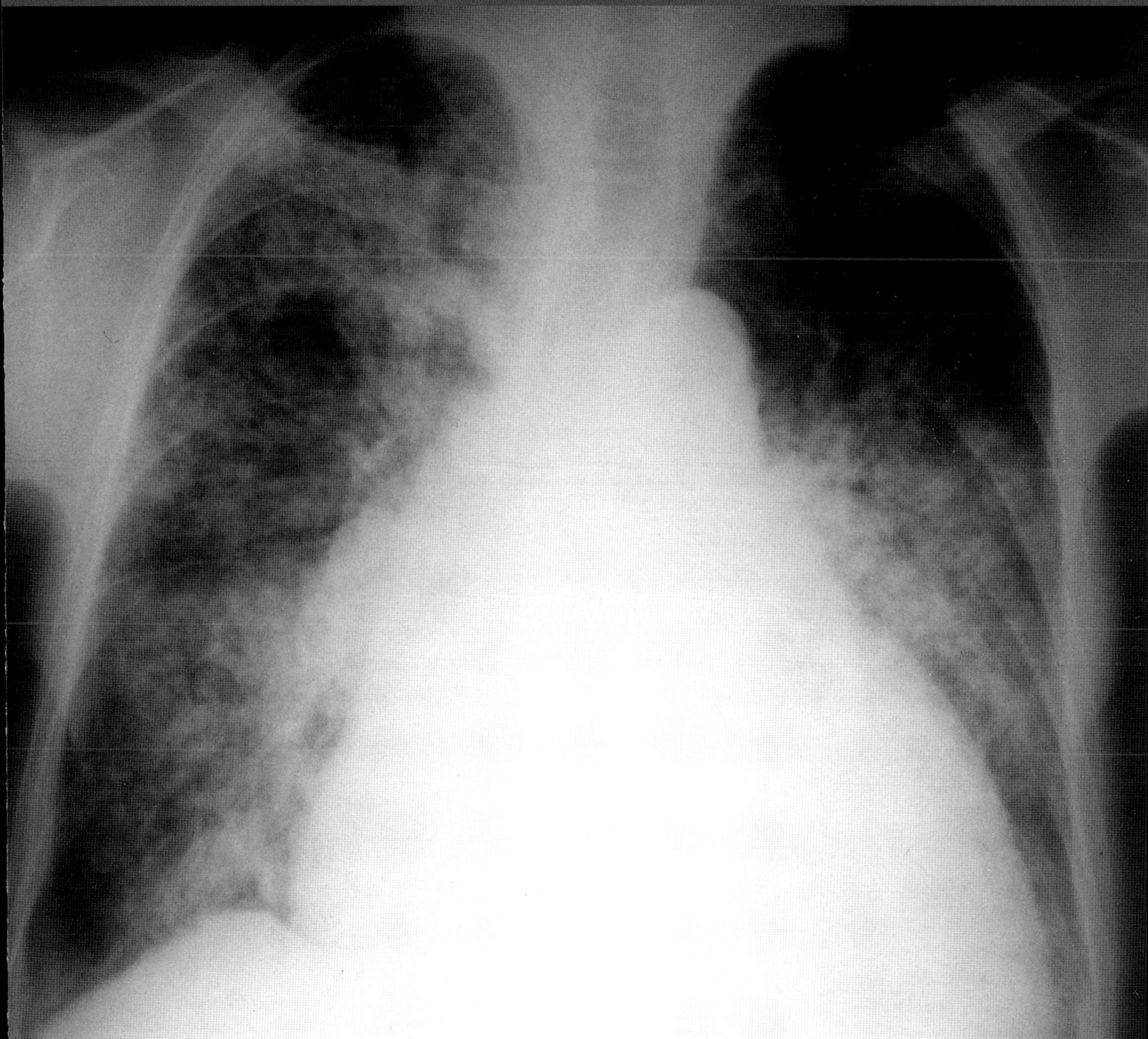

Keywords of this section

Butterfly shadow
Pulmonary edema
Peribronchial cuffing
Kerley's line
Vanishing tumor
Acute respiratory distress syndrome (ARDS)
Diffuse alveolar damage (DAD)
Paraquat
Pulmonary alveolar proteinosis
Crazy-paving appearance
Acute eosinophilic pneumonia due to smoking

Pulmonary edema, reverse pulmonary edema shadow

Masamitsu Nakajima
Faculty of Health Sciences, Hiroshima International University, Hiroshima, Japan

Chest radiographic findings of pulmonary edema may show air-space consolidation indicating alveolar space lesions and small irregular round nodular shadows and linear shadows indicating interstitial lesions. This type of shadow typically appears as a shadow distributed in the perihilar areas. However, pulmonary edemas have different onset mechanisms and show different types of shadow and distribution. This section describes the characteristic chest radiographic findings and the points for differential diagnosis from other diseases with similar radiographic findings.

Case 1 Pulmonary edema due to renal failure
79-year-old female

Chief complaints: Shortness of breath, dyspnea
Medical history: Hypertrophic cardiomyopathy
Present illness:
Dialysis was scheduled due to renal failure but before that dyspnea appeared and the patient was hospitalized. Hemodialysis and other procedures were performed, and hypoxemia improved.

A chest radiograph (P.69) shows perihilar patchy shadow, air-space consolidation, ground glass opacity and small round or irregular nodular shadows with indistinct boundaries that tend to fuse, referred to as a butterfly shadow.

Enlarged cardiac shadow due to previous hypertrophic cardiomyopathy is observed. In this case, because dialysis improved the shadow (*Fig. 1*) rather than body fluid removal, uremic pulmonary edema was diagnosed.

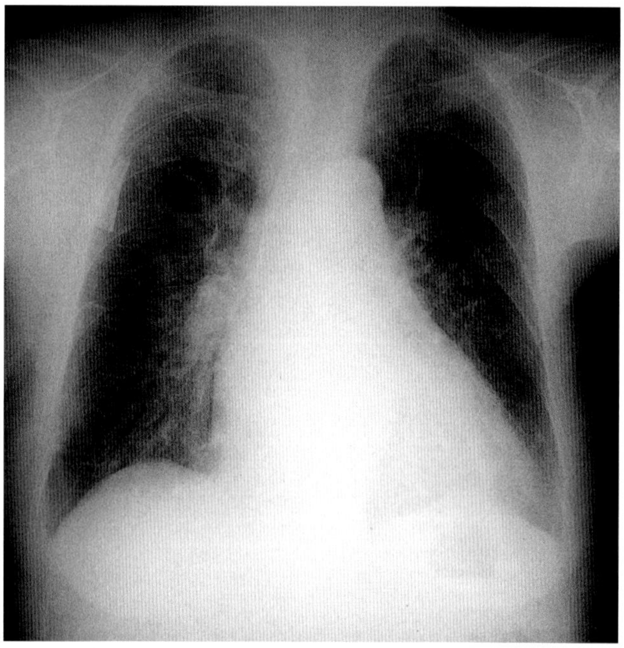

Figure 1. **Chest radiograph**: after improvement

What is a pulmonary edema?

Pulmonary edemas can be broadly classified by the two mechanisms of elevated pulmonary venous pressure and increased pulmonary capillary membrane permeability (*Table 1*). There are characteristic radiographic findings of pulmonary edema for both mechanisms. In actual clinical cases, however, due to a combination of various factors depending on the length of time after the onset and degree of severity of the pulmonary edema, chest radiographic findings and also pathological findings differ.[1–3)]

Regarding the pathological findings of pulmonary edema, the first stage is interstitial edema leading to the alveolar spaces filling with exudative fluid. Then, the radiographic findings are influenced by the degree of this intra-alveolar space exudative fluid's protein concentration, amount of fibrin, inflammatory cell count, organized pneumonia and fibrosis.

Increased pulmonary venous pressure:	Diseases causing left heart failure Mitral insufficiency etc. Fluid overload
Increased pulmonary capillary vessel permeability:	Diseases that cause acute respiratory distress syndrome (ARDS) Respiratory tract burn Severe infections, sepsis Aspiration pneumonia Shock Drugs (paraquat)
Other distinctive pulmonary edemas:	High-altitude pulmonary edema Cardiogenic pulmonary edema Re-expansive pulmonary edema

Table 1. **Major diseases causing pulmonary edema**

Since biopsies are generally not performed, most histopathological findings of pulmonary edemas are

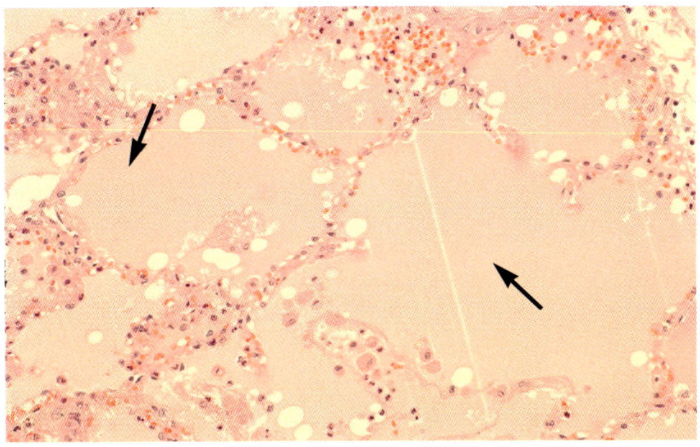

a. HE stain: Exudative fluid (→) filling alveolar spaces

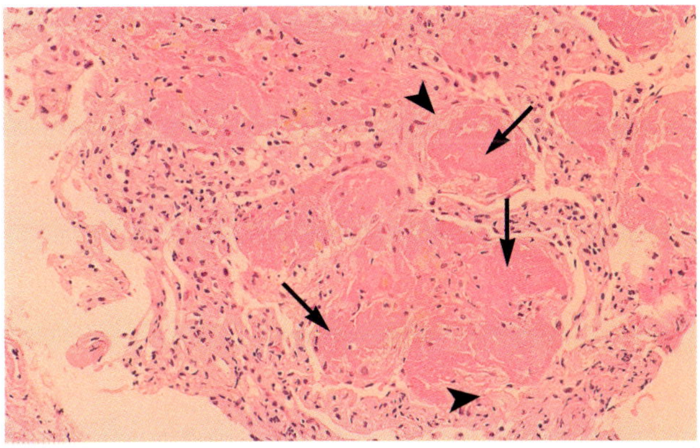

b. HE stain: Fibrin deposits (→) noticeable in alveolar spaces. Partial fibrosis (➤) can also be seen

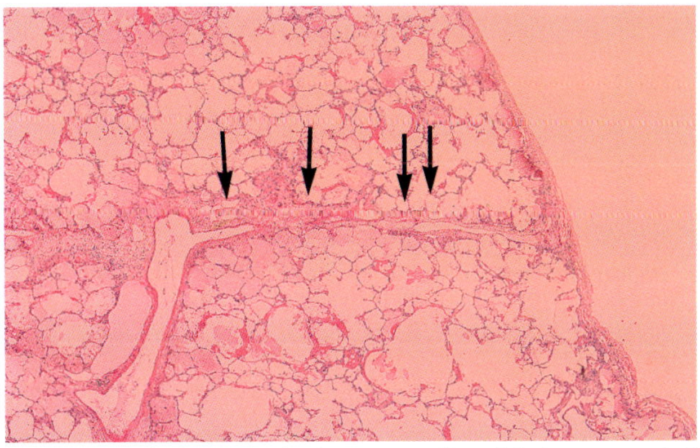

c. Edematous thickening and enlargement of interlobular septum (→) seen as Kerley's line

Figure 2 a–c. **Pathological findings**

obtained at times such as during autopsies. Pathological findings (HE stain) in *Figure 2 a* are an example of pulmonary edema at an autopsy showing exudative fluid in the alveolar spaces shortly before becoming filled. Mild edema can be seen in the alveolar wall, with mild infiltration of inflammatory cells. A suggested cause of this case was increased capillary membrane permeability. In an other case with uremic lung (HE stain) in *Figure 2 b* shows fibrin deposits in alveolar spaces.

One characteristic chest radiographic finding of pulmonary edema is bilateral perihilar shadow (butterfly shadow). There are also unilateral cases, with reports of them accounting for 4.5 % of all cases (Case 5). Here follow more detailed explanations (*Fig. 3*). As an indication of the development of edema in the interstitium, there is edematous thickening of the bronchial wall, exudation in alveolar spaces and edema in the interstitium surrounding the bronchial wall. In chest radiographic findings this bronchial wall may show a ring shadow, and is particularly easily seen in the B^3b bronchial wall when chest radiographic findings of the B^3b bronchial wall are thickening with indistinct peripheral boundaries and peribronchial cuffing. Interlobular septum enlargement in (*Fig. 2 c*) is seen as the linear shadows in the lung field know as Kerley's lines, with the location determining whether they are called Kerley's A, B or D lines (Case 7). Indistinct borders of hilar shadow (hilar haze), and pleural thickening seen as interlobular lines are also observed.

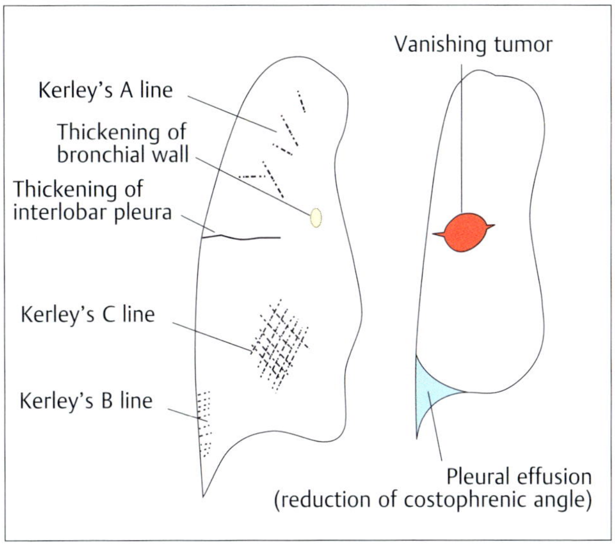

Figure 3. **Characteristic shadows in pulmonary edema**

In general, intrapleural fluid is absorbed from the visceral pleura and eliminated by intrapulmonary lymph ducts, but there is pleural effusion retention from the early stage of pulmonary edema. In addition, localized pleural effusion retention between lobes looks like a tumor. If treatment is conducted to reduce this pleural effusion, the tumor-like shadow disappears, which is why this is known as a vanishing tumor.

If edema progresses in the alveolar spaces it appears as alveolar pattern such as air-space consolidation, irregular small and round nodular shadows, and air bronchogram with ground glass opacity. Since this pattern of shadow is characteristically distributed[1)] in the perihilar area, it is expressed as butterfly shadow, bat-wing shadow and perihilar consolidation (Cases 1, 2). Depending on changes in the alveolar spaces the shadow becomes stronger to a certain degree, changes in surrounding alveolar lesion making air in the bronchial lumen easier to see to provide a radiographic finding called an air bronchogram (Case 5).

Differentiating chest radiographic findings

The characteristics of chest radiographic findings for cases of elevated pulmonary venous pressure and cases of increased pulmonary capillary membrane permeability differ, and so discriminatory points are given for both (*Table 2*).[2, 4]

With elevated pulmonary venous pressure, radiographic findings are clear wall thickening (ring shadow), peribronchial cuffing, cardiac contour enlargement, superior lung field vascular enlargement (Case 3), enlarged space between the border of the superior vena cava and border of the aorta (*Fig. 4*), Kerley's lines and pleural effusion. In contrast to this, in cases of increased pulmonary capillary membrane permeability, an air bronchogram tends to be visible, while the shadow tends to be distributed from the hilum to the periphery. Pulmonary edema is often due to a combination of infection, cardiac failure, shock and neurological disease (raised intracranial pressure, head trauma and seizure). In many cases, it is not possible to differentiate between elevated pulmonary venous pressure and increased permeability of pulmonary capillary membrane. Furthermore, in cases of elevated pulmonary venous pressure due to acute myocardial infarction, idiopathic arrhythmia and other causes, even in the absence of cardiac enlargement, shadow due to edema may be initially visible.

	Elevated pressure	Increased permeability
Cardiac enlargement	+	–
Kerley's lines	+	–
Pleural effusion	+	–
Air bronchogram	–	+
Peribronchial cuffing	+	–

Table 2. **Chest radiograph points that differentiate between cases of elevated pulmonary venous pressure and cases of increased pulmonary capillary permeability.**

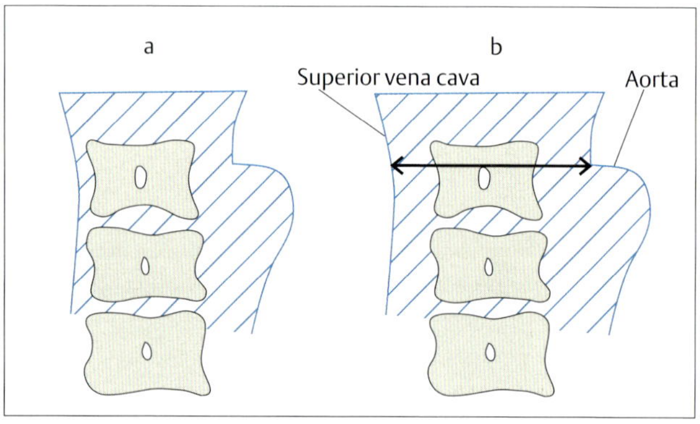

Figure 4 a–b. **(a) Normal, (b) Increased space between the border of the superior vena cava and the border of the aorta**

Case 2 Pulmonary edema due to contrast medium

52-year-old female

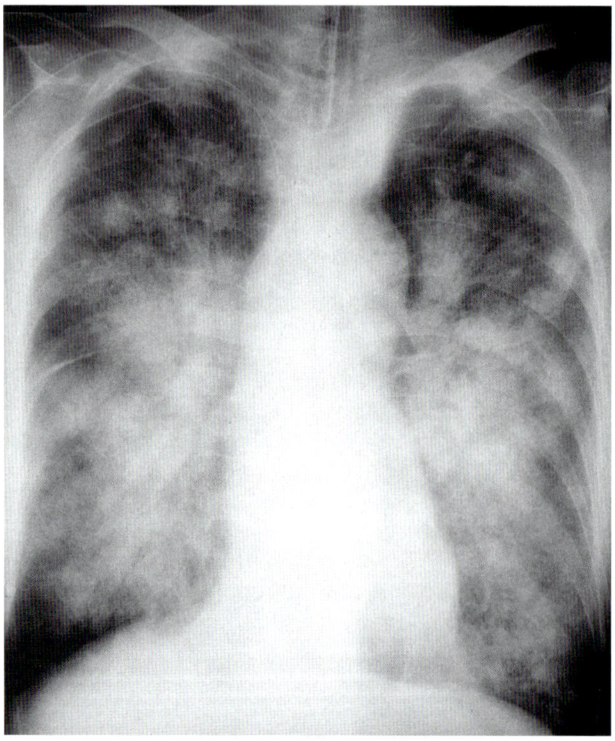

Figure 5. **Chest radiograph**

Chief complaint: Dyspnea

Allergy history: No drug or food allergies, no notable allergies

Medical history: Diagnosed with Parkinson's disease

Present illness:

Difficulty walking seven years ago. Gait disorder worsened. The patient was diagnosed with Parkinson's disease at our hospital, and received treatment. Drip infusion pyelography was conducted to examine for vesicorectal disorder. A previous iodine test was negative but after performing the pyelography, the patient began to feel ill, and exhibited symptoms such as dyspnea and decreased blood pressure.

Chest radiographic findings show a shadow in the perihilar area resembling the outstretched wings of a butterfly or bat. This shadow is referred to, among other names, as a butterfly or bat-wing shadow.

Diagnosis: Decreased blood pressure, dyspnea and other symptoms observed after using contrast medium. No abnormal shadows were observed in chest radiographic findings before performing pyelography, but a typical butterfly shadow suddenly appeared in the center of the hilum in chest radiographic findings after pyelography. From this course, pulmonary edema due to contrast medium was diagnosed.

Case 3

Pulmonary congestion

48-year-old male

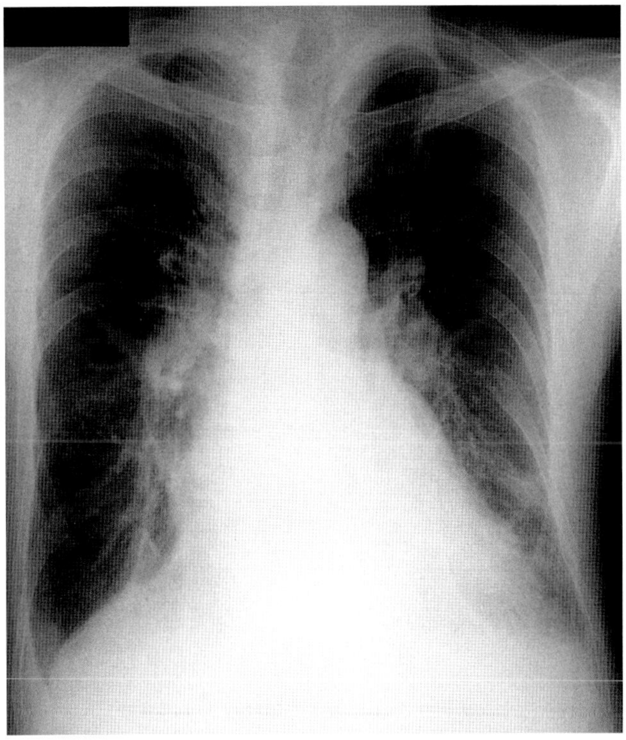

Figure 6. **Chest radiograph**

The patient was suffering from Marfan syndrome. Marfan syndrome is often associated with diseases of the aorta and heart, but this was a case of pulmonary congestion resulting from mitral insufficiency associated with mitral valve prolapse.

Although it is actually more difficult to see and interpret thin vascular shadows, bilateral enlarged vascular shadows in the upper lung field can be observed reaching comparatively peripheral areas.

Thickening of the bronchial wall, enlargement of the pulmonary artery and enlarged cardiac contour are also visible. Deformation of the diaphragm can also be seen, but this is a previous shadow and is not related to the pulmonary edema.

Case 4

Acute respiratory distress syndrome (ARDS)

63-year-old female

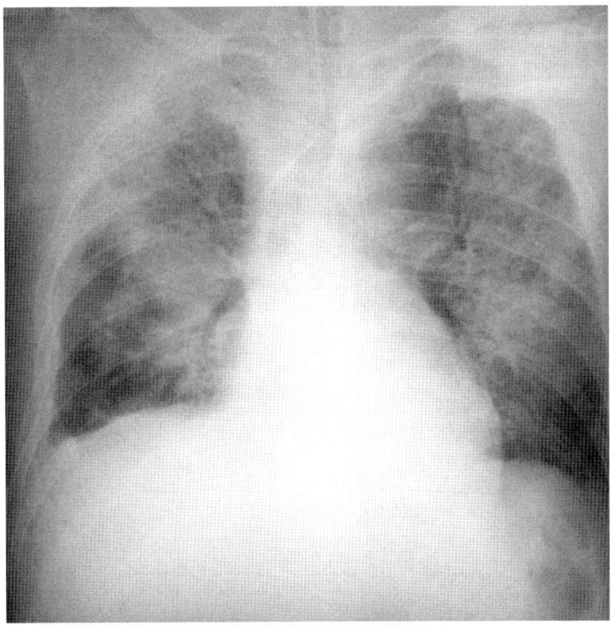

Figure 7. **Chest radiograph**

A case of pulmonary edema associated with sepsis.

A chest radiograph (*Fig. 7*) at the time of onset shows bilateral diffuse alveolar pattern, ground glass opacity and linear shadow, with shadow distribution featuring indistinct borders up to peripheral areas, as well as what could be thought of as distribution in the perihilar area, indicating acute respiratory distress syndrome (ARDS).

ARDS histopathological findings

As can be understood from the diagnostic criteria for ARDS[5)] (*Table 3*), this case is a combination of multiple causes. Furthermore, although the same can be said for many inflammatory pulmonary diseases, ARDS histopathological findings change significantly during the course of the disease.

The histopathological findings (*Figs. 8 a–e*) show pulmonary edema and diffuse alveolar damage (DAD). Due to partial alveolar wall damage (alveolar mouth), DAD results in the appearance of exudative fluid and the start of hyaline membrane formation (*a*, →). From this membranous state, a hyaline membrane forms (*b, c*). When

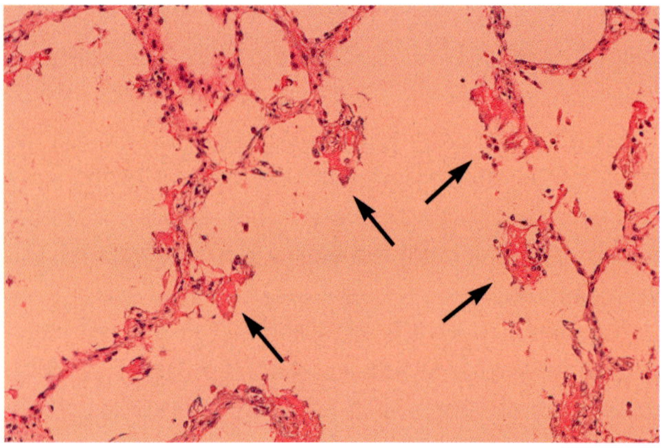

a. HE stain: Damage to alveolar mouth (→) leading to the beginning of hyaline membrane formation.

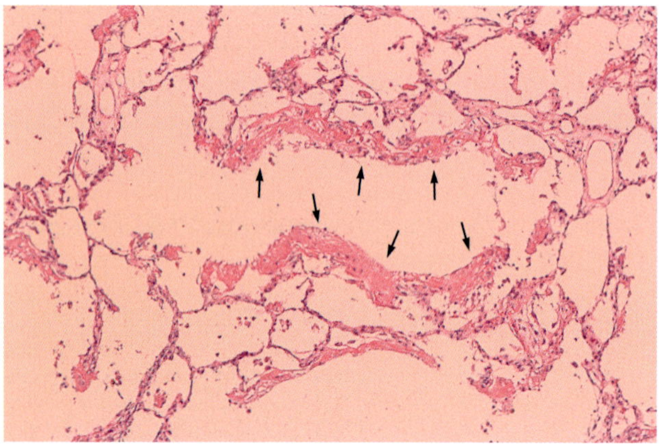

b. HE stain: Hyaline membrane (→)

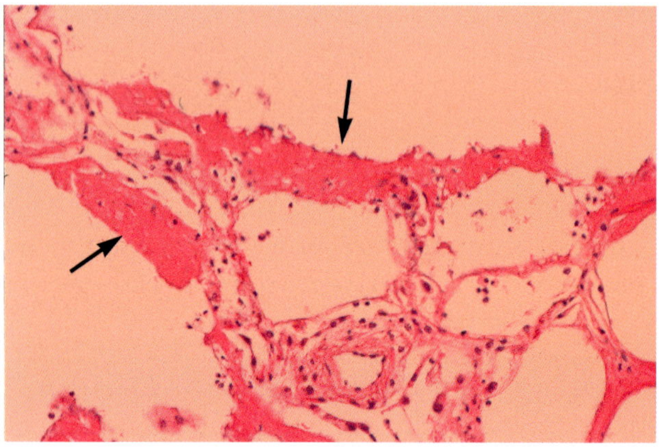

c. HE stain: (high magnification) hyaline membrane (→)

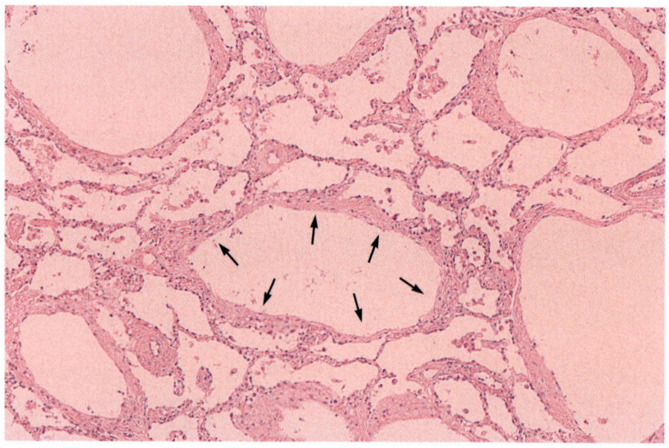

d. HE stain: Membranous fibrosis (→)

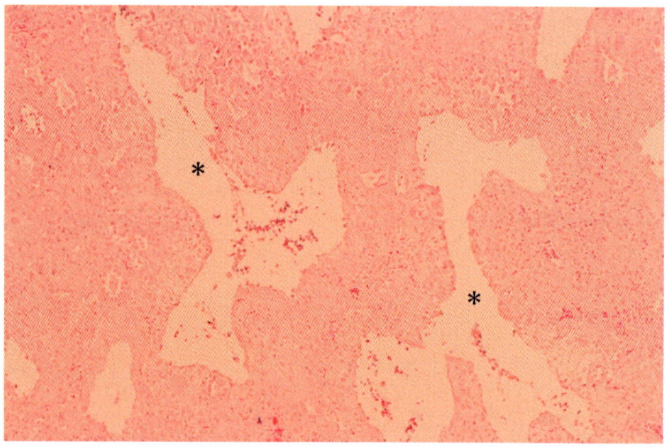

e. HE stain: Fibrosis throughout alveolar wall and alveolar duct (∗) enlargement.

Figure 8 a–e. **Pathological findings**

this membrane comes into contact with the alveolar mouth, there is fibroblast infiltration leading to a proliferative stage, and then the hyaline membrane becomes membranous fibrosis (*d*). In another proliferation stage, DAD histopathological findings show damage to the entire alveolar wall, with overall fibrosis formation in some cases (*e*).[3, 6]

Type of injury	Oxygenation (PaO_2/FiO_2)	Chest radiograph (frontal view)
ALI	≤300 mmHg (regardless of PEEP)	bilateral infiltrates
ARDS	≤200 mmHg (regardless of PEEP)	bilateral infiltrates

Type of injury	PCWP	Timing
ALI	≤18 mmHg (no clinical evidence of left heart failure)	acute onset
ARDS	≤18 mmHg (no clinical evidence of left heart failure)	acute onset

PCWP = pulmonary capillary wedge pressure
PEEP = positive end-expiratory pressure

Table3. **Criteria for acute lung injury (ALI) and ARDS** [5]

Case 5 Unilateral pulmonary edema

67-year-old male

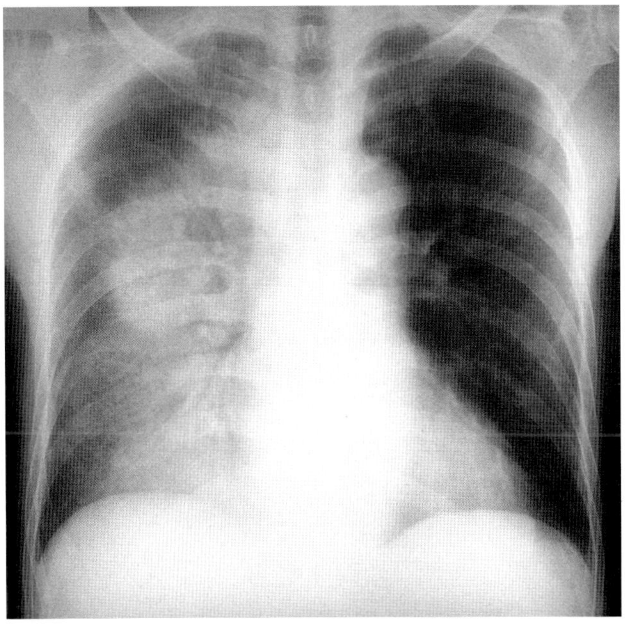

Figure 9. **Chest radiograph**

Pulmonary edema due to hemorrhagic shock.

Chest radiographic findings show a shadow in the perihilar area on the right side. An air bronchogram can be observed at the lower right of the hilum, with conspicuous linear vascular shadows outside the surrounding main shadow. Mild vascular enlargement is also seen in the left lung. After taking this radiograph, a similar central hilar shadow began to appear on the left lung, and eventually there were shadows on both lungs. Unilateral pulmonary edema is occasionally seen but its incidence seems to differ depending on the statistical methods used in reports and the time after onset.

Causes of unilateral pulmonary edema include unilateral pulmonary vascular occlusive disease, long-term side-lying, re-expansive pulmonary edema and following aorta-to-pulmonary artery anastomosis.

Case 6 Localized interlobar pleural effusion retention

66-year-old male

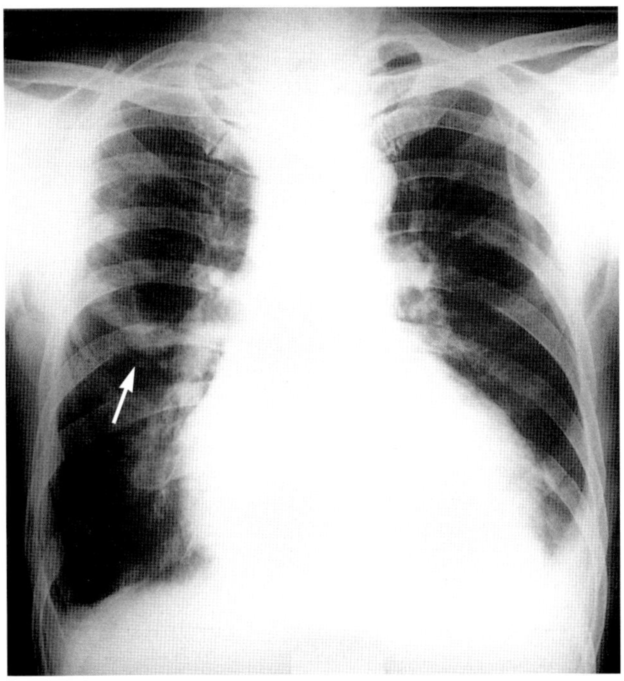

Figure 10. **Chest radiograph**

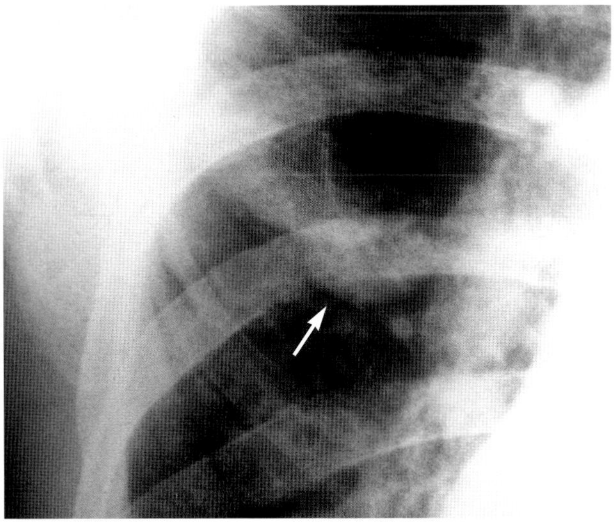

Figure 11. Chest radiograph

Localized pleural effusion between the lobes on the right side (→) which shows as a nodule-like tumor. As this localized retention of pleural effusion disappears with treatment, it is called a vanishing tumor.

Case 7 Kerley's A and B lines

48-year-old female

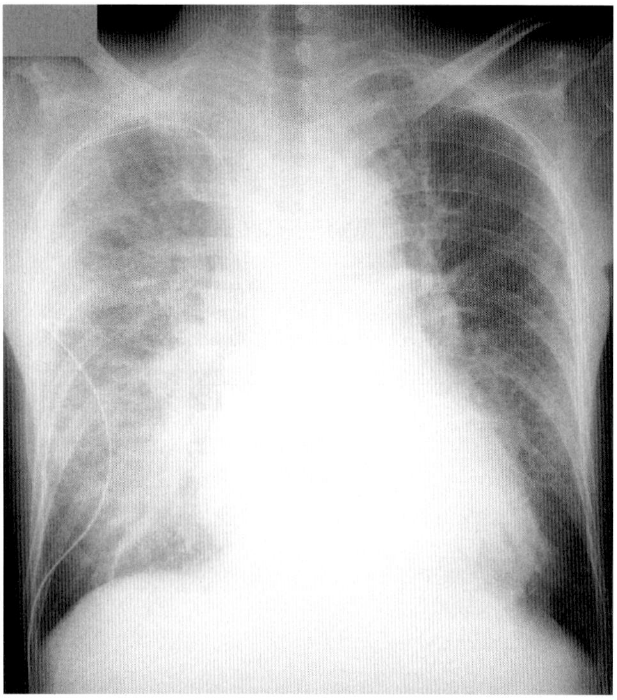

Figure 12. **Chest radiograph: Kerley's A and B lines**

The roughly 1 mm-thick and 1.5 to 2.0 cm-long shadow located in the lateral lower lung field is called a Kerley's B line. The linear shadow from the hilum to the upper lung field is called a Kerley's A line. This is a case of pulmonary edema due to cardiac failure with visible cardiac enlargement, indistinct hilar shadow (hilar haze), enlarged pulmonary artery, and Kerley's A and B lines (*Fig. 12*). Enlarged shadows between the border of the superior vena cava and the border of the aorta can also be seen. Kerley's B lines (→) are seen as linear shadows stretching horizontally towards the pleura (*Fig. 13*). Kerley's A lines (*Fig. 14*, →) are seen as linear shadows stretching from the hilum to peripheral lung.

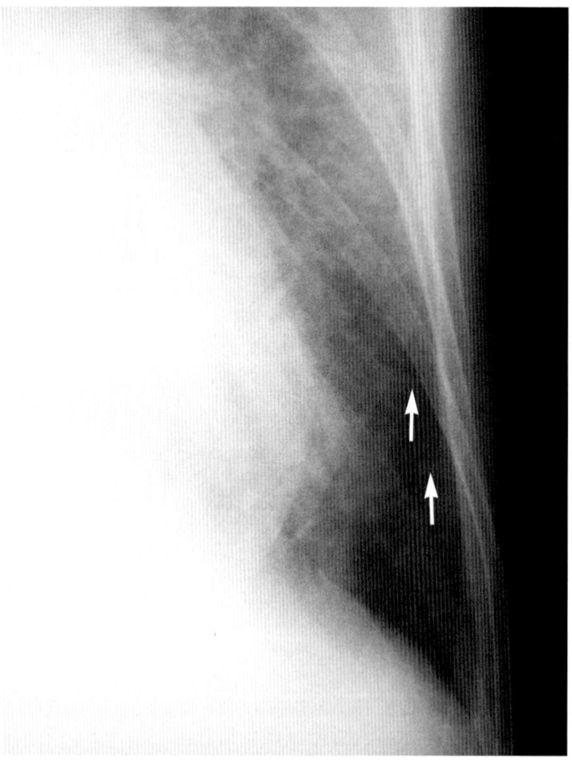

Figure 13. **Chest radiograph: Kerley's B line in the left lower lung field**

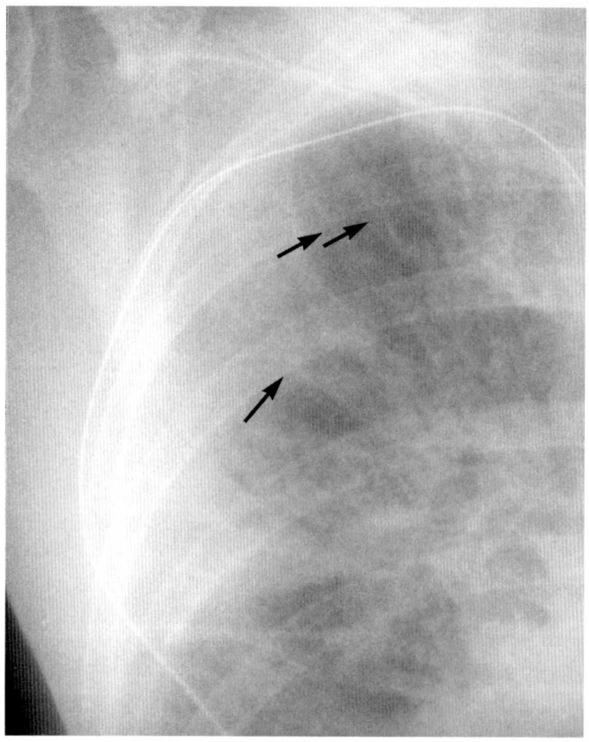

Figure 14. **Chest radiograph: Kerley's A line in the right upper lung field**

Case 8 Extensive burn, respiratory tract burn

65-year-old female

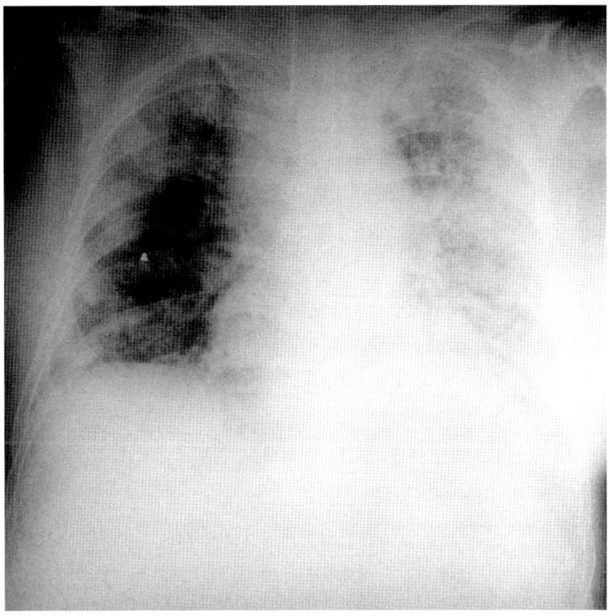

Figure 15. **Chest radiograph**

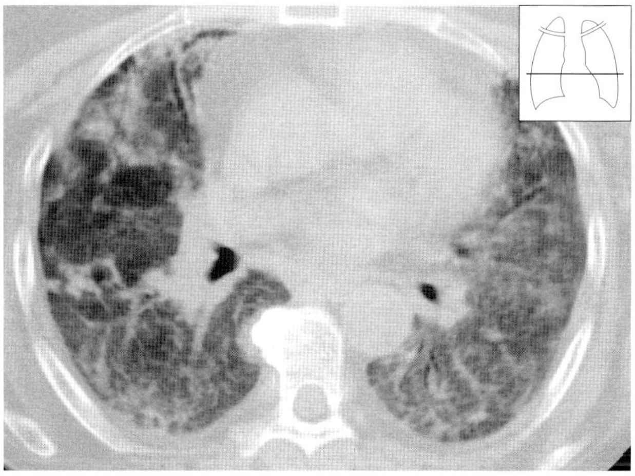

Figure 16. **Chest CT**

The patient's clothing was set alight by a bonfire. She was hospitalized with extensive burn and respiratory tract burn.

A chest radiographic finding 2 days after hospitalization shows bilateral diffuse shadow and predominantly peripheral alveolar pattern, with ground glass opacity.

A chest CT shows bilateral diffuse shadow with airspace consolidation and ground glass opacity, with thickening of the interlobular septa.

In this case, the patient's life was saved with mechanical ventilation care and treatment with steroids and antibiotics, but even after treatment pulmonary fibrosis remained.

Case 9 ARDS due to paraquat

75-year-old male

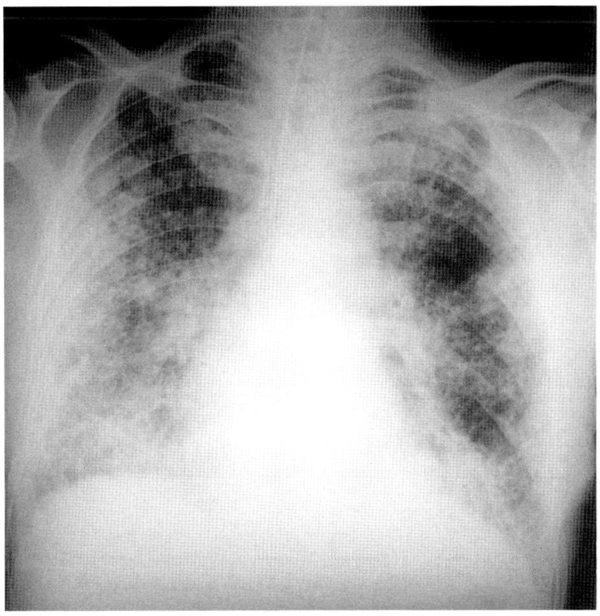

Figure 17. **Chest radiograph**

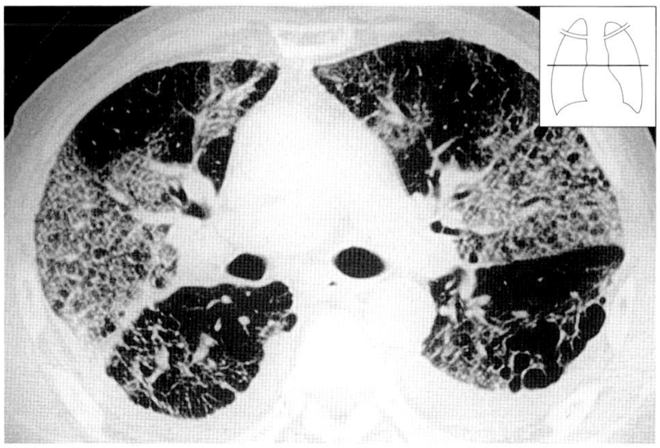

Figure 18. **Chest CT**

The patient was hospitalized after attempting suicide by drinking the weedkiller paraquat. Gastric lavage and dialysis were performed and other measures taken but severe hypoxemia led to clinical deterioration.

A chest radiograph shows diffuse alveolar pattern particularly in peripheral areas of the lungs, with linear shadows and ground glass opacity.

A chest CT shows thickening of the bronchial wall and interlobular septum with ground glass opacity and diffuse alveolar air-space consolidation and bilateral pleural effusion. Emphysematous lesions, which were probably present before the ingestion of paraquat, are also visible.

For diagnosis, proof that paraquat has been ingested in the clinical history and qualitative and quantitative blood and urine tests are important. It is also important to be aware that the symptoms related to paraquat are due to progressive renal failure, gastritis, and esophagitis.

Case 10 Pulmonary alveolar proteinosis

39-year-old male

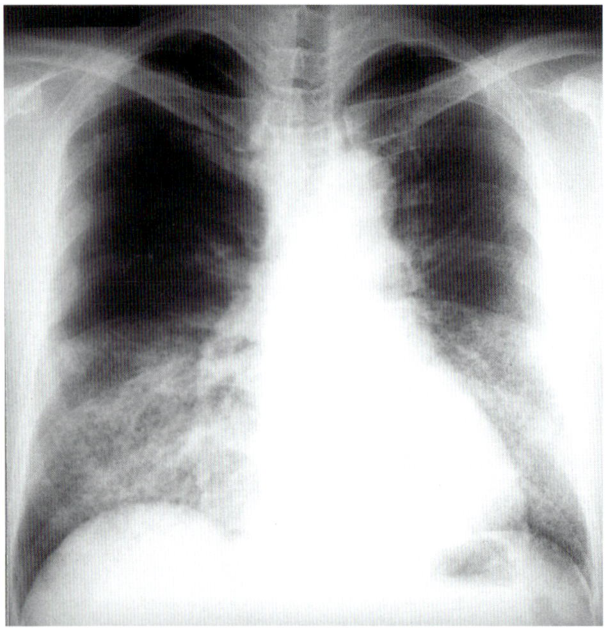

Figure 19. **Chest radiograph**

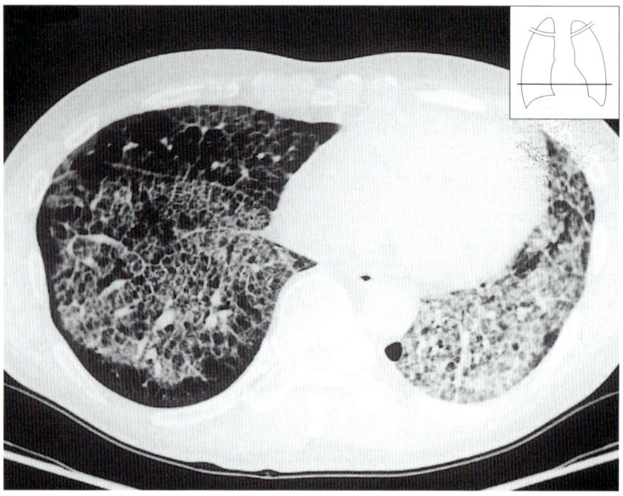

Figure 20. **Chest CT**

The patient had dyspnea while working and was hospitalized. There was no fever, sputum or cough.

A chest radiograph shows ground glass opacity predominantly in the perihilar area and the lower lung fields, there is air-space consolidation tending to partially fuse and boundaries are indistinct. This pattern is similar to pulmonary edema.

A chest CT shows a fine linear shadow forming polygonal shapes superimposed on an area of ground glass opacity. This combination gives an appearance that has been described a "crazy-paving appearance". It should be noted that crazy-paving appearance can also be seen in a variety of other conditions, including bacterial pneumonia and pulmonary hemorrhage.[7)]

Alveolar lavage fluid is white and turbid, resembling water that has been used to wash rice.

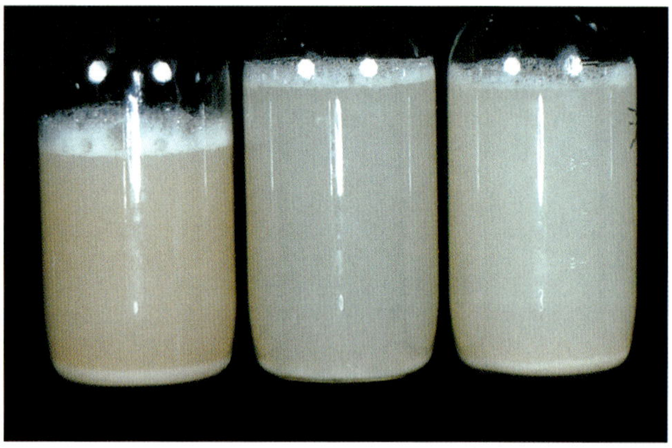

Figure 21. **White, turbid alveolar lavage fluid.** There is layered white material at the bottom.

Differentiation points

Chest CT findings are characteristic. However, it is also useful for diagnosis that symptoms are mild compared with the degree of shadow, and the serum KL-6 level is high.[8)]

Case 11 Smoke-induced acute eosinophilic pneumonia (peripheral type, reverse pulmonary edema)

18-year-old male

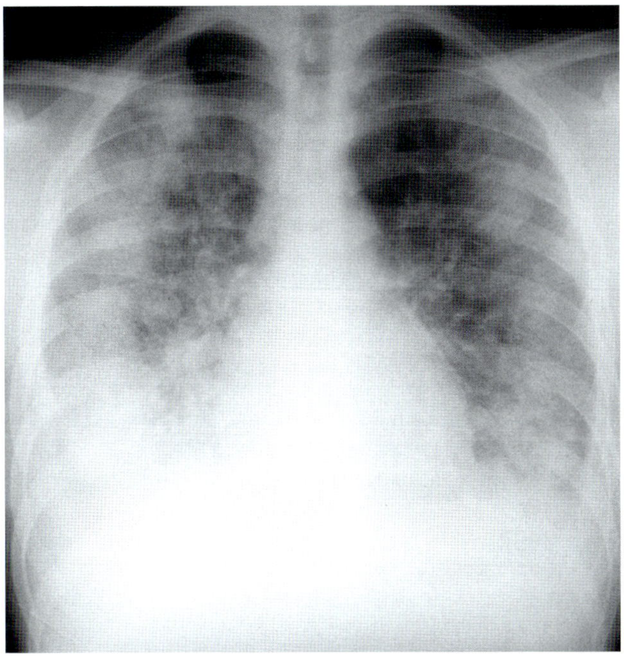

Figure 22. **Chest radiograph**

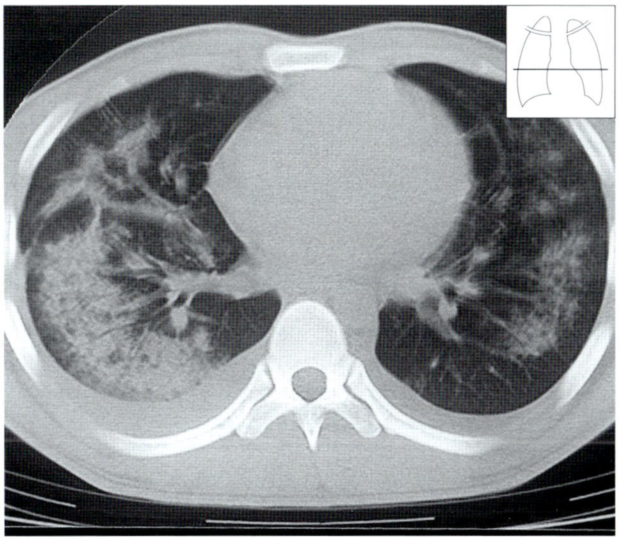

Figure 23. **Chest CT**

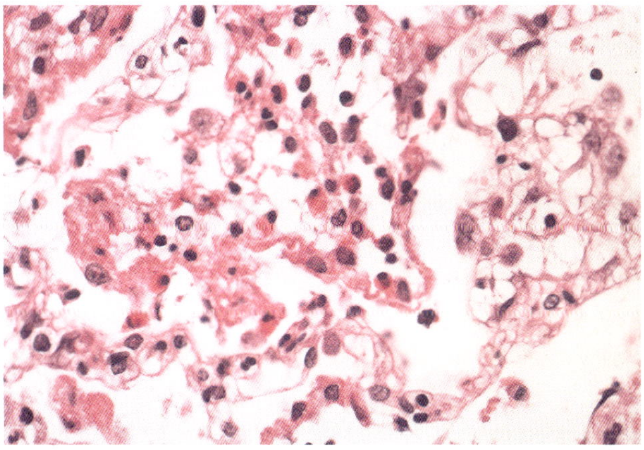

Figure 24. **Pathological findings in a transbronchial lung biopsy tissue (HE stain)**: alveolar air space filled with numerous eosinophils, proliferation of type II alveolar pneumocytes, and macrophages and fibrin observed in alveolar spaces.

The patient was hospitalized for acute onset of cough and dyspnea after smoking for the first time in his life.

A chest radiograph shows predominantly peripheral air-space consolidation, ground glass opacity and bilateral pleural effusion. Since distribution is the opposite to that of perihilar distribution in pulmonary edema, it is called reverse pulmonary edema pattern.

A chest CT shows air-space consolidation with predominantly peripheral distribution accompanied by air bronchogram, ground glass opacity, Kerley's B line and bilateral pleural effusion. No swelling of lymph nodes was observed.

A transbronchial lung biopsy indicated eosinophilic pneumonia, and an increased number of eosinophils in bronchoalveolar lavage fluid was observed.

Differentiation points

Characteristics of acute eosinophilic pneumonia include 1) fever, cough, dyspnea, 2) crackles on chest auscultation, 3) chest radiographic finding showing diffuse infiltration shadow, pleural effusion and Kerley's lines, 4) normal or slightly increased eosinophils in peripheral blood, 5) 28 to 50% increase in eosinophils in bronchoalveolar lavage fluid, 6) duration from onset of acute respiratory failure is less than 1 week, 7) steroids are markedly effective, with improvement in most cases seen within 8 days, and 8) no recurrence. As for the cause of respiratory failure, it is also important to test for serum antibodies for *Chlamydia psittaci, Chlamydia pneumoniae, Mycoplasma pneumoniae, Legionella,* viruses and other agents to rule out infection. A characteristic of smoke-induced AEP is that in many cases it occurs in young people with onset after smoking for the first time.[9, 10]

In this section, pulmonary edema was classified into cases of increased pulmonary venous pressure and increased pulmonary capillary membrane permeability and explanations were provided from the viewpoint of image findings and pathological findings.

At the beginning of pulmonary edema due to elevated pulmonary venous pressure, thickening of the bronchial wall (peribronchial cuffing) is observed with indistinct borders. Edematous thickening of the interlobular septa and vascular enlargement are seen as Kerley's lines. Indistinct perihilar shadow (hilar haze), pleural thickening and localized pleural effusion (vanishing tumor), and pleural effusion are also observed.

After development of interstitial edema in interlobular septum, bronchial wall, alveolar wall and other interstitial areas, exudation and inflammatory cell reaction are seen in the alveolar spaces.

As edema in the alveolar spaces proceeds, ground glass opacity and air-space consolidation are seen. In the case of elevated pulmonary venous pressure, this shadow is distributed in the perihilar area and has a characteristic shape which is referred to as a butterfly shadow.

The characteristics of increased pulmonary venous pressure are Kerley's lines, peribronchial cuffing, pleural effusion, and shadow with distribution in the perihilar area. Other characteristics are enlarged vascular shadow in the upper lung fields, enlarged cardiac shadow, and increased space between the border of the superior vena cava and the aorta.

Differentiating from other diseases

Some diseases show similar shadows to the chest radiographic findings of pulmonary edema. It is necessary to distinguish between pulmonary edema and infections or other diseases by symptoms, clinical course and laboratory findings.

References

1) Toshiharu Matsushima: Interpreting Chest Radiographs, second edition. Kinpodo Inc., Kyoto, 1992
2) Imaging of Diseases of the Chest, second edition. Armstrong P., Wilson A. G., Dee P., Hansell D. M., eds. Mosby, 1990
3) Toshiaki Manabe: Diagnosis of Inflammatory Pulmonary Diseases Using Tissue Patterns, Kinpodo Inc., Kyoto, 1991
4) Smith R. C., et al.: Radiological differentiation between different etiology of pulmonary edema. Invest. Radiol. 22: 859–863, 1987
5) Bernard GR, et al.: Report of the American-European Consensus conference on acute respiratory distress syndrome: definitions, mechanisms, relevant outcomes, and clinical trial coordination. Consensus Committee
6) Masamitsu Nakajima: Pathological Images of Pulmonary Fibrosis in ARDS, Progress in Medicine 20: 2145–2152, 2000
7) Johkoh T., et al.: Crazy-paving appearance at thin-section CT: Spectrum of disease and pathologic findings. Radiology 211: 155–160, 1999
8) Nakajima M, et al.: Serum KL-6 level as a monitoring marker in a patient with pulmonary alveolar proteinosis. Thorax. 53: 809–11, 1998
9) Nakajima M., et al.: Cigarette smoke-induced acute eosinophilic pneumonia. Radiology 207: 829–831, 1998
10) King M. A., et al.: Acute eosinophilic pneumonia: Radiologic and clinical features. Radiology 203: 715–719, 1997

6. Nodular shadow:

Solitary nodular shadow 1

[Pattern classification IV-D-1]

●Authors — Kenji Eguchi, Nobuhiko Seki

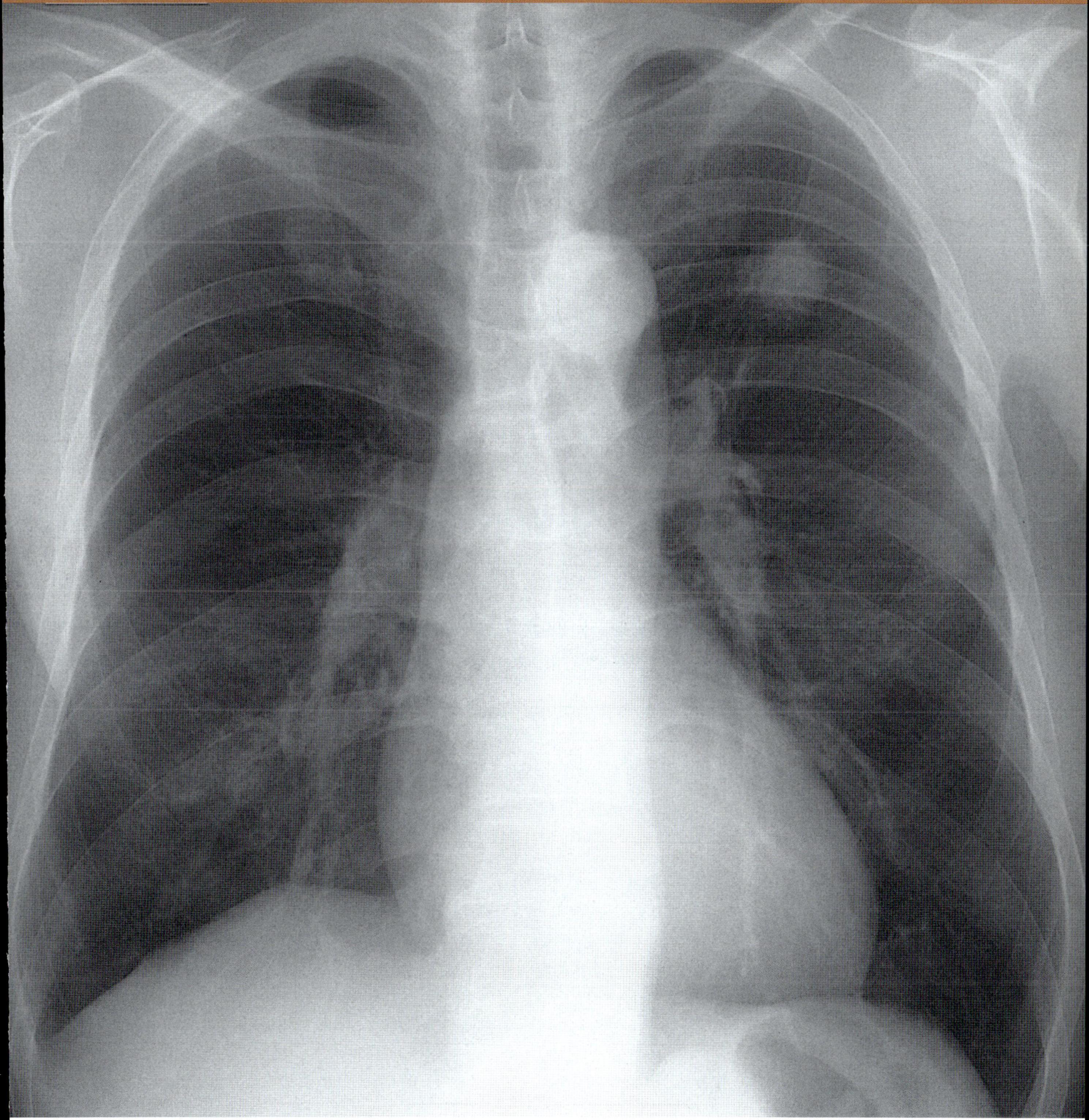

Keywords of this section

Lung segmental anatomy
Solid-type adenocarcinoma
Silhouette sign
Notch
Thin slice CT
Lung window setting
Mediastinal window setting
Lobulation
Peripheral-type lung adenocarcinoma
Segment
Subsegment
Secondary pulmonary lobule
Pleural retraction
Air bronchogram

Solitary nodular shadow 1

Kenji Eguchi, Nobuhiko Seki
Division of Medical Oncology, Tokai Oncology Center, Tokai University School of Medicine, Kanagawa, Japan

When interpreting solitary nodular shadow, rather than paying attention to just the superficial characteristics of the shadow, having a three-dimensional understanding of the involvement of surrounding structures based on lung segmental anatomy provides clues for interpreting the evolution and extension of lesions. This section covers imaging diagnosis of typical solid-type adenocarcinoma, focusing on its differentiation.

Case 1 65-year-old male

Chief complaint: Bloody sputum
Medical history: Gastric ulcer operation at age 40
Family history: Father had stomach cancer, elder brother had rectal cancer, paternal aunt had uterine cancer
Smoking history: 30/day for 45 years
Present illness:
Patient became aware of bloody sputum on bathing and received a medical examination at a local hospital. A chest radiograph revealed an abnormal shadow and he was referred to this hospital for a detailed examination.
Physical findings on admission:
Weight loss of 3 kg in 3 months, nothing else of note
Laboratory data on admission:
No particular abnormalities
Imaging findings:
A chest radiograph (P. 81) shows a 25 mm diameter nodule with slight peripheral irregularity and a comparatively defined border at the point where the second anterior rib and sixth posterior rib intersect in the left upper lung. Vascular shadows can just be seen inside the shadow but the shadow and its silhouette sign are negative, and are simply superimposed. However, there are a comparatively large number of vascular shadows surrounding the shadow in both lungs.

Chest CT (*Figs. 1 a–r*) shows shadow characteristics of bronchial patency inside the shadow with homogeneous density. Borders are distinct but there is notch formation (*f, g*) (➤) due to the presence of peripheral bronchi and blood vessels. The area of the shadow in thin slice (2 mm thick, 2 mm intervals) CT in the lung window setting (WL -500, WW 1,500) (*n*) and in the mediastinal window setting (WL 40 HU, WW 400 HU) (*m*) is almost the same, pointing to probable solid-type shadow.[1]

To look at the relationship with surrounding structures, here is an analysis combining chest CT and thin slice CT. First, there is involvement of the bronchi, but the chest CT (*e*) shows B^{1+2}a+b touching the inner side of the shadow and ascending.

Bearing this in mind, looking at thin slice CT starting

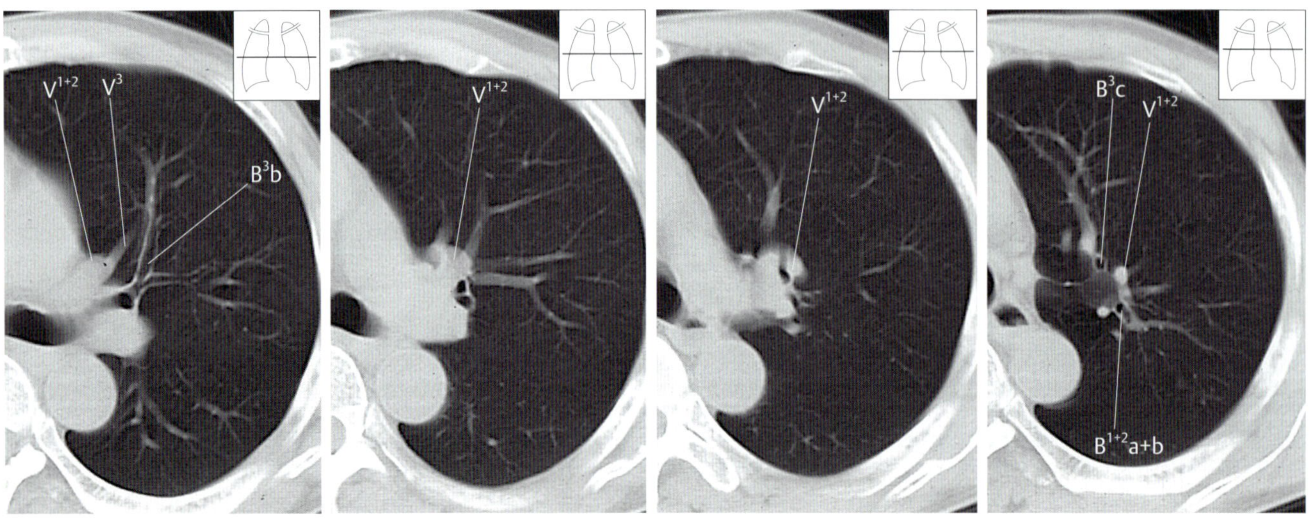

a *b* *c* *d*

Figure 1 a–r. **Chest CT**: (i–r) Thin slice CT

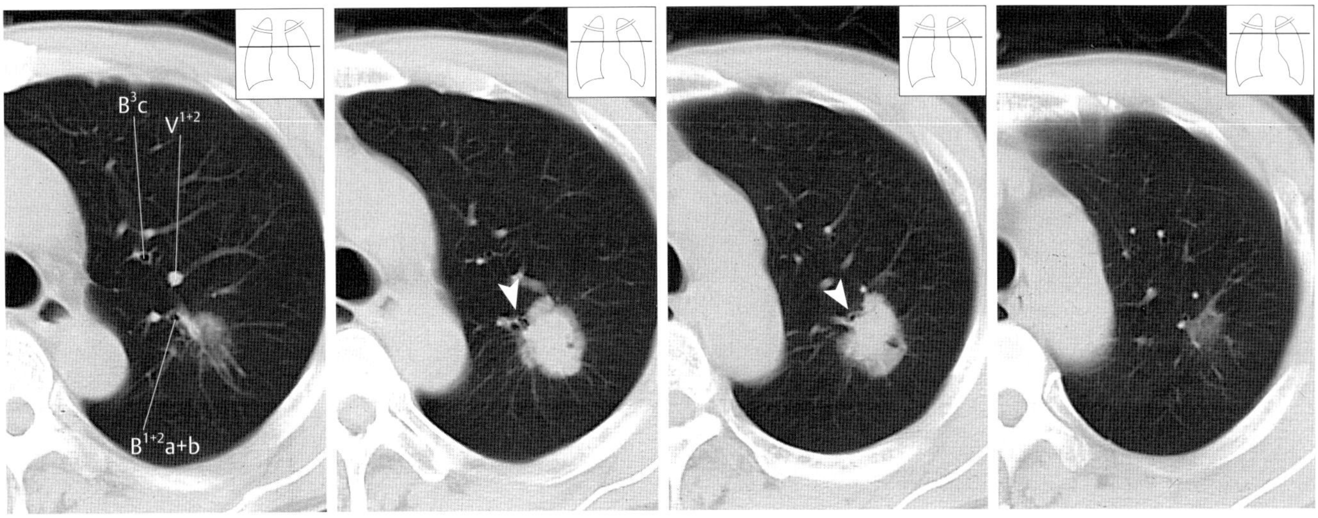

e *f* *g* *h*

<i-r. Thin slice CT >

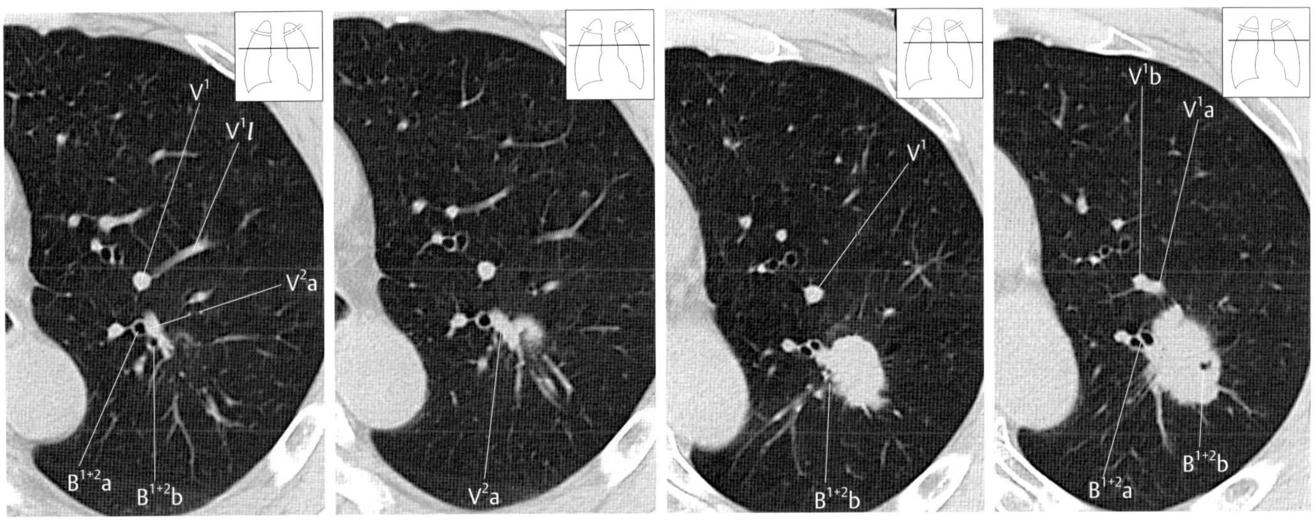

i *j* *k* **l**

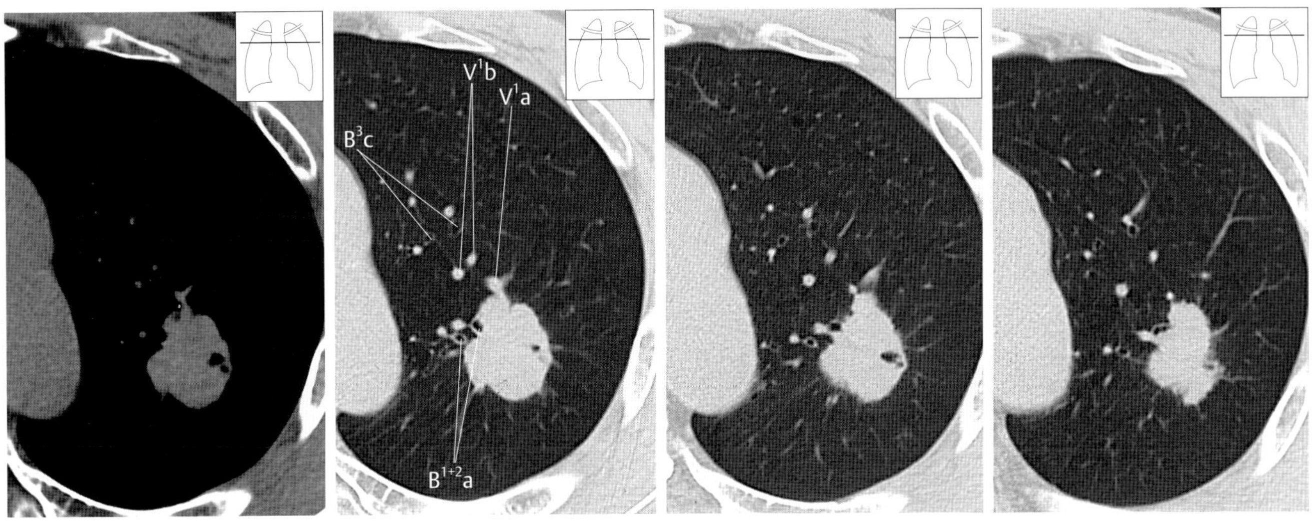

m *n* *o* *p*

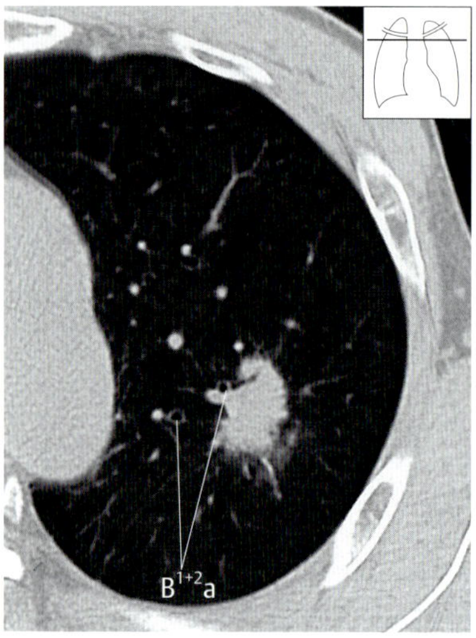

q

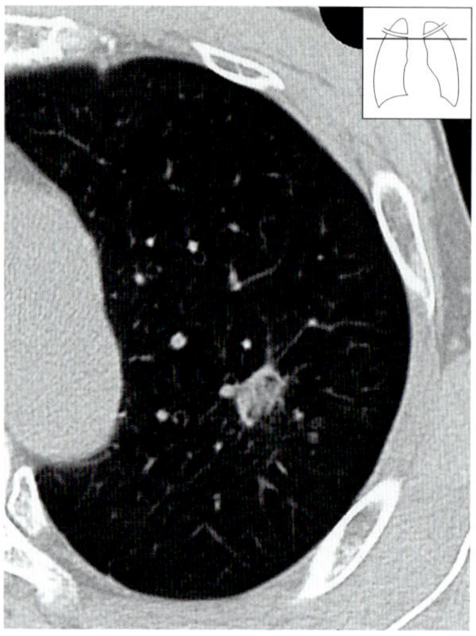

r

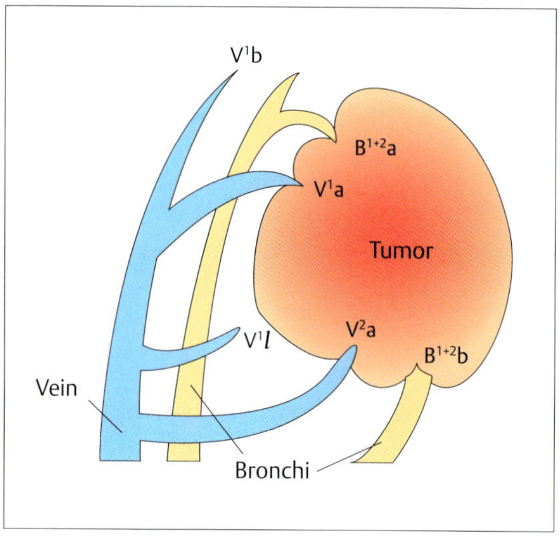

Figure 2. **Illustration of reconstruction**

from the lower border of the shadow, after separation of B^{1+2}a+b into B^{1+2}a and B^{1+2}b (*i*), B^{1+2}a touches the inner side of the shadow and ascends (*l*), and the outer side branch of the bifurcation is involved in the upper edge of the shadow (*q*). After B^{1+2}b has been incorporated into the lower border of the shadow (*k*), inside the shadow, the previous bifurcated bronchi are made patent (*l*), indicating that they are involved bronchi.

A look at venous involvement. Following the left upper pulmonary vein from the center to the periphery in a chest CT, the single thick vein V^{1+2} (*a*) that bifurcate at the inner side of B^3b ascends between B^3c, which turns around towards the outer anterior border of B^3b (*b, c*), and B^{1+2}a+b (*d, e*). This variation is classified as V^{1+2} (semi-central vein type) (*Fig. 7 I*).

Looking at venous involvement segmentally with thin slice CT from the lower border of the shadow, first V^2a on the border between the S^{1+2}a and S^{1+2}b segments bifurcates from V^{1+2}(*i*) and ascends along the outer side of B^{1+2}a and B^{1+2}b (*j*), and can be seen to converge from the lower border of the shadow into the shadow (*k, l*). V^1l abutting on the lower border between S^3c and S^{1+2}a bifurcates from V^1 after the V^2a bifurcation (*i*). Furthermore, V^1a on the border between S^{1+2}ai and S^1 + 2aii and V^1b on

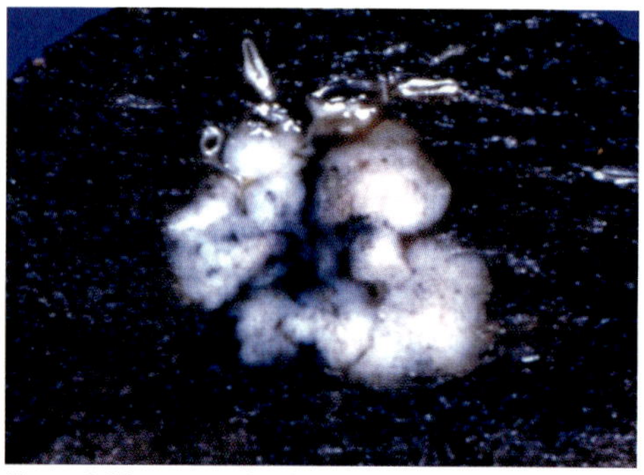

Figure 3. **Macroscopic picture**

the border between S^3c and S^{1+2}a bifurcate from V^1 (*l*). Compared to V^1a, which is pulled into the shadow from the anterior border, V^1b ascends between B^3c and B^{1+2}a (*n*).

In this case, chest CT and thin slice CT indicate the solid-type shadow characteristics of distinct border with accompanying notches, and involvement of B^{1+2}b and part of B^{1+2}a surrounding structures, and V^1a and V^2a. Consequently, it was suspected that solid-type adenocarcinoma had progressed from S^{1+2}b to beyond the S^{1+2}a segment (*s*). These are typical CT findings of peripheral lung adenocarcinoma.

Diagnosis

On interpretation of the CT, solid-type lung adenocarcinoma was strongly suspected, and after bronchial brushing cytology was performed from left B^{1+2}b during a bronchoscopy, lung adenocarcinoma was diagnosed. As a result, with the clinical classification being cT1N0M0 Stage IA cancer, a resection of the upper lobe of the left lung was conducted. Postoperative stage was pT2N0M0, with a 35 x 28 x 26 mm moderately differentiated papillary adenocarcinoma.

Macroscopic findings of a resection sample (*Fig. 3*) show not only notching due to blood vessels but also a tumor with distinct borders showing lobulation, which was not revealed by thin slice CT. The involvement of bronchi and blood vessels inside and surrounding the tumor can also be clearly seen.

What is a solid-type solitary nodular shadow?

According to the definition of Fraser et al., a solitary nodular shadow is a shadow with a maximum diameter of 3 cm completely surrounded by normal lung, regardless of whether borders are distinct or not.[2] We perform imaging diagnosis in line with this definition.

Radiographs of solitary nodular shadows are broadly classified depending on differences in peripheral lung lesion density and the volume of air in a lung as indicated by differences in density of the radiograph. It is easier to understand if solitary nodular shadows are classified as solid-type, part-solid-type or nonsolid-type. It was reported by Tanaka et al. that using HRCT, it is useful for classification to compare the shadow area in the lung window setting and mediastinal window setting, with a reduction in shadow size of less than 50% in the mediastinal window setting indicating solid-type, and a reduction of more than 50% indicating part-/nonsolid-type.[1]

In lung adenocarcinoma showing as a solid-type solitary nodular shadow, air is eliminated by the advanced part of the tumor growing to fill bronchi and alveolar spaces, resulting in a shadow with uniform density and distinct borders that contrasts strongly with neighboring normal lung. In many cases notching is also seen (*Fig. 4*) due to lobulation or bronchial and vascular compression resulting from nonuniform growth rates at the periphery of the tumor.

Types of lung cancer that can be discerned with these kinds of radiographs include moderately and poorly differentiated adenocarcinoma, peripheral squamous cell carcinoma and small cell lung adenocarcinoma, large cell carcinoma and mucus producing differentiated adenocarcinoma.[3]

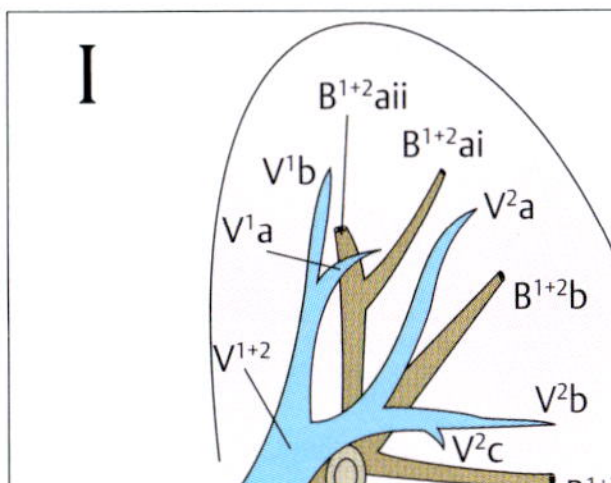

Figure 4.

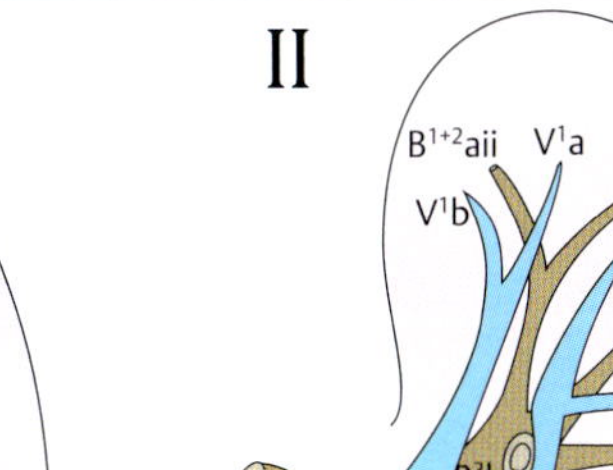

Figure 5.

Interpreting solid-type nodular shadows based on lung segmental anatomy[3-5]

In terms of the way in which it progresses, the biggest difference between lung adenocarcinoma and inflammatory lung diseases is that since it forms tumors regardless of the lung structural units of segments, subsegments and secondary pulmonary lobules, multiple bronchi and pulmonary arteries and veins in neighboring segments are also involved.

Located at the top of the area where segmental bronchi begin below the pulmonary pleura, lung segments are conical in shape. Compared to segmental bronchi and segmental arteries which almost always run together towards the periphery, segmental veins run along the borders of the two neighboring lung segments (*Fig. 5*). As a result, when interpreting a radiograph, looking at the involvement of segmental veins enables judgment of whether a tumor extends through two lung segments, providing a hint for discerning if it is benign or malignant.

Based on an understanding of lung segmental anatomy including veins, gaining a three-dimensional idea of involvement in surrounding structures requires effort but it is an effort that should be made.

An attempt to interpret shadows based on segmental analysis is made for just two cases of small lung adenocarcinoma in the left upper lobe.

The left upper lobe segmental vein paths (*Fig. 6*) and simplified representations of variations (*Fig. 7*) are for reference when interpreting the two cases.

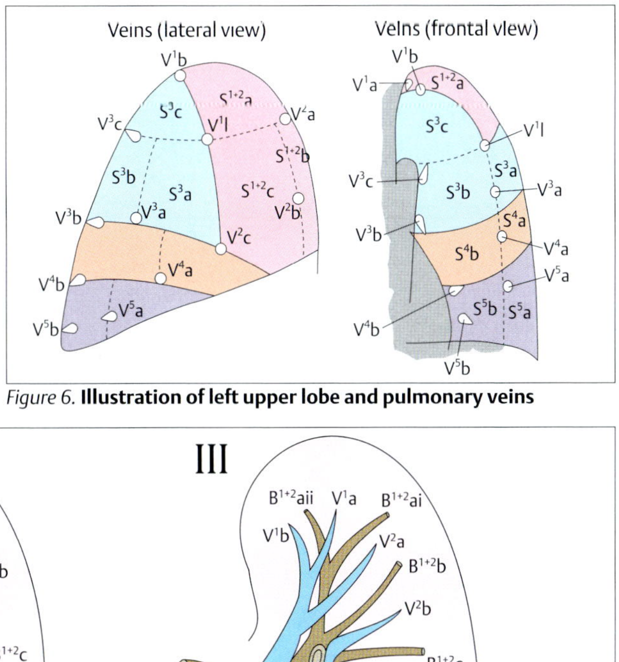

Figure 6. **Illustration of left upper lobe and pulmonary veins**

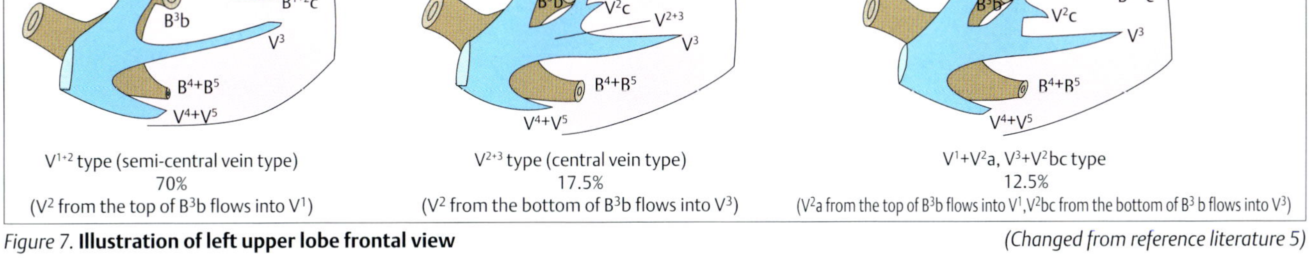

Figure 7. **Illustration of left upper lobe frontal view**

(Changed from reference literature 5)

Case 2 60-year-old male

Chief complaint: Nothing in particular
Medical history: Ureter stone at age 53
Family history: Nothing of note
Smoking history: 10/day for 20 years (up to age 40)
Present illness:
Patient was referred to this hospital for examination after chest radiographs taken at an annual health examination revealed an abnormal shadow.
Physical findings on admission:
No weight loss, nothing else of note
Laboratory data on admission:
No particular abnormalities
Imaging findings:
Chest radiographs show a faint nodular shadow with indistinct border coinciding with the lower pulmonary arteries in the left hilar area. A lateral chest radiograph shows a 25 mm diameter, nodular shadow with uniform internal density and distinct border directly under the chest wall at the same height as the orifice to the left upper lobe bronchus.

Chest CT shows the periphery of the shadow to be almost regular with a distinct border and uniform internal density, together with pleural retraction and lobulation. The pleural surface on the visceral side is also separated from the pleural surface on the wall side and lung has entered the space from above and below (➤) (*c*). Another finding revealed by thin slice CT is air bronchogram. In the thin slice CT, the shadows in the lung window setting and mediastinal window setting were almost the same as those in Case 1, pointing to probable solid-type.

Looking at the relationship with surrounding structures, a shadow can be seen in a chest CT of the B^3b peripheral area (*b, c*) indicating bronchial involvement. Looking at the path of B^3b in thin slice CT, it has bifurcated up and down at the periphery, and it can be understood from the lower border (*g, h, i*) and upper border (*i, j, k, l*) of the shadow that there is involvement.

Venous involvement can be understood by following

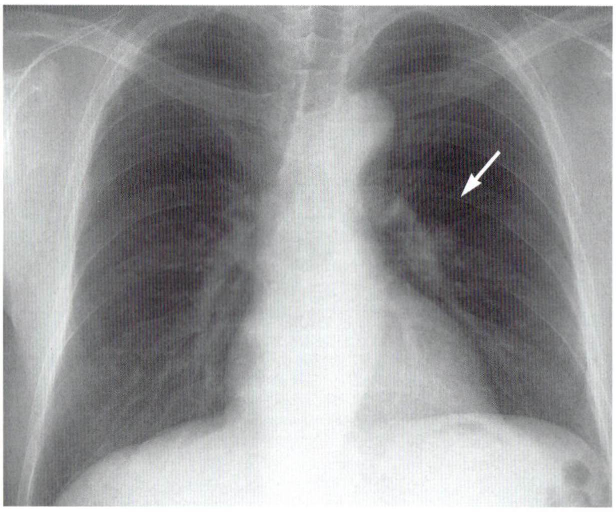

Figure 8. **Chest radiograph**

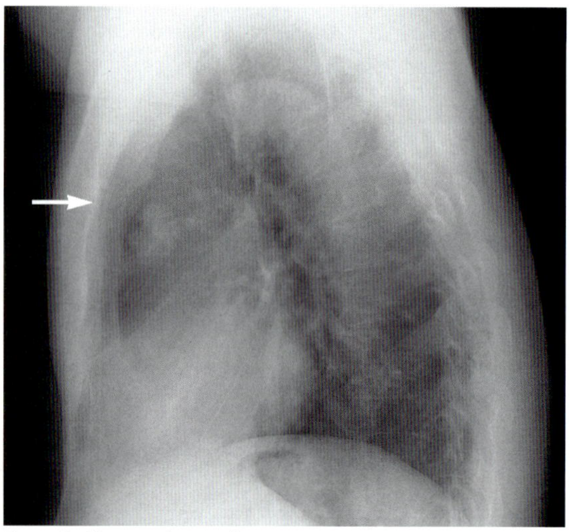

Figure 9. **Chest radiograph**

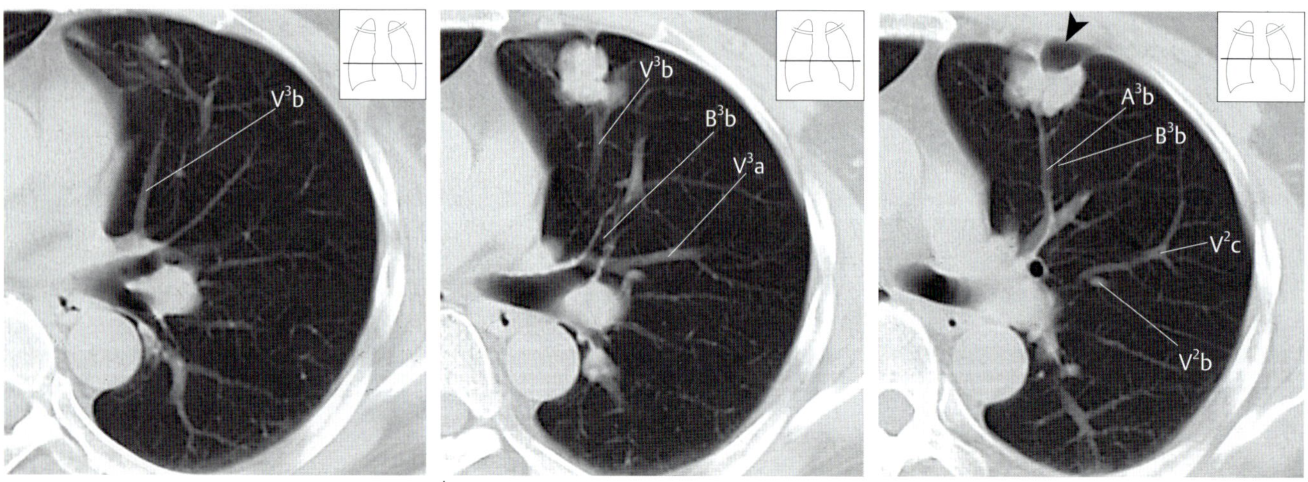

a *b* *c*

Figure 10 a–m. **Chest CT:** (g–m) Thin slice CT

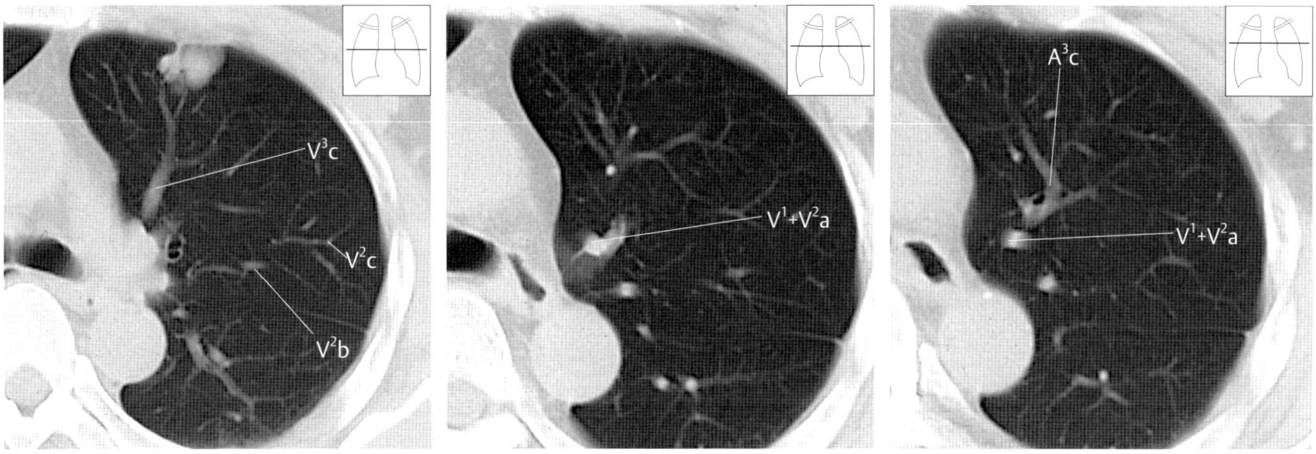

d *e* *f*

<g-m: Thin slice CT>

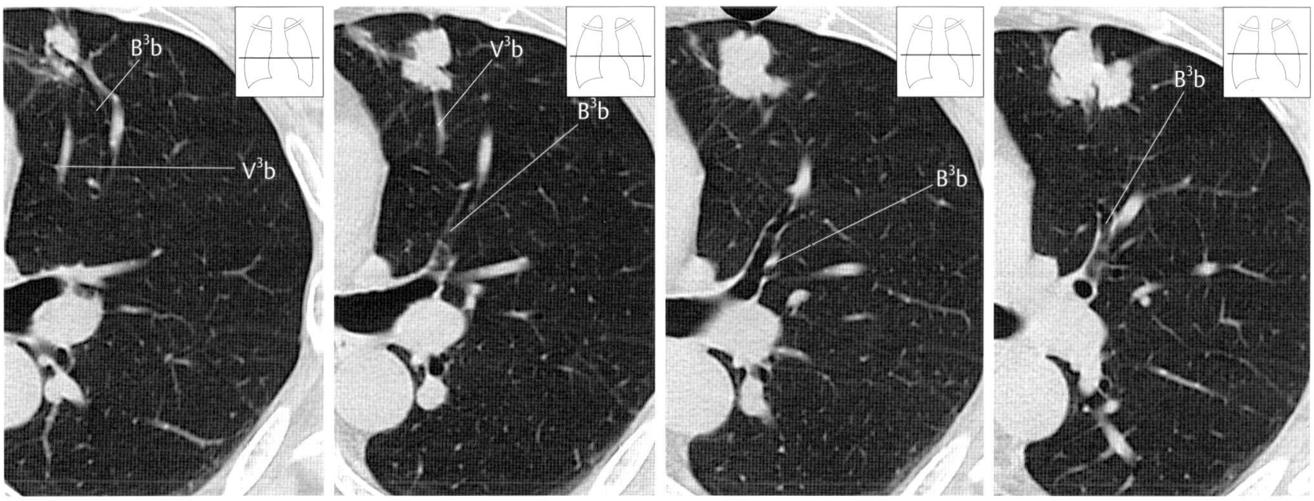

g *h* *i* *j*

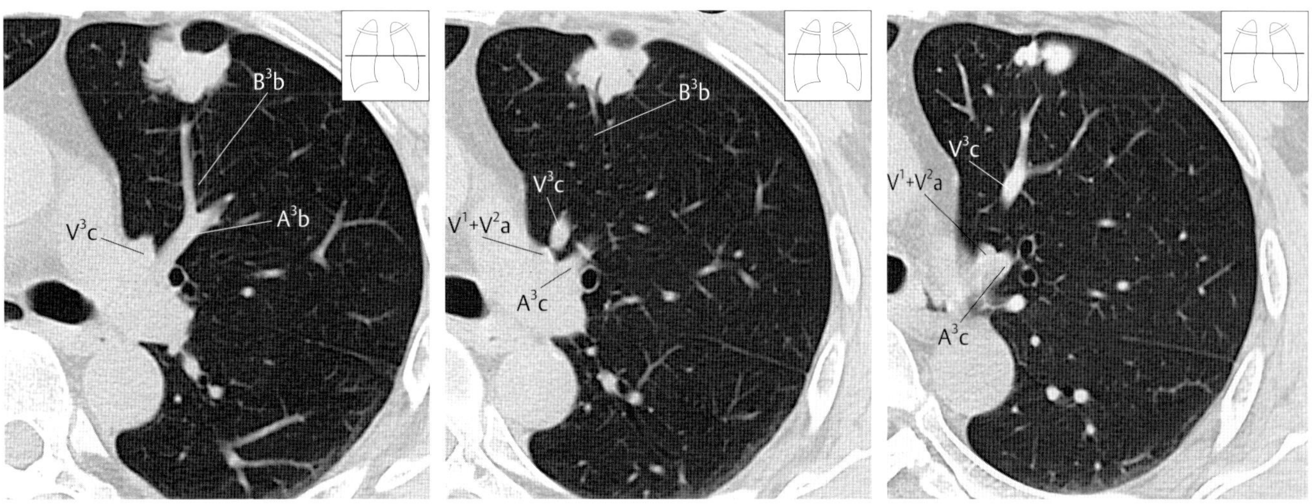

k *l* *m*

the path of left upper pulmonary veins from the center to the periphery in chest CT. After bifurcation of V^3c (*d*) at the border between S^3b and S^3c, one vein on the inner side ascends higher than B^3b (*e, f*), and on the outer side of B^3b at the border between $S^{1+2}c$, S^3a and S^4a there is bifurcation from V^3a (*b*) into two ascending veins (*c, d*). Having understood these variations, taking into consideration bifurcation of ascending veins inside and outside B^3b, $V^1 + V^2a$ and $V^3 + V^2bc$ types could be possible as patterns of venous distribution.

Looking at segmental venous involvement with thin slice CT, after bifurcation of V^3c at the inner side of A^3b (*k*), $V^1 + V^2a$ ascends on the inside of A^3c (*l, m*). V^3c is partially involved at the very top border of the shadow (*m*).

With regard to involvement from the lower border of the shadow, V^3b at the border of S^3b and S^4b runs through the inner part of B^3b, and is converging in from the bottom of the shadow with B^3b (*g, h*).

In this case, chest CT and thin slice CT indicate a solid-type shadow with a distinct border, pleural retraction and lobulation, and with the pleural surface separated from the chest wall. Surrounding structures involved in the shadow were thought to have been two B^3b peripheral branches, V^3b and part of V^3c. Consequently, progressive solid-type lung adenocarcinoma centered in S^3b extending to S^4b and part of S^3c and traversing segments was suspected (*Fig. 11*).

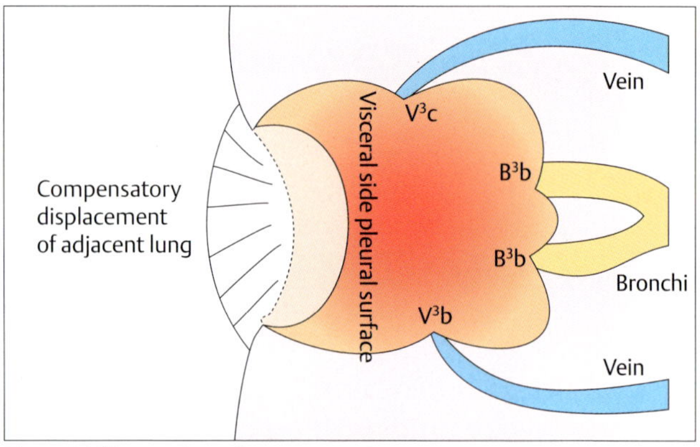

Figure 11. **Illustration of reconstruction**

Diagnosis

In the light of radiographic findings, solid-type lung adenocarcinoma was strongly suspected. A sample from left B^3b and a bronchoscopy revealed it was adenocarcinoma. With the clinical classification being cT1N0M0 Stage IA cancer, a resection of the upper lobe of the left lung was conducted. Postoperative stage was pT2N0M0, with a 35 x 28 x 15 mm poorly differentiated papillary adenocarcinoma.

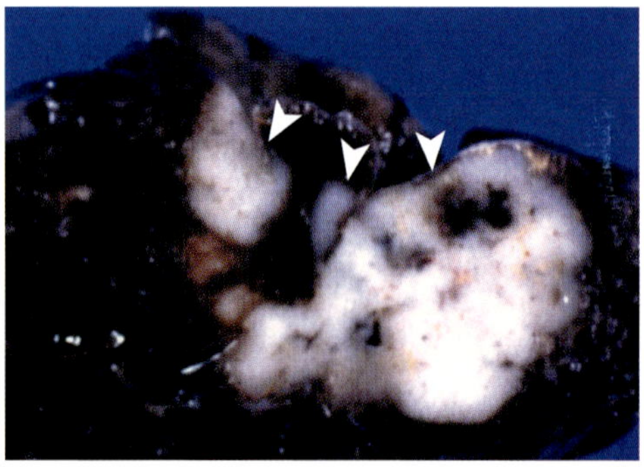

Figure 12. **Macroscopic picture**

Macroscopic findings of a resection sample (*Fig. 12*) show a tumor with a distinct border and lobulation. Furthermore, the characteristic of the entire pleural surface on the visceral side being retracted by the tumor (➤) is easily understood. The involvement of bronchi and blood vessels inside and surrounding the tumor can also be clearly seen.

Conclusion

When conducting qualitative imaging diagnosis of solitary nodular shadows, attention should be paid to shadow characteristics, but it has also been outlined that clarification of the involvement of surrounding structures and discerning whether progression traverses segments are also important considerations. From the two cases here, it is probably clear that it is important to interpret segmental veins.

However, it has also been pointed out that to interpret segmental veins, after having grasped the fundamental pathways of veins from chest CT to gain a basic understanding of existing vein pathway patterns, it is also important to identify the same veins in thin slice CT and then apply painstaking effort to trace veins that bifurcate from them. Another major point to remember when identifying veins is that arteries and bronchi run together whereas veins run between bronchi.

Although there is a tendency for the interpretation of shadow characteristics to be conducted using only planar images, taking full advantage of segmental analysis to gain a three-dimensional idea of the involvement of surrounding structures offers useful hints for diagnosis.

This section focused on the characteristics of shadows associated with solid-type lung adenocarcinoma, but the next section explains how to interpret shadows associated with part-solid and nonsolid-type lung adenocarcinoma.

Acknowledgment: With regard to the cases presented in this section, we would like to express our deep appreciation for the cooperation provided by the doctors in the Respiratory Organ Group at the Cancer Center, Shikoku National Hospital.

References

1) Manabu Tanaka, et al.: Study of CT and Pathologic Correlation of Small Peripheral Lung Carcinomas of 15 mm Diameter or Less. Clinical radiology. 44: 1–10, 1999
2) Fraser, R. S., et al.: Synopsis of Diseases of the Chest. Saunders, Philadelphia, 1994
3) Kenji Eguchi, et al.: Diagnostic radiography for Early Stage Discovery of Lung Cancer. Kyowa Kigaku Tsushin, Tokyo, 1995
4) Kenji Eguchi, at al.: Cancer Imaging Diagnosis 2. Lung Cancer and Mediastinal Tumor. Medical View, Tokyo, 1997
5) Yamashita, H.: Roentgenologic Anatomy of the Lung. Igaku-Shoin, Tokyo, 1978

Chapter 4

Radiographs of intrapulmonary lesions with decreased radiolucency

7. Nodular shadow:

Solitary nodular shadow 2

[Pattern classification IV-D-2]

●Authors — Kenji Eguchi, Nobuhiko Seki

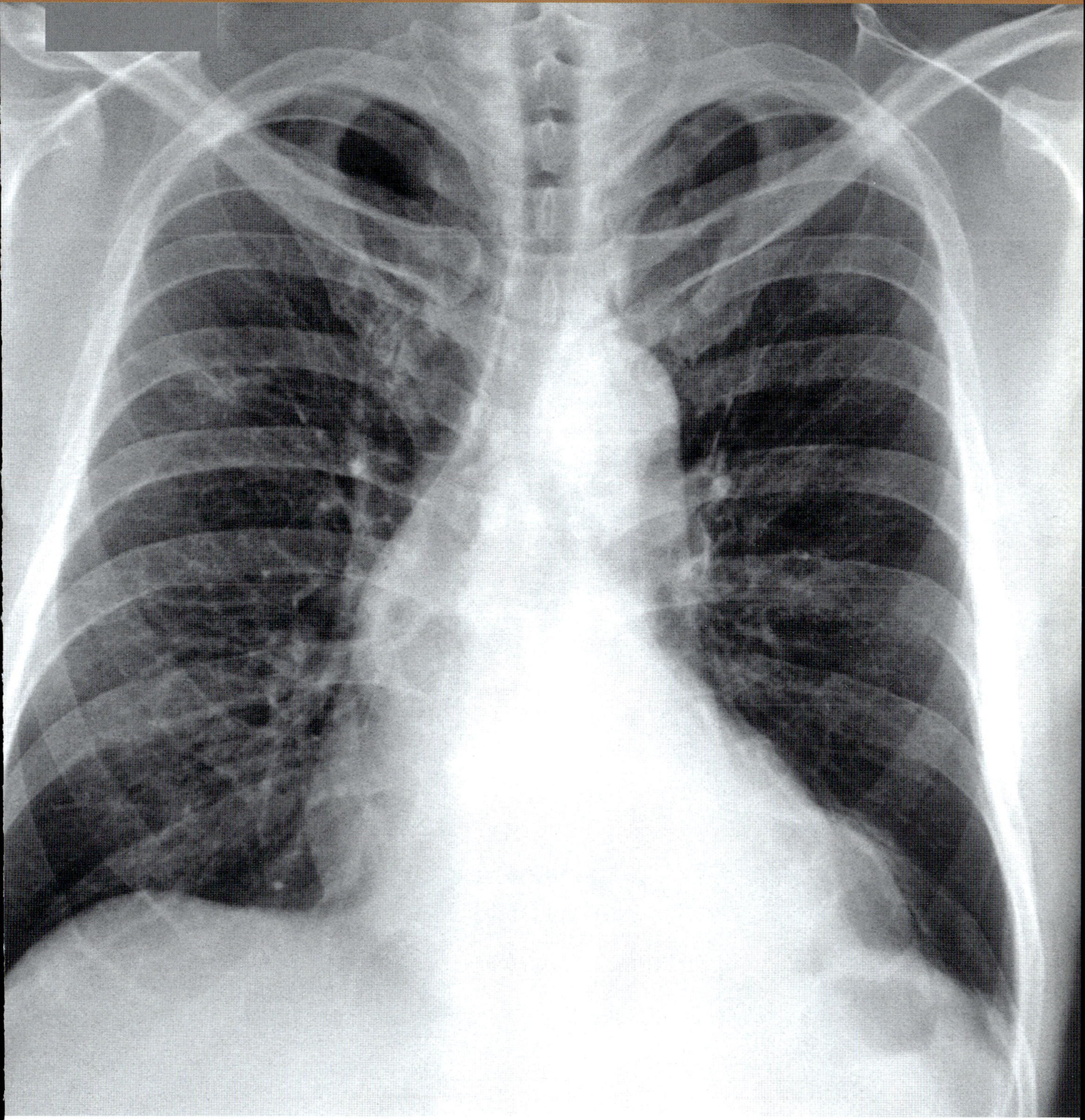

eywords of
is section

Solitary nodular shadow
Small air spaces
Ground glass opacity (attenuation)
Spicula
Part-solid or nonsolid nodular shadow
WHO classification of tumors (2003 update)
BAC *in situ*
BAC with microinvasion
Lepidic growth of cancer cells
Circumvascular connective tissue
Interlobular septa
Fibrotic scarring
Atypical adenomatous hyperplasia
Localized organizing pneumonia
Alveolar collapse
High attenuation area
Low attenuation area

Solitary nodular shadow 2

Kenji Eguchi, Nobuhiko Seki
Division of Medical Oncology, Tokai Oncology Center, Tokai University School of Medicine, Kanagawa, Japan

Having a three-dimensional understanding of shadows based on lung segmental anatomy also provides hints for differential diagnosis and pathological analysis when interpreting part-solid and nonsolid solitary nodular shadow. This section covers imaging diagnosis of typical part-/nonsolid lung adenocarcinoma, focusing on lung differentiation as in the previous section. At the same time, this section aims to deepen understanding of the significance of the pathological morphology that results in these images, and diagnoses over time.

Case 1 64-year-old male

Chief complaint: Nothing in particular
Medical history: Facial paralysis at the age of 51
Family history: Father had colon cancer
Smoking history: None
Present illness:
The patient had received annual medical examinations but this year there was an abnormal shadow in a chest radiograph, and he was referred to this hospital for a detailed examination.
Physical findings on admission:
Including neurological findings, nothing of note
Laboratory data on admission:
No particular abnormalities
Imaging findings:
In a chest radiograph (P. 89), a faint nodular shadow of about 15 mm diameter, with indistinct and irregular border can be observed in the area of the right upper lung where the upper border of the third anterior rib and the lower border of the sixth posterior rib intersect. From the orifice to the right upper lobe bronchus there are three reticular shadows heading towards the lesion but no reduction in volume is observed in the upper lobe.

To investigate the shadow characteristics and the involvement of surrounding structures, here is a look at interpretation using both chest CT and thin slice CT (*Figs. 1 a–q*).

The shadow characteristics indicated by a chest CT (*b*) are a high attenuation area above a concentric circle composed mainly of small air spaces, and an 18 x 15 mm diameter nodular shadow with extensive ground glass attenuation (GGA). However, looking at a thin slice CT (*i*) that reflects actual pathological macroscopic findings, at the tip of blood vessels in the central part there are air spaces of 4 mm in diameter surrounded by extensive diffuse GGA including punctate and linear structures. The slice under this (*j*) shows a comparatively high attenuation area and numerous small air spaces. Spicula and pleural retraction are also seen at the periphery of irregular, extensive shadows.

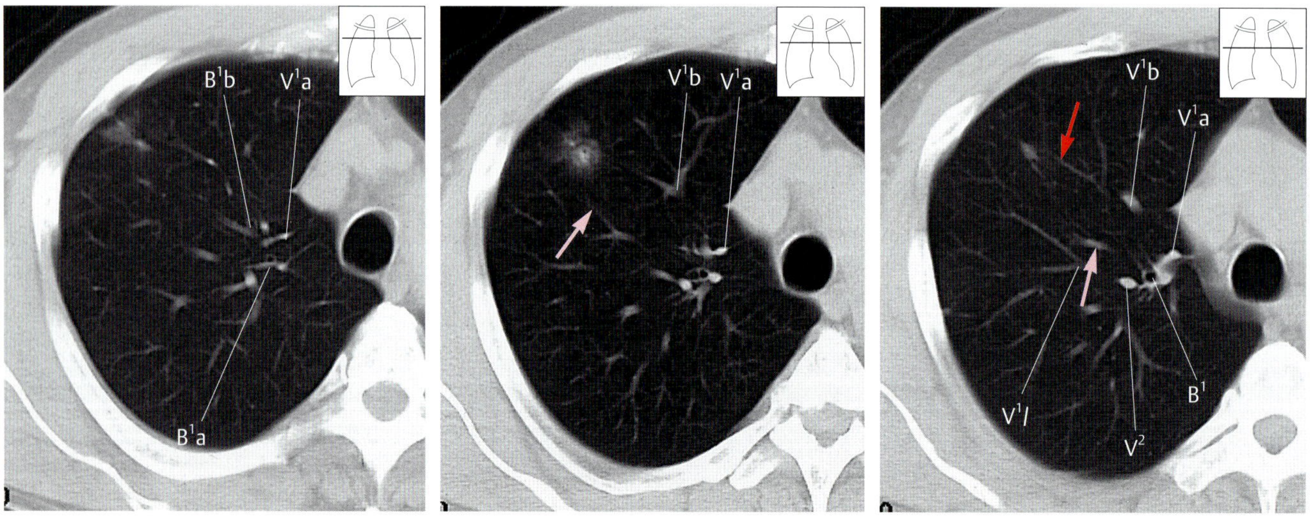

a *b* *c*

Figure 1 a–q. **Chest CT**: (g–q) Thin slice CT

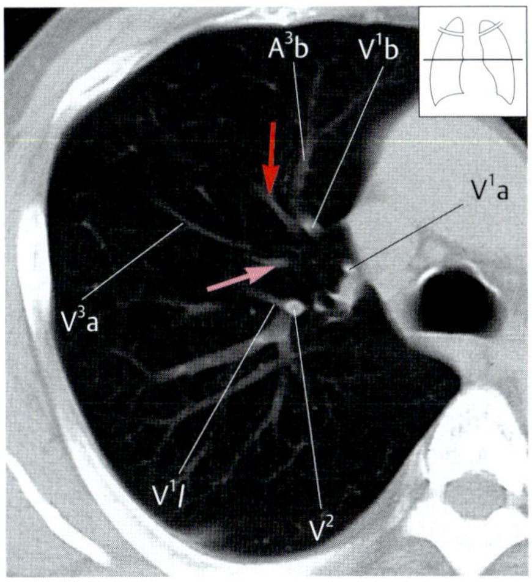

d

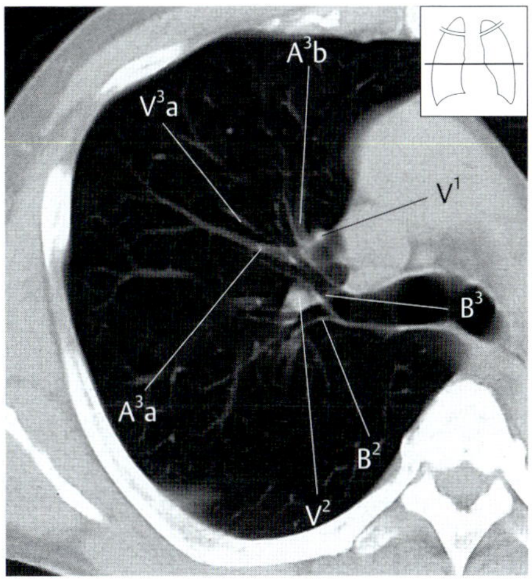

e

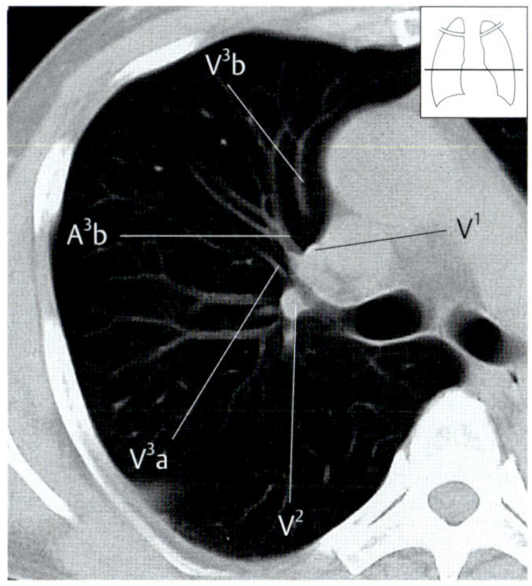

f

<g-q. Thin slice CT>

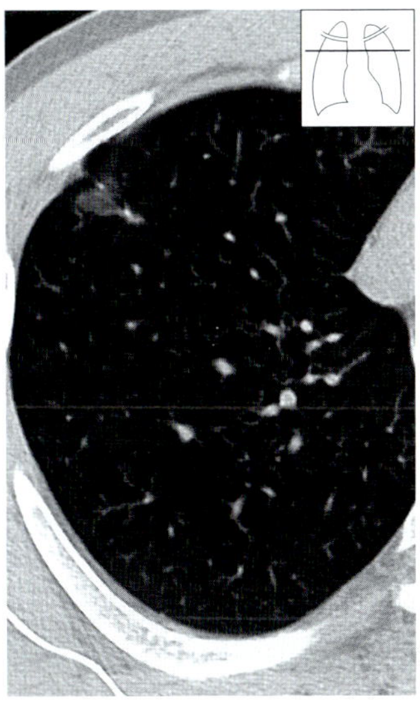

g

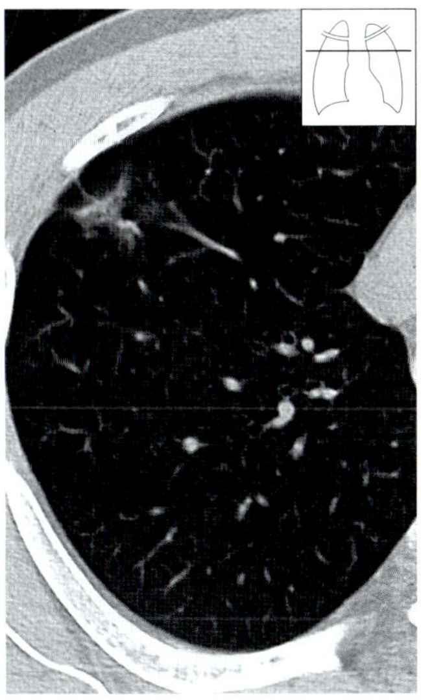

h

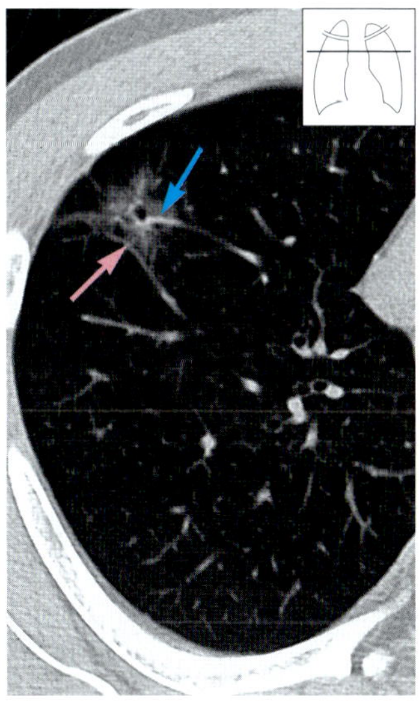

i

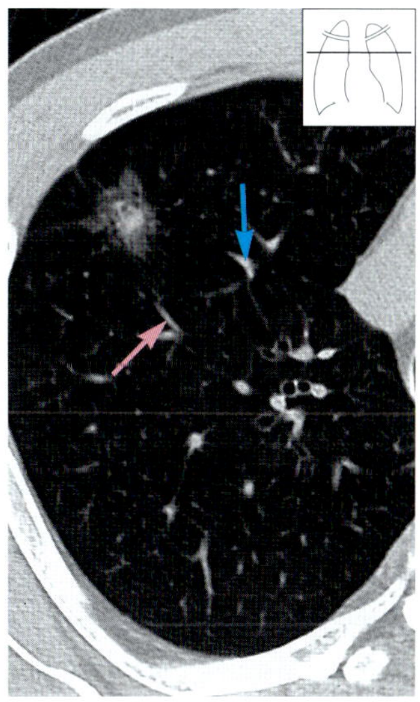

j

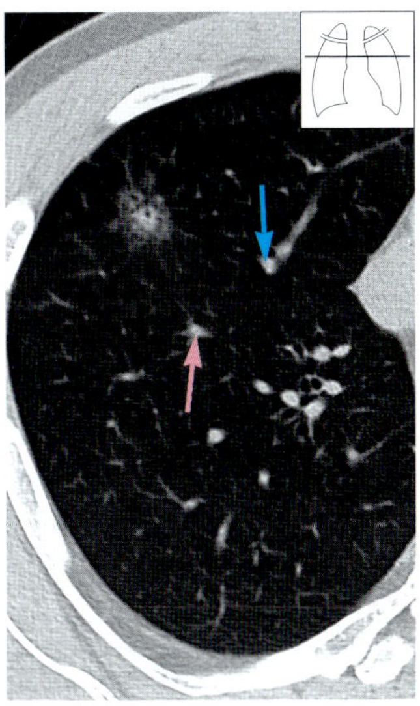

k

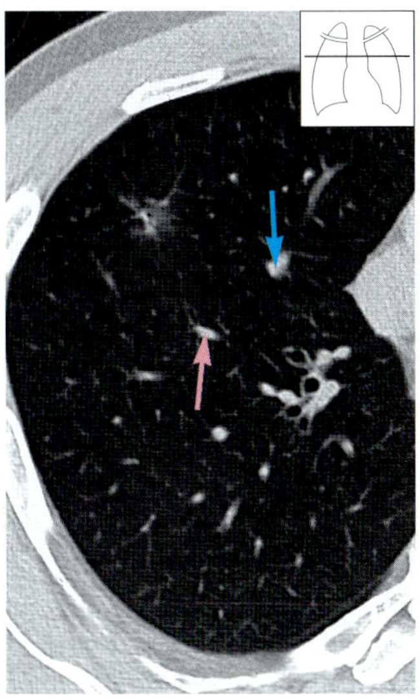

l

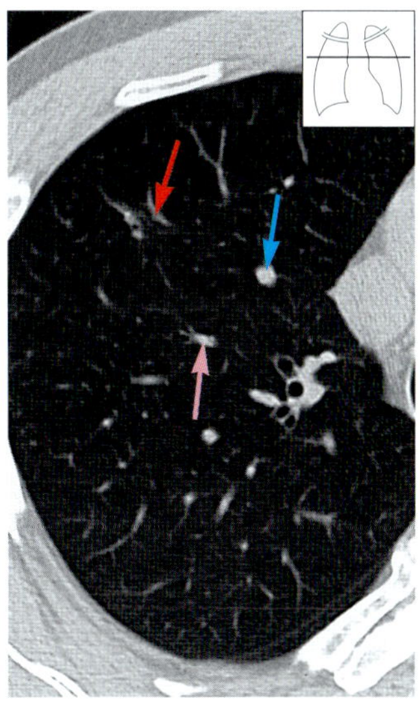

m

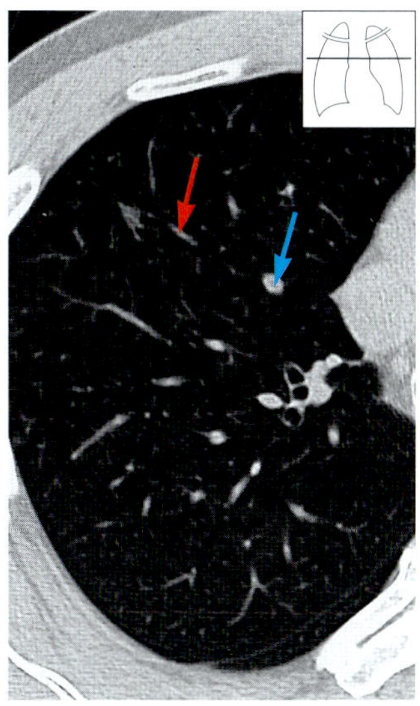

n

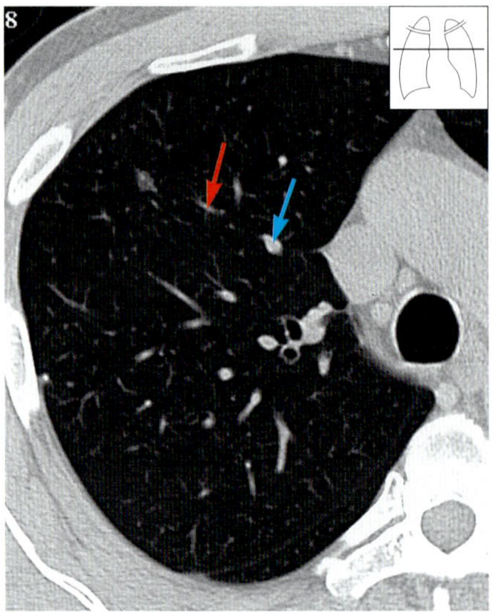

o

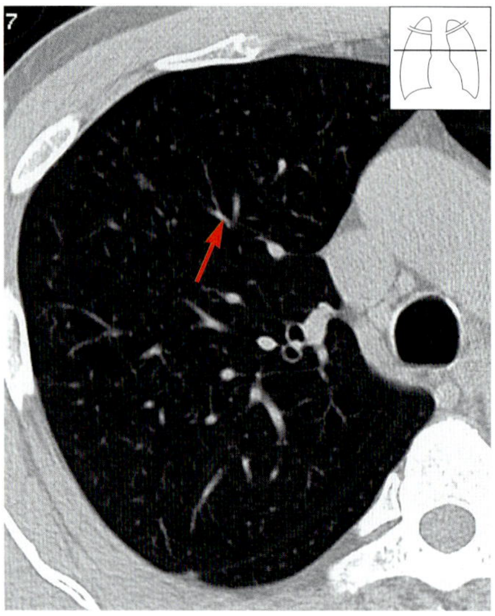

p

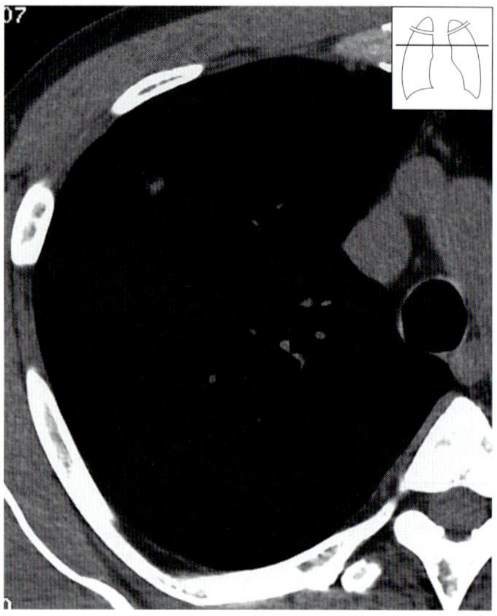

q

Furthermore, thin slice CT at the mediastinal window setting (WL 40HU, WW 400HU) (*q*), shows that the shadow area is less than 50% that of the shadow area at the lung window setting (WL -500, WW 1500) (*j*), indicating probable part-solid or nonsolid shadow type.

Regarding the relationship with surrounding structures, there is involvement of the bronchi, but this involvement is in the shadows in both chest CT and thin slice CT, and no clear images of bronchi are observed. However, a thin slice CT (*i*) shows vascular involvement in the shadow (→), and if this is traced through to the center (*j, k, l*) a blood vessel can be seen running along the bronchus (*m*), and it can be discerned to be an artery. In addition, if this blood vessel (→) is traced in CT with a blood vessel on the same level (→) (*b*) to the central part (*c, d*), it can be ascertained that they join at A^3a (*e*) as peripheral branches of A^3a.

In the same way, if the small blood vessel involved at the caudal border of the shadow in the thin slice CT (→) is traced towards the center (*n, o*), it can be seen that it runs along the bronchus (*p*). Furthermore, if this blood vessel (→) and another blood vessel on the same level (→) (*c*) are traced to the center on CT (*d*), it can be ascertained that they join at A^3b (*e*) as peripheral branches of A^3b.

On the other hand, if the blood vessel (→) involved in the central part of the shadow in thin slice CT (*i*) is traced (*j, k, l*), it does not run along the bronchus and is therefore a vein.

To identify this vein, in CT the right upper pulmonary vein is traced from the center to the periphery. As for variations, after bifurcation of the vein V^1 ascending from the inner side of B^3b (*f* through *b*) and V^3 (V^3b [*f*] running along the upper medial interlobular surface, and V^3a [*f, e, d*] running along the border of S^3a and S^3b) at the caudal side of B^3b, vein V^2 ascending along the outer side of B^1 from the bifurcated part of B^2B^3 can be seen, and it could be a V^1,V^{2+3} type (central vein type) (*Fig. 3 l*)

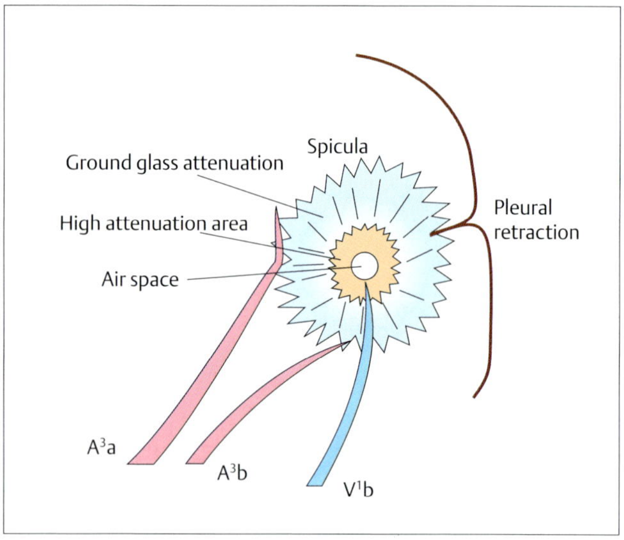

Figure 2. **Illustration of image reconstruction**

Bearing this in mind, if attention is paid to following the path of V^1 with CT, it can be understood that V^1 (*e*) bifurcates into V^1a (*d* through *a*) bordering S^1a and S^1b and ascending between B^1a and B^1b, and V^1b bordering on S^1b and S^3 and ascending on the ventral side. In addition, if V^1b in CT (*c*) is verified with a thin slice CT image of the same level (*o*), it can be discerned that the leading blood vessel is V^1b (→), pointing to direct involvement in the shadow of the peripheral branch of the V^1b vein.

Since V^1a (*b, a*) and V^1*l* (*c*) are not involved in the shadow, it can also be understood that there has been no progression into S^1a.

The chest CT and thin slice CT findings for this case were the shadow characteristics of GGA with a high attenuation area mainly in the center of the shadow, scattered small air spaces inside the shadow, spicula at

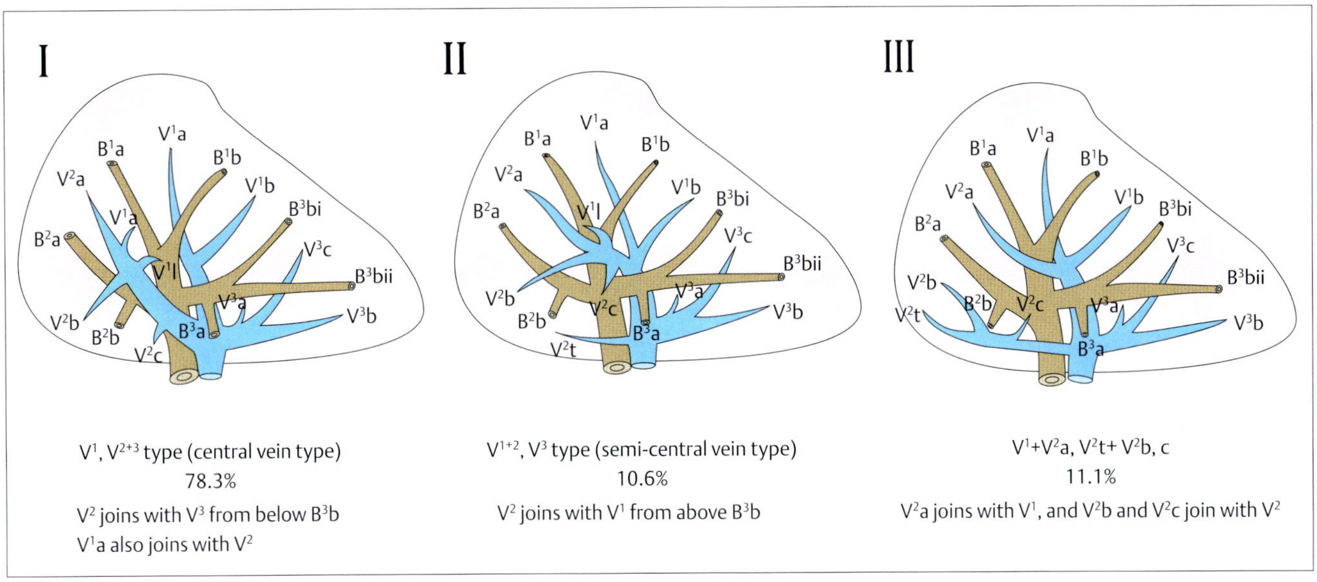

Figure 3. **Illustration of right upper lobe lateral view:** Changed from reference literature 6

the peripheral zone and part-solid or mixed GGA indicating pleural retraction. There was also involvement of the surrounding structures of B^3a, B^3b and V^1b. Consequently, also taking into consideration the relationship with V^1a and V^1l, part-solid lung adenocarcinoma extending into the S^1b, S^3a and S^3b subsegments was suspected (*Fig. 2*).

When these veins are involved in the focus, and there are indications that the lesion or lesions extend to two segments or subsegments, they become very important for the diagnosis of malignancy (*Fig. 4*).

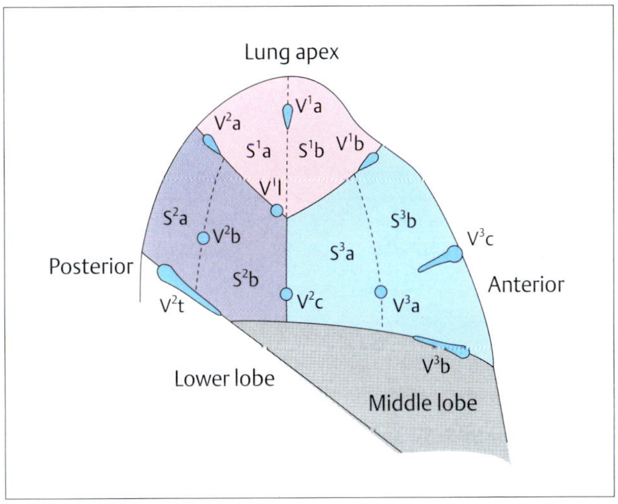

Figure 4. **Illustration of lateral view of right upper lobe and pulmonary veins**

Diagnosis

From imaging findings, cT1N0M0 stage IA part-solid lung adenocarcinoma was strongly suspected. Since a diagnosis of lung adenocarcinoma was reached after performing a rapid thoracoscopic biopsy diagnosis, the procedure continued with resection of the right upper lobe. Postoperative stage was pT1N0M0 with an 18 x 15 x 11 mm well-differentiated papillary adenocarcinoma.

Pathohistological findings of a resection sample (*Fig. 5*) show incomplete disappearance of air due to lepidic growth of cancer cells in the peripheral areas of the tumor. This area could correspond to the GGA in the thin slice CT.

Moving from the peripheral areas towards the center, cancer cell proliferation and interstitial thickening are seen, with gradual fibrotic scarring in the center. A large degree of lost volume is observed. This area could correspond to the comparatively high attenuation area in the thin slice CT (*Fig. 6 a*).

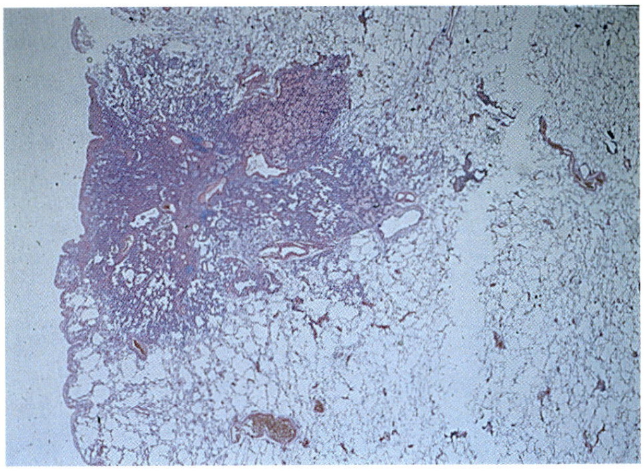

Figure 5. **Histopathological picture**

What is a part-solid solitary nodular shadow?

As indicated in solitary nodular shadow 1 (P. 81), a part-solid solitary nodular shadow is a shadow with distinct or indistinct borders 3 cm or less in diameter,[1] with high-resolution CT indicating that the shadow area at the mediastinal window setting is reduced by 50% or more compared to the shadow area at the lung window setting.[2]

The WHO classification of tumors (2003 update) broadly classifies lung cancer as papillary adenocarcinoma and nonmucus-producing bronchioloalveolar carcinoma (the so-called bronchioloalveolar cell carcinoma *in situ*: BAC *in situ*) and many kinds of mixed-type adenocarcinoma (BAC with microinvasion). In particular, with the recent rise in the opportunity to perform chest CT, there has been an increase in the discovery of BAC with microinvasion. It is hoped that the following explanation, which looks at the correlation between the radiological features and histopathologies of the two types will be well understood because having a clear idea of the pathological progression makes it easier to understand the imaging findings.[3,4]

As indicated in *Figure 3*, progression involves continued lepidic growth of cancer cells along alveolar walls in the peripheral areas of the tumor. As a result, air in the same area does not completely disappear and localized GGA is seen in CT, which causes shadows to disappear when using high-resolution CT at the mediastinal window setting. Whether GGA can be observed in a plain chest radiograph depends very much on the amount of air.

Furthermore, since progression appears to involve cancer cells moving from lobulus to lobulus, traversing structural units of the adjacent bronchoalveolar system, 70% of the adenocarcinomas are about 3 cm in diameter, and extend to two adjacent subsegments. This is why it is important to understand segmental anatomy.

The shadow of a linear structure radiating from the periphery of the tumor into the surrounding areas (spicula) is circumvascular connective tissue and/or interlobular septal thickening due to cancer cells or interstitial reaction.

In papillary adenocarcinoma, lepidic growth spreading at the peripheral areas to close to the center, and interstitial thickening are observed, gradually leading to fibrotic scarring in the central area. As a result, images of surrounding structures converging towards tumors are seen together with pleural retraction and converging bronchovascular involvement. These are the cause of the high attenuation areas seen at the lung window setting and shadows observed at the mediastinal window setting with thin slice CT.

On the other hand, with BAC *in situ* and BAC with microinvasion, cancer cell proliferation and mild interstitial thickening are observed but lepidic growth is basically preserved, and fibrotic scarring in the central area may or may not be observed (even if it is, it is comparatively mild). Consequently, convergence of surrounding structures towards tumors is comparatively weak, and even if high attenuation areas are seen at the lung window setting with thin slice CT, shadows are rarely observed at the mediastinal window setting.

In both types, irregular enlargement of bronchi and cavities inside tumors is sometimes seen, but this is due to destruction of alveolar structure by cancer cells in the same area or contraction of the tumor tissue itself.[5]

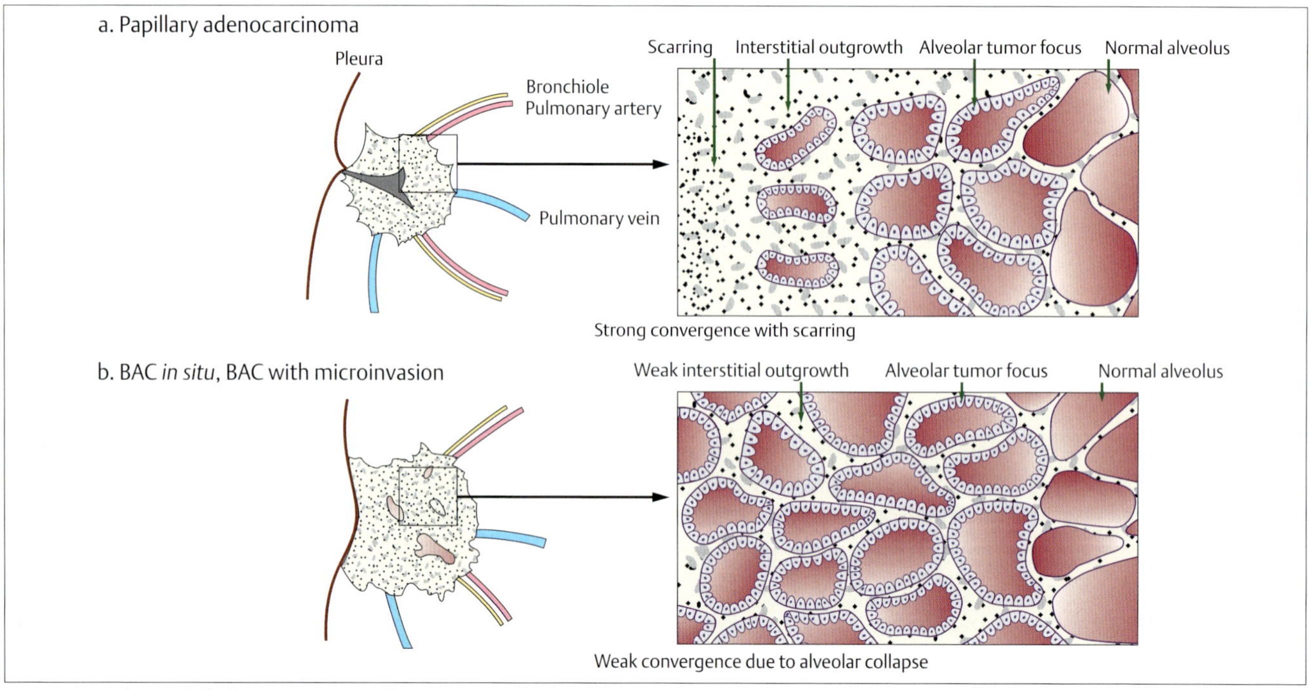

Figure 6. **Part-/nonsolid adenocarcinoma schematic**

Differential diagnosis of part-/nonsolid solitary nodular shadow

In addition to the tissue type mentioned earlier, there are two major differential diseases, namely atypical adenomatous hyperplasia and localized organizing pneumonia. There remains room for discussion concerning the difference between atypical adenomatous hyperplasia and nonmucus-producing bronchioloalveolar carcinoma (BAC *in situ*), but as a noninvasive lesion it is a neoplastic disease and consequently its differentiation between localized organizing pneumonia is a problem in everyday clinical situations.

Concerning this point, as well as investigating targeted thin slice CT characteristics and the involvement of surrounding structures, observation over a few months is another important procedure for differentiation. With localized organizing pneumonia, the shadow may be seen to shrink or disappear whereas with neoplastic diseases it remains unchanged or becomes enlarged.

However, with targeted thin slice CT, even if localized GGA is seen at the lung window setting, when high attenuation areas are observed inside it is often due to fibrotic scarring and/or alveolar collapse resulting from adenocarcinoma, indicating the invasive nature of the tumor. The current view is that only uniform internal GGA differentiates localized organizing pneumonia, and so observation over time is required.

The thin slice CT imagings (*Figs. 7, 8*) are of a case with uniform internal GGA diagnosed as localized organizing pneumonia after observation over time. Although it is difficult to assess subtle changes when simply comparing shadow size before and after observation over time, gaining an understanding of the locational relationship with surrounding structures is also useful here. Rather than comparing shadows themselves, comparing distances between the shadows and surrounding structures, that is vessels and bronchi, enables assessment of subtle changes.

In this section, interpretation of shadows based on segmental analysis is attempted for just one case of right upper lobe small lung denocarcinoma. The paths of right upper lobe segmental veins (*Fig. 4*) and variations[6] (*Fig. 3*), and solitary nodular shadow differential findings[7] (*Table 1*) are indicated for reference when interpreting the shadows of the case.

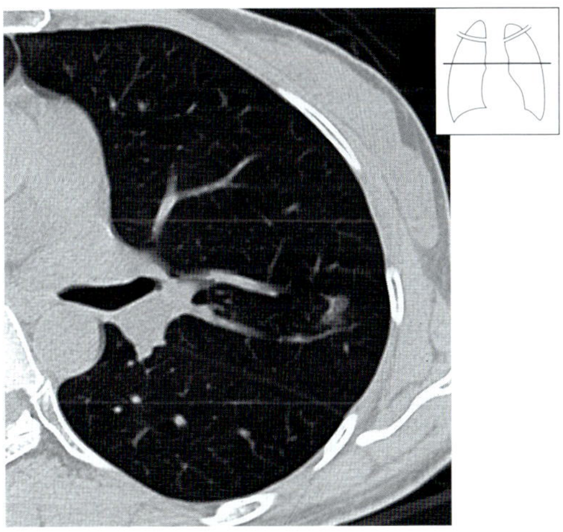

Figure 7. **Thin slice CT:** before observation over time

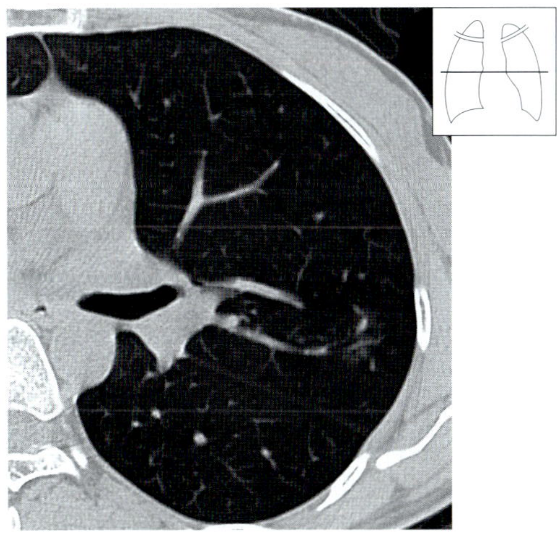

Figure 8. **Thin slice CT:** after 2 months of observation

			Lung adenocarcinoma		Old inflammation
			Part-/nonsolid type	Solid type	(Tuberculoma, granuloma, etc.)
Bronchi vessels and pleura	Involved bronchi		No central thickening/enlargement		Central thickening/enlargement
	Involved blood vessels	Pulmonary artery	Clear involvement in focus		Scarce
		Pulmonary vein	Clear involvement in focus		Rare
	Extent of vascular image		Normal, Increased		Shadow surroundings also become scarce
	Pleural retraction		Yes	A little	Yes (thickening broadly)
	Scattered foci		No		Yes
Shadow characteristics	Periphery		Indistinct	Distinct	Distinct or indistinct
	Spicula		Yes	A little	Rare
	Notch		A little	Yes	No
	Image of latent bronchiole inside focus		Yes	A little	Sometimes observed
	Calcification		Rare		Sometimes observed

Table 1. **Solitary nodular shadow differential findings**

Case 2 74-year-old female

Chief complaint: Nothing in particular
Medical history: Cholecystectomy due to gall stones at the age of 53
Family history: Nothing of particular note
Smoking history: None
Present illness:
During treatment for a gastric ulcer, a plain chest radiograph taken at an annual medical examination indicated an abnormal shadow and the patient was referred to this hospital for detailed examination.
Physical findings on admission:
No weight loss, nothing else of particular note
Laboratory data on admission:
No particular abnormalities
Imaging findings:
In a frontal chest radiograph, a faint nodular shadow of roughly 12 mm diameter, with slightly irregular periphery and indistinct border can be observed in the area where the upper border of the right second anterior rib and the upper border of the right fifth posterior rib intersect.

In a chest CT (*Fig. 10 c*), a circular shadow about 15 mm in diameter with slightly irregular periphery and comparatively distinct border can be seen, with comparatively faint density increase and a core with areas of mixed high and low attenuation. With thin slice CT (*Figs. 10 k–o*), GGA and a shadow with high attenuation are visible to the same degree, with small air spaces scattered throughout the shadow. A spicula can also be observed at the periphery together with retraction of surrounding small blood vessels. As with Case 1, with thin slice CT at the mediastinal window setting, almost no shadow is observed, pointing to possible part-/nonsolid solitary nodular shadow.

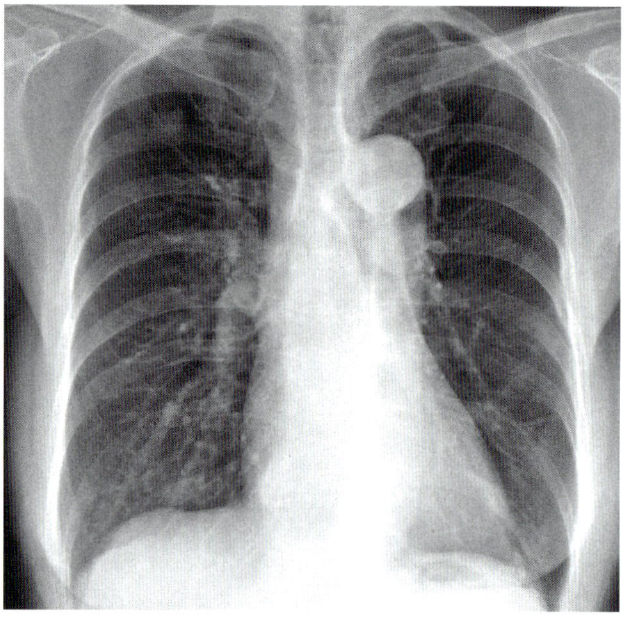

Figure 9. **Chest radiograph**

The relationship between the shadow and surrounding structures can be understand by looking at the involvement of the bronchi. With chest CT, the involvement of the bronchi can not be clearly identified. However, a thin slice CT (*m*) shows a bronchus at the side of the shadow (→) with an artery running along it (→), and from that artery a thin artery can be seen being retracted into the shadow (→), indicating that this bronchus is involved. If this bronchus is traced to the center (*n* through *q*), thin slice CT range ends at (*q*). If this bronchus (→) is then traced to the center (*e, f*) with CT on the same level (*d*), it can be seen to be B^2a (*g*).

Furthermore, if the blood vessel (→) traversing the shadow on the ventral side is traced with thin slice CT

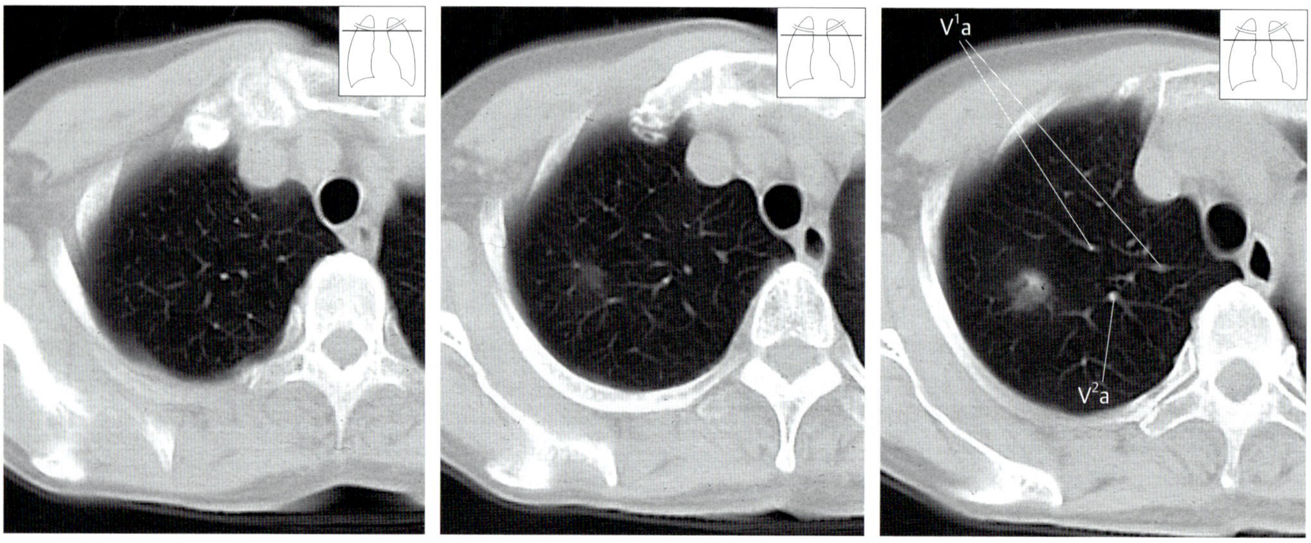

a *b* *c*

Figure 10 a–q. **Chest CT**: (k–q) Thin slice CT

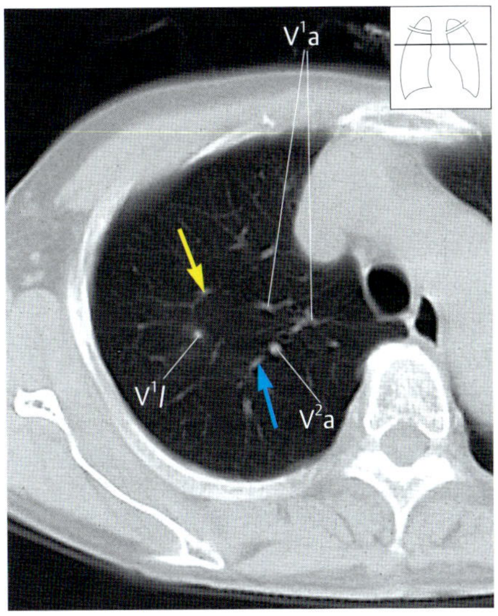

d

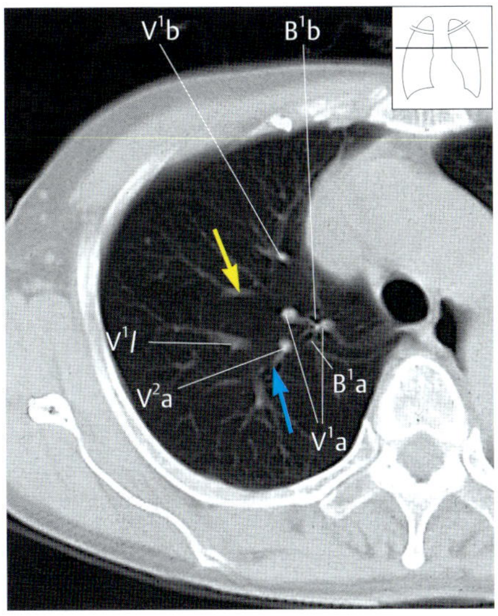

e

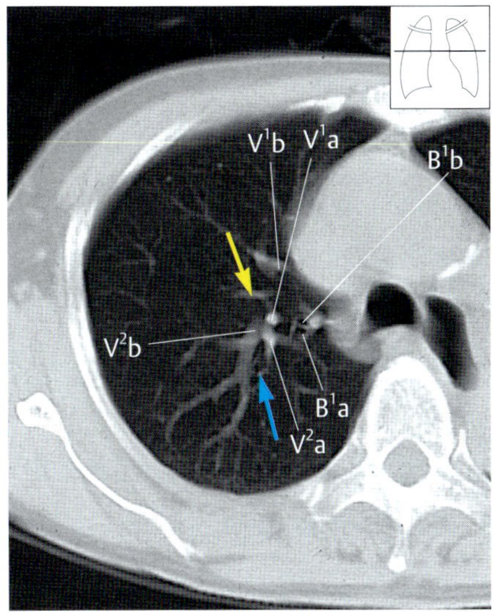

f

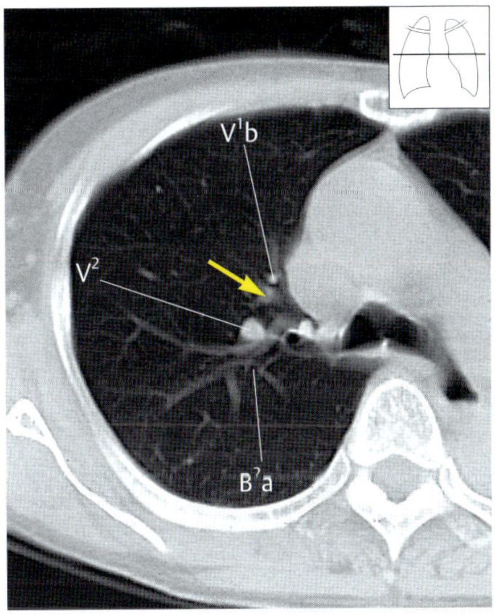

g

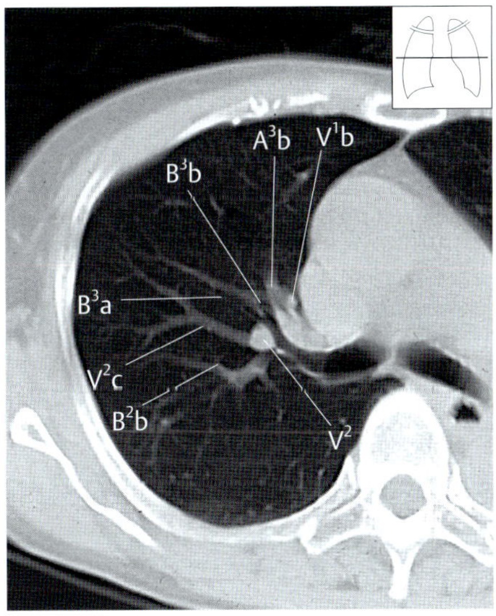

h

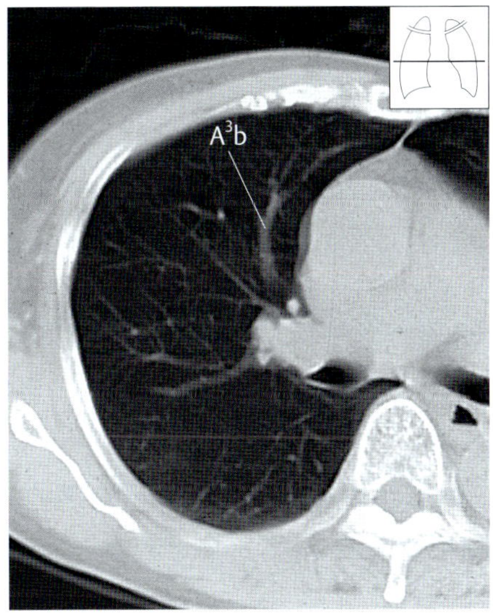

i

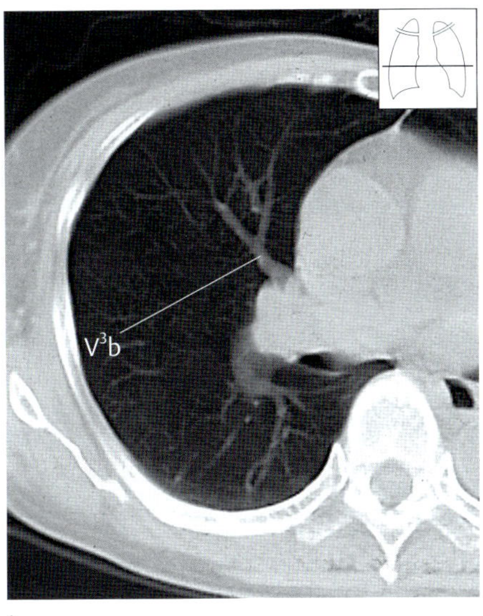

j

(*o*), it can be seen to join with the blood vessel running along with the bronchus (*q*), indicating that it is an artery. If this artery is traced to the center (*e, f*) with CT (*d*) on the same level, it can be seen to be A^3a (*g*). On the other hand, with thin slice CT (*q*), there is a comparatively thick blood vessel (→) in the shadow that does not run along with the bronchus, and this is interpreted as indicating that the shadow extends as far as the vein separating segments. Consequently, it is possible that at the very least, the shadow has also progressed to the area in which A^3a is involved.

To identify the veins directly involved with the shadow, in CT the right upper pulmonary vein is traced from the center to the periphery. The variations that can be seen are a single vein V^1b (*h* through *e*) ascending from the inner side of A^3b more towards the ventral side than B^1b, V^3b running along the upper middle interlobular surface more caudally than B^3b before bifurcating (*j*), and vein V^2

<k-q. Thin slice CT>

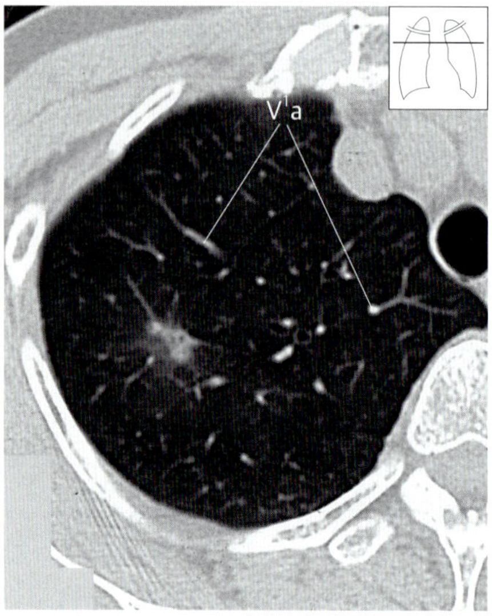

k

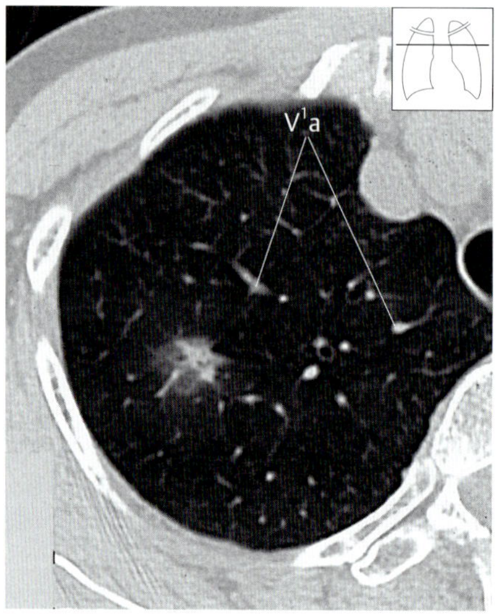

l

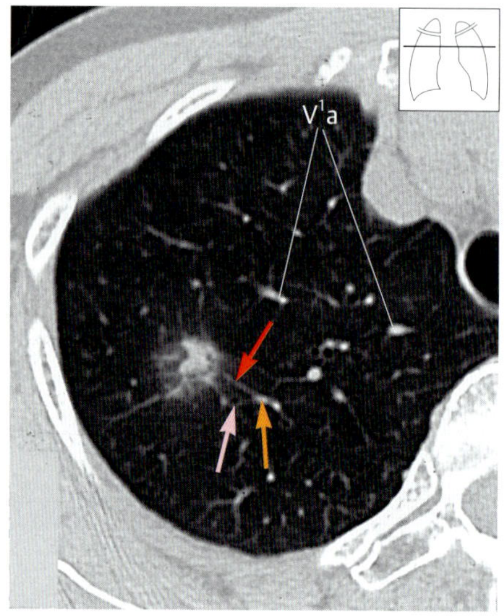

m

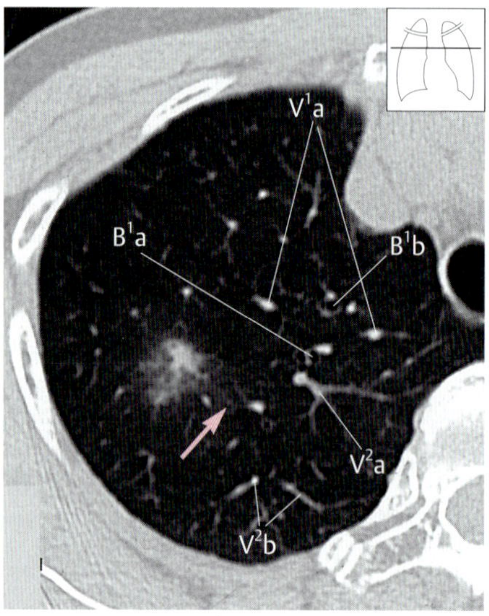

n

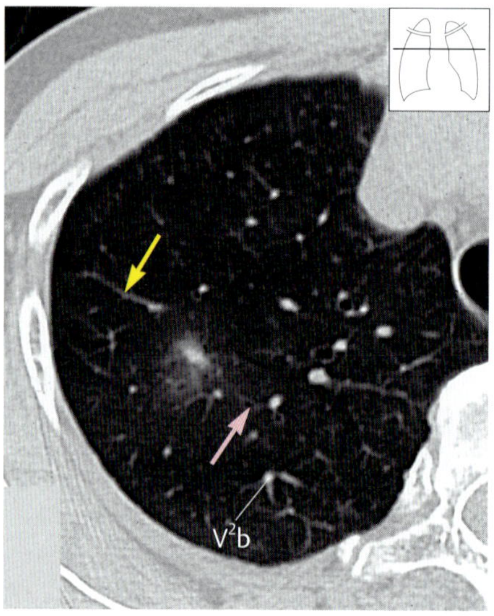

o

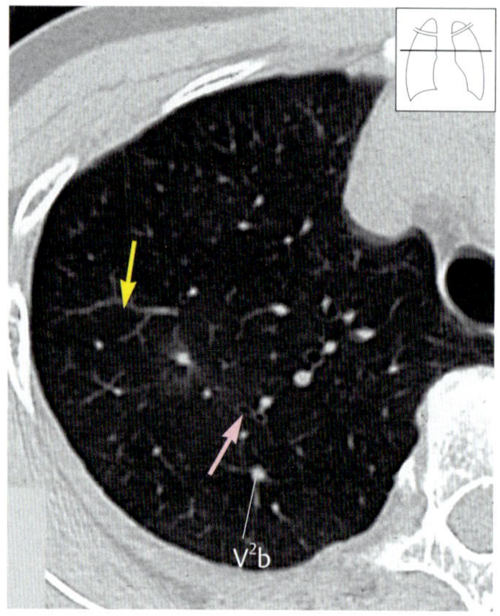

p

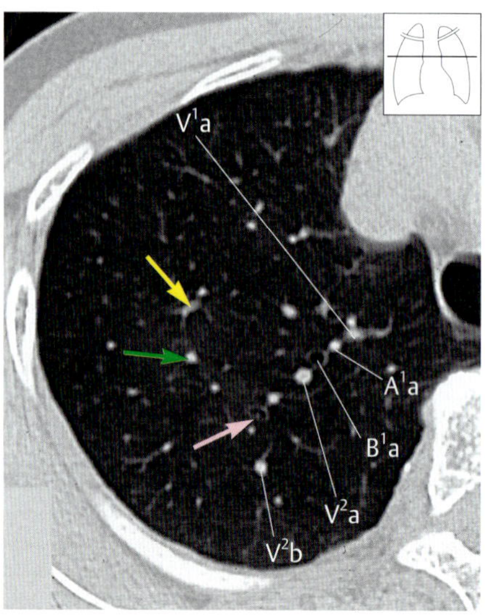

q

(*h*) ascending between B^3a and B^2b, indicating a possible V^1, V^{2+3} type (central vein type) (*Fig. 3 I*).

If V^2 is traced to the periphery in CT, first V^2c (*h*) bordering S^1a and S^1b bifurcates. After that it branches into three, with V^2b (*f*) bordering S^2a and S^2b, and two branches ascending on the inner and outer sides between B^1a and B^1b, V^1a (*f*) bordering S^1a and S^1b, and V^2a (*f*) bordering S^2 and S^1a, ascending dorsally from the outer side of B^1a (*e* through *c*).

From V^2b (*f*) a thick vein bifurcates towards the outer side again, and could be V^1l bordering S^1, S^2 and S^3 running along the outer side of the lower border of S^1. V^1l then once more bifurcates vertically upwards, and this invades the central part of the shadow (*d*).

If V^1a is once again traced to the periphery, the outer branch is located on the ventral side of the shadow (*c*), and it can be seen that inside S^1 the shadow exists only in S^1a. This can be clearly seen in thin slice CT (*n* through *k*).

If V^2a is once again traced to the periphery with thin slice CT, a branch bordering S^2 and S^1a is sent out (*n*). And since V^2b bordering B^2a (→) and S^2a and S^2b can also be seen in the same slice, it can be understood that from the inner side of the shadow caudal side border, the dorsal side part is S^2a, and from the dorsal side the outer side part is the S^2b area.

The chest CT and thin slice CT findings for this case were the shadow characteristics of GGA with a high attenuation area mainly in the center of the shadow, scattered small air spaces inside the shadow, spicula at the peripheral zone and retraction of small blood vessels indicating a part-solid shadow. Furthermore, involvement in the shadow of the surrounding structures of B^2a, A^3a and V^1*l* was indicated. As a result, taking into consideration the relationship of V^1a, V^2a and V^2b, part-solid lung adenocarcinoma with progression extending to the four subsegments of S^1a, S^2a, S^2b and S^3a was suspected (*Fig. 11*).

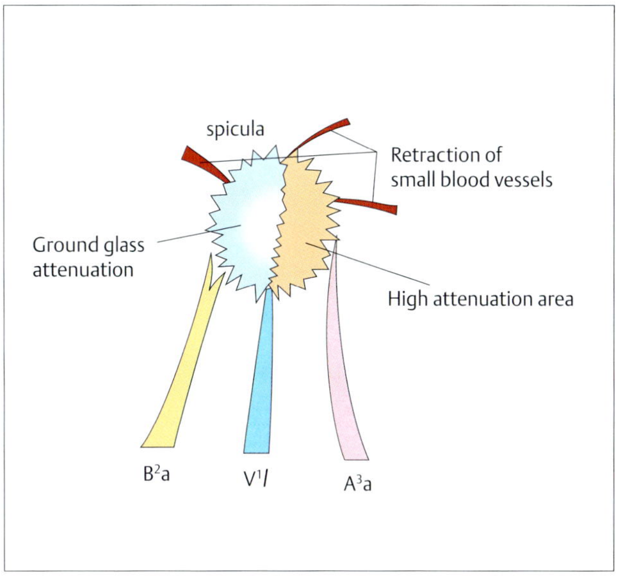

Figure 11. **Illustration of image reconstruction**

Diagnosis

From imaging findings, cT1N0M0 stage IA part-solid lung adenocarcinoma was strongly suspected. Since a diagnosis of lung adenocarcinoma was reached after performing a rapid thoracoscopic biopsy, the procedure continued with resection of the right upper lobe. Postoperative stage was pT1N0M0, with a 15 x 10 x 8 mm invasive-type bronchioloalveolar carcinoma (adenocarcinoma with BAC component).

Pathohistological findings of a resection sample (*Fig. 12*) show incomplete disappearance of air due to lepidic growth of cancer cells in the peripheral areas of the tumor. This area could correspond to the GGA in the thin slice CT.

In the central area, cancer cell proliferation and mild interstitial thickening are observed, but unlike Case 1, no strong interstitial proliferation or fibrosis are observed, lepidic growth is also preserved, and a comparatively large volume of air remains. This area could correspond to the comparatively high attenuation area in the thin slice CT (*Fig. 6 b*).

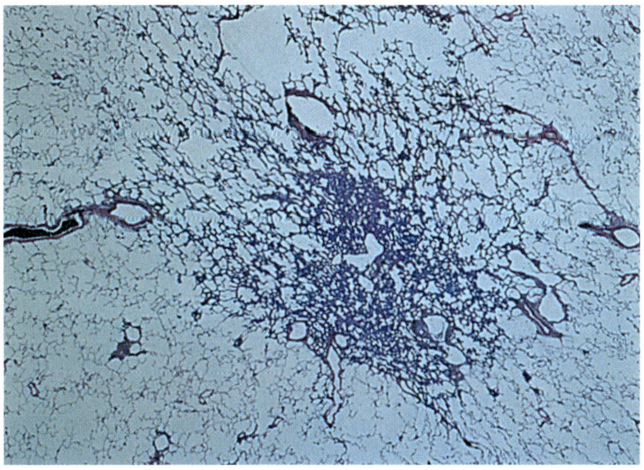

Figure 12. **Hisotopathological picture**

In addition, there is irregular enlargement of bronchioles and extensive small air cavities due to destruction of alveolar structure which could correspond to the small air spaces scattered throughout the shadow.

Conclusion

It has been reiterated that having a grasp of the three-dimensional involvement of surrounding structures based on lung segmental analysis is also important when conducting a qualitative diagnosis of part-/nonsolid solitary nodular shadows. Involvement of veins on HRCT indicates lesions that extend over more than two respiratory segments and tend to be malignant. Convergence of vessels, bronchi and pleural retraction toward the central part of a nodule on HRCT strongly indicates peripheral adenocarcinoma.

A clear understanding of the pathomorphological images that comprise part-/nonsolid lung adenocarcinoma images when analyzing shadow characteristics also makes interpretation easier.

It has also been noted that when conducting differential diagnosis of uniform internal GGA, observation over a set period enables differentiation of localized organizing pneumonia and neoplastic lesions.

This and the previous section covered interpretation of solitary nodular shadows focusing on segmental analysis.

Acknowledgement: We would like to express our deep appreciation for the cooperation with this section provided by the doctors in the Respiratory Organ Group at the Cancer Center, Shikoku National Hospital.

References

1) Fraser, R.S. et al.: Synopsis of Diseases of the Chest. Saunders, Philadelphia, 1994
2) Gaku Tanaka et al.: Study of CT Images and Pathologic Correlation of Small Peripheral Carcinomas of the Lung with a Diameter of 15 mm or Less. Clinical radiology. 44: 1–10, 1999
3) Harumi Ito et al.: Chest Image Diagnosis in Consideration of Peripheral Lung Structure. Kinpodo Inc., Kyoto, 1995
4) Kenji Eguchi et al.: Chest X-ray Diagnosis. Kyowa Kikaku Tsushin, Tokyo, 1985
5) Kuriyama, K. et al.: Prevalence of air bronchogram in small peripheral carcinomas of the lung on thin section CT: Comparison with benign tumors. A.J.R. 156: 921–24, 1991
6) Yamashita, H.: Roentgenologic Anatomy of the Lung. Igaku-Shoin, Tokyo, 1978
7) Masahiro Fukuoka et al.: Practical Internal Medicine Series 1 Lung Cancer, Nankodo, Tokyo, 1998

Chapter 4

Radiographs of intrapulmonary lesions with decreased radiolucency

8. Nodular shadow:

Solitary nodular shadow 3

[Pattern classification IV-D-1]

●Author — Hitoshi Tokuda

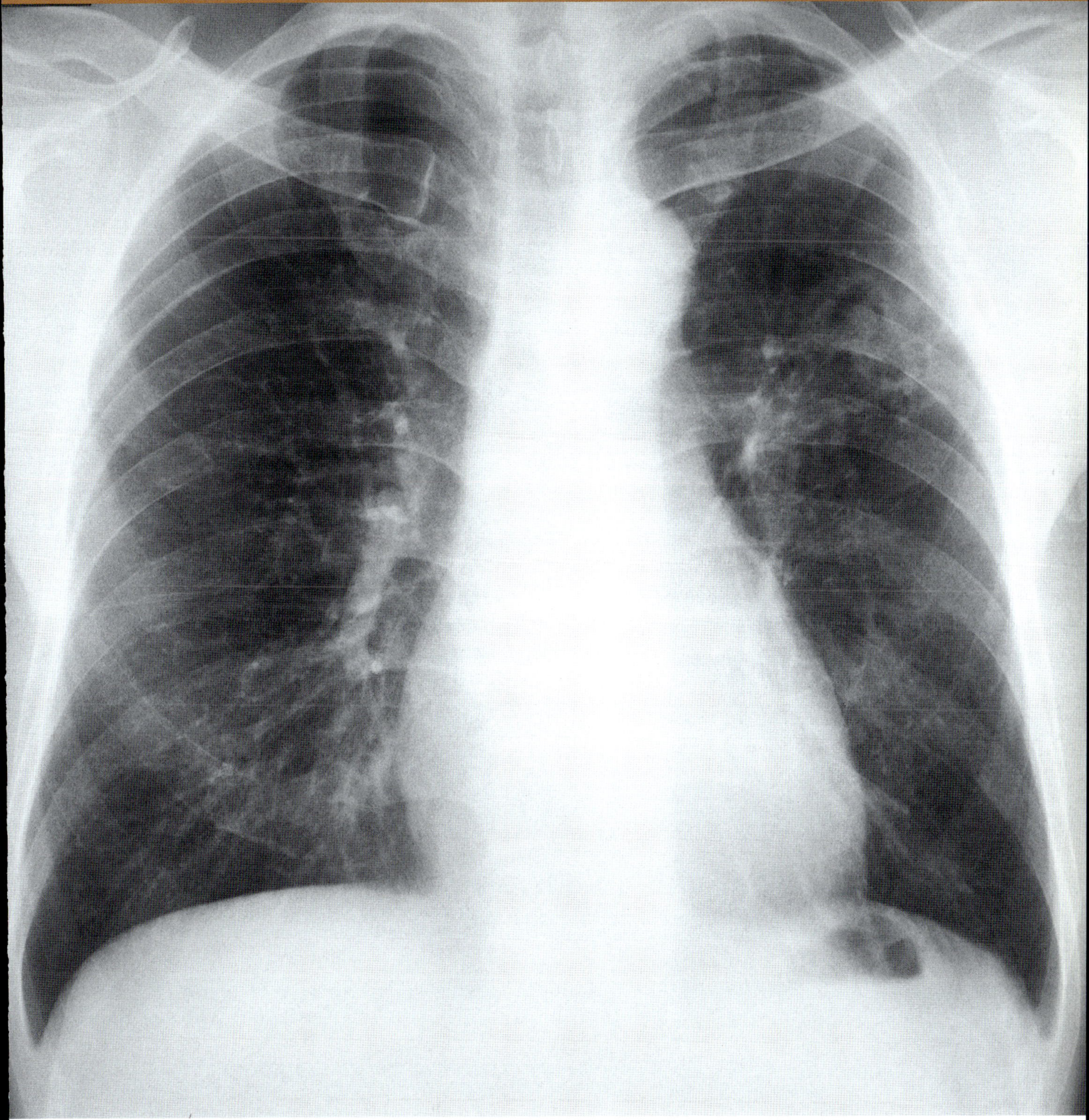

eywords of
is section

Solitary nodular shadow
Infectious disease
Pulmonary cysts
Fungus ball
Aspergilloma
Localized shadow
Tuberculoma
Centrilobular
Tree-in-bud appearance
Localized organizing pneumonia
Lung abscess
Pulmonary suppuration
Rounded atelectasis
Mycobacterium infection
Pulmonary tuberculosis
Pulmonary mycosis

Solitary nodular shadow 3

Hitoshi Tokuda
Department of Internal Medicine, Respiratory Medicine, Social Insurance Central General Hospital, Tokyo, Japan

This section provides discussions concerning nodular shadows formed by inflammation (infection in many cases). It is not unusual for infections to form a solid focus in a single location which shows as a solitary nodular shadow in chest radiographs. However, with infections, when a glance at a plain chest radiograph indicates a solitary nodular shadow, it often occurs that the shadow breaks up into pieces when CT is conducted, and an analysis of those surrounding lesions provides clues for accurate diagnosis. This is the reason why imaging diagnosis is expected to play a useful role in this situation.

Case 1 51-year-old male

Chief complaint: Bloody sputum

Medical history: Received a medical examination 7 years ago for bloody sputum. A cyst containing fluid was found in the left upper lobe S^4, and a diagnosis of infected bulla was made. An antimicrobial agent was administered for 2 weeks and the symptoms disappeared. The patient had not visited a hospital since that time.

Smoking history: 30/day for 24 years. Stopped smoking 7 years previously.

Present illness:

From the end of October, the patient had bloody sputum for several consecutive days. There were no other respiratory symptoms or fever.

Laboratory data:

WBC 4,100/μL, CRP 0.1 mg/dL, ESR 12/h, CEA 2.0 ng/mL, CYFRA 1.9 ng/mL, NSE 4.5 ng/mL, aspergillus antigen (–), beta-D-glucan 5.1 pg/mL.

Chest radiograph on admission (P. 101, *Fig. 1*) shows a thin walled cavitary lesion (➞) in the left middle lung field, inside of which a spherical structure (➞) can be seen. Scattered nodular shadows (➤) are found at the periphery of the lesion.

Chest CT (*Fig. 2*) shows a cavitary lesion (➞) in left upper lobe S^4, and a ball-like structure (➤) inside it. Blood vessels and bronchi are involved, indicating, along with traction of the pleura, the strong shrinking nature of this lesion. This lesion is formed in the same location as the cyst found in a plain chest radiograph (*Fig. 3*) and chest CT (*Fig. 4*) taken 7 years previously. It could be a predisposing lesion for this new disease.

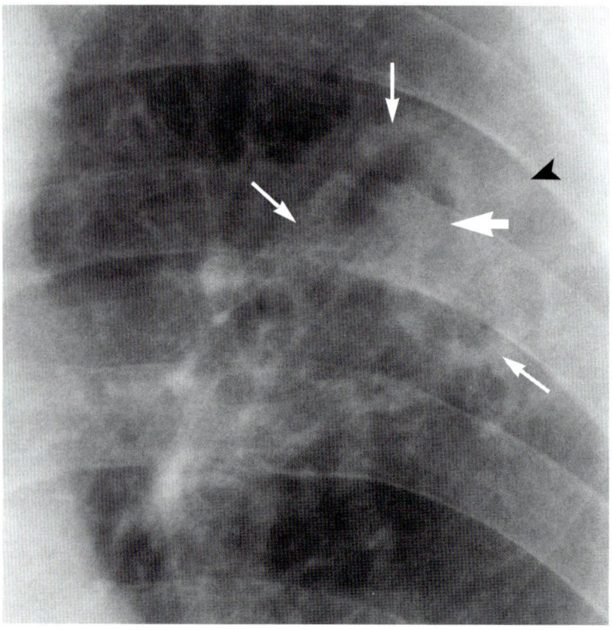

Figure 1. **Chest radiograph**

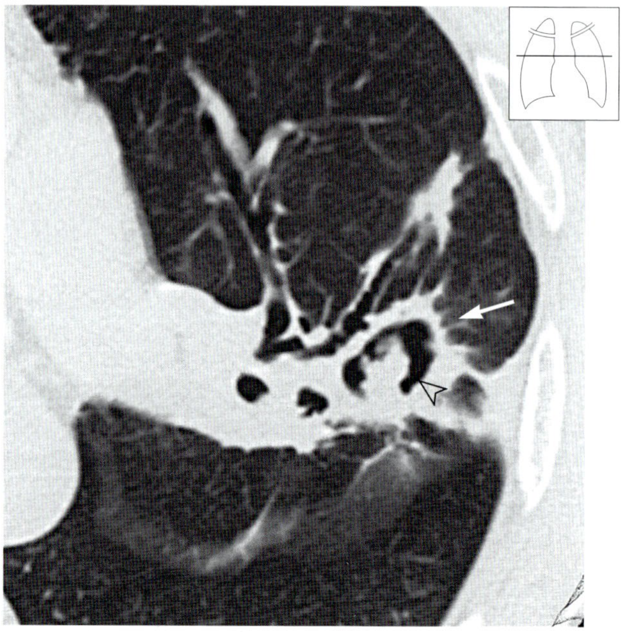

Figure 2. **Chest CT**

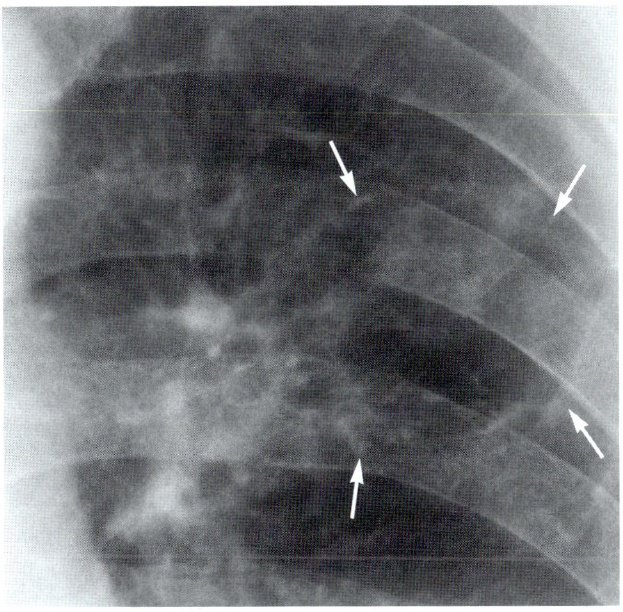

Figure 3. **Chest radiograph:** After treatment for an infected bulla 7 years ago. A thin-walled cyst resided (→).

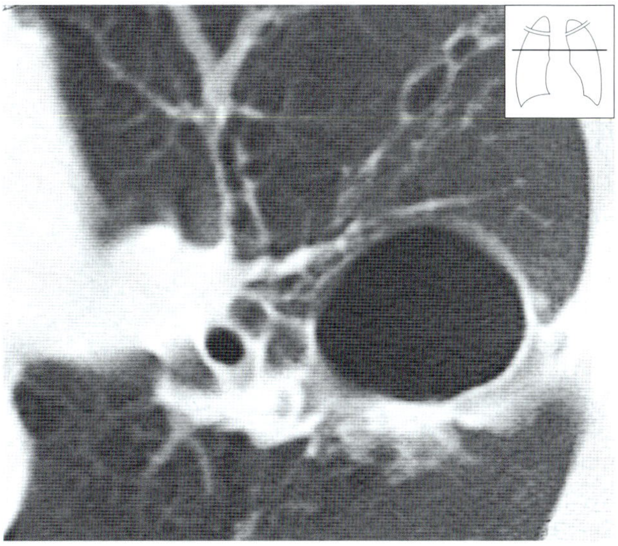

Figure 4. **Chest CT:** A CT taken at the same time. This cyst probably afforded a suitable site for the fungus ball formation.

Diagnosis
Fungus ball (aspergilloma)

Aspergillus is a fungus that is present everywhere in the environment but it is relatively rare that it causes pulmonary lesions in healthy individuals. Aspergillosis is divided into four known types, that is fungus ball, chronic necrotizing aspergillosis, allergic bronchopulmonary aspergillosis and invasive aspergillosis, the last of which is seen in patients with suppressed immunity. With fungus ball type, the fungus invades the lungs in residual cavities after treatment of tuberculosis, bronchiectasis or other conditions such as the cyst in this case, and forms a saprophytic fungal ball taking an apparently benign course. However, since this condition is often complicated with bloody sputum and gradually destroys the neighboring lung over an extended period, appropriate diagnosis and treatment are mandatory.

An essential point of imaging diagnosis for aspergilloma is to detect a spherical structure (fungus ball) in a cavity. Thickening of the adjacent pleura is often observed, confirming the diagnosis. As can be seen in this case, serological tests, that is to say for the serum aspergillus antigen beta-D-glucan, are not useful in many cases. A positive result for precipitation antibody for *Aspergillus* may contribute to the diagnosis. *Aspergillus* should be verified from the content of the cavity. In this case a definite diagnosis was made through a CT-guided percutaneous fine-needle biopsy (*Fig. 5*).

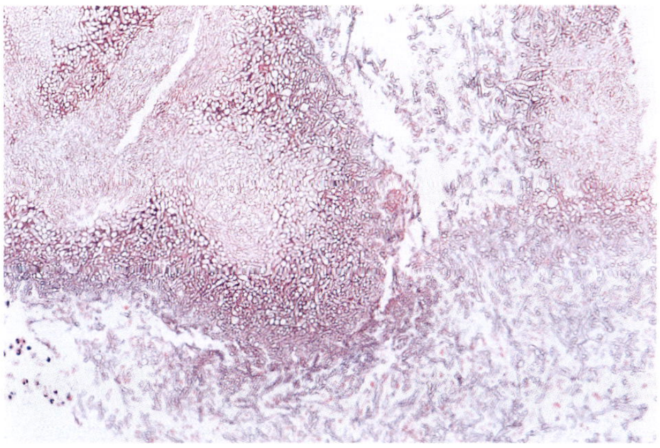

Figure 5. **Histopathology: Percutaneous fine-needle biopsy**

Inflammatory solitary (localized) shadows and their differentiation

When an inflammatory mass is viewed in CT, in many cases it appears as a complex shadow comprising a main focus with surrounding subfoci, or a conglomerate of microfoci without a main focus. The name "localized shadow" would be more suitable.

Various infectious diseases are encountered as localized shadows in chest radiographs. Acute infections usually respond to treatment and may disappear rapidly. In such cases clinical differentiation is not problematic. However, even in some cases of acute infection absorption may be protracted and the lesion may remain as a nodular shadow for a while, causing the clinical problem of differentiation from malignancies (organizing pneumonia).

Chronic infections showing as localized shadows cause clinical problems. These include pulmonary tuberculosis, pulmonary nontuberculous mycobacteriosis, pulmonary mycosis and chronic lung abscess.

Clinical symptoms are absent or mild in these cases, and serological tests are also useless. Along with utilizing chest radiographs, one should also make every effort to detect the causative organism through sputum examination, bronchoscopy and other means in order to differentiate from malignancies and also to treat the disease appropriately.

In pulmonary mycobacteriosis (pulmonary tuberculosis, pulmonary nontuberculous mycobacteriosis) characteristic patterns are often found in CT, making CT an extremely useful tool for diagnosis of this disease, especially in cases of negative sputum study.

The morphology of Pulmonary mycobacteriosis

To understand the image findings of pulmonary mycobacteriosis (hereafter taking pulmonary tuberculosis as a typical example), it is necessary to understand its pathology (*Fig. 6*). The most important characteristic is the tendency for foci to become encapsulated due to specific immunity against the mycobacterium, forming a tubercular nodule, a so called tubercle. Inside this tubercle, caseous necrosis occurs while at the periphery a chronic inflammatory process results in fibrosis to create a defined border for each focus. After further time has elapsed, a natural healing mechanism causes tubercles to contract and become polygonal.

When caseous necrosis occurs in one or a few neighboring lobuli, the encapsulated nodule may be 1 to 3 cm in diameter. If solitary, it is called a tuberculoma, since it evokes a differentiation problem between malignancies. Macroscopic findings of a tuberculoma are shown in *Figure 7*, low magnification microscopic findings are shown in *Figure 8*, and a contracted tubercle (HE stain) is shown in *Figure 9*. In the contraction stage, thickened interlobular septa (→) are linked at each corner of the polyhedron which may be observed in CT as spicula.

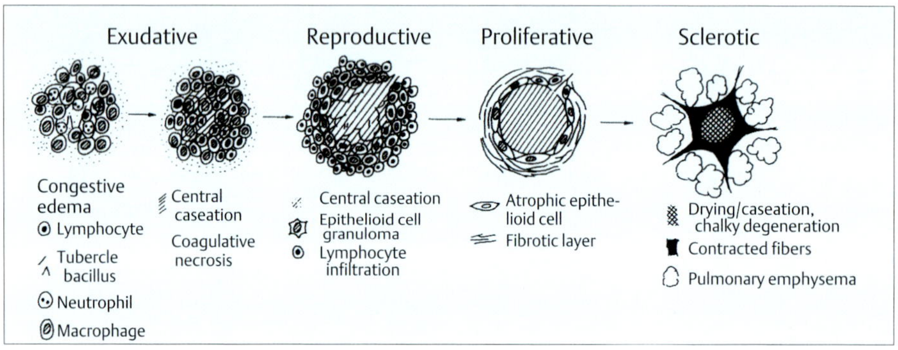

Figure 6. **Phases of tubercular lesion**

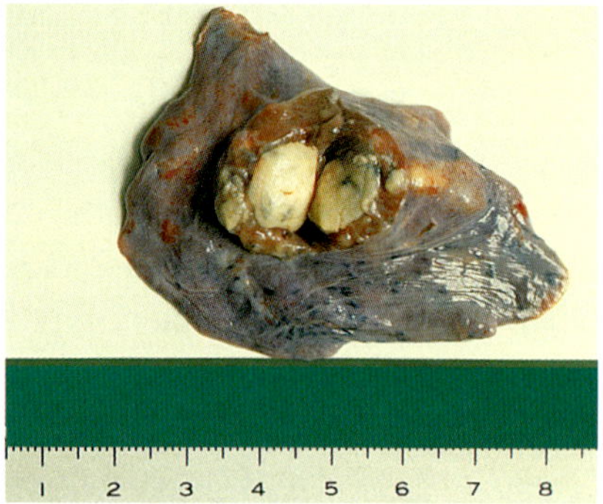

Figure 7. **Macroscopic findings:Tuberculoma**

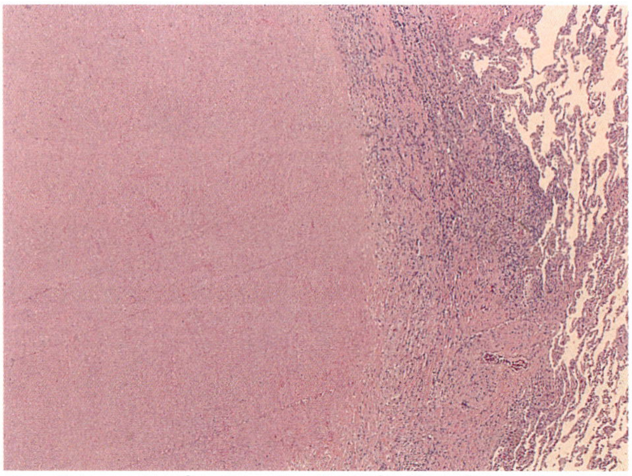

Figure 8. **Low magnification microscopic findings: Tuberculoma**

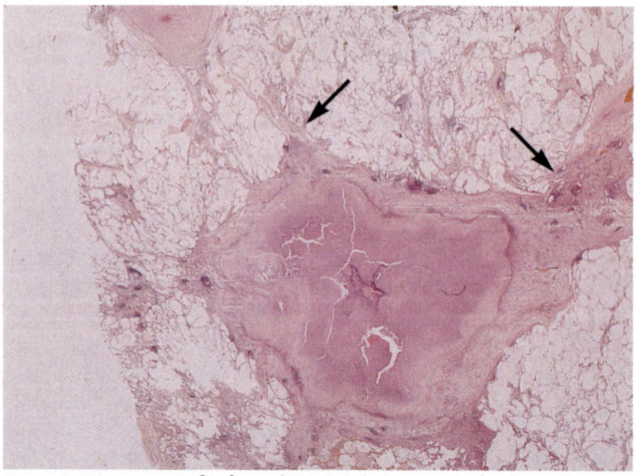

Figure 9. **Microscopic findings (HE stain): Contracted tuberculoma**

Case 2 Tuberculoma

38-year-old male

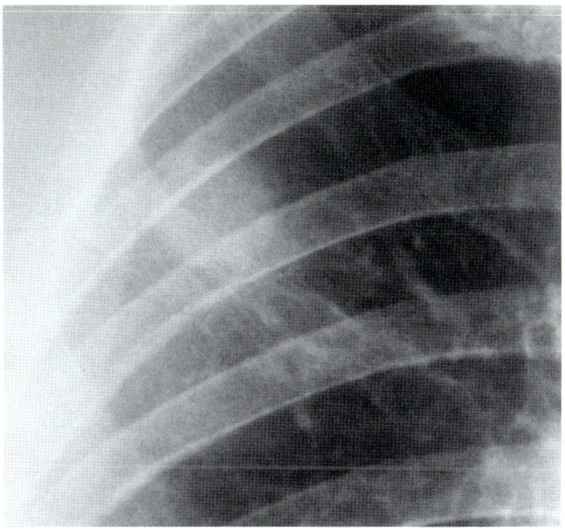

Figure 10. **Chest radiograph**

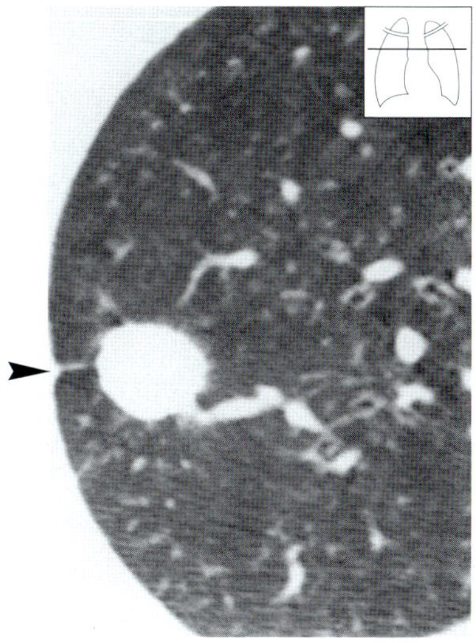

Figure 11. **Chest CT**

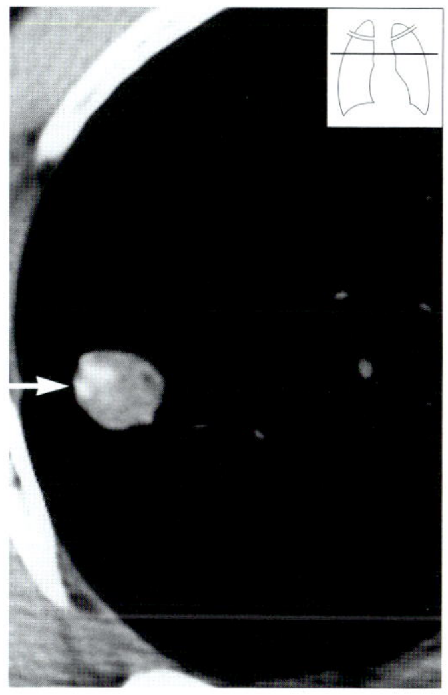

Figure 12. **Chest CT: Mediastinal window setting**

Asymptomatic, found on regular checkup.

Plain chest radiograph (*Fig. 10*): Solitary nodular shadow in the right upper lung field.

Chest CT (*Fig. 11*): Nodular shadow with comparatively distinct border. No surrounding scattering. Pleural indentation (➤) can be observed. This finding is seen not only in cancer but also frequently in chronic inflammation. Coarse calcification (→) is seen in the mediastinal window setting (*Fig. 12*).

Note: Tuberculomas may appear as various images which will be shown in *Figures 13 and 14*.

Tuberculoma exhibiting polygonal shape (*Fig. 13*). Spicula (➤) can be seen at the corners, which correspond to thickened interlobular septa. That is easy to understand when compared with pathological findings (*Fig. 9*).

Tuberculoma exhibiting notching (*Fig. 14*). Blood vessels are strongly attracted toward the lesion, making differentiation from cancer a problem. However, CT at the cranial level 4 mm higher (*Fig. 15*) shows adjacent fine granular shadows (➤). This is an important point for suspecting an infectious disease, particularly tuberculosis.

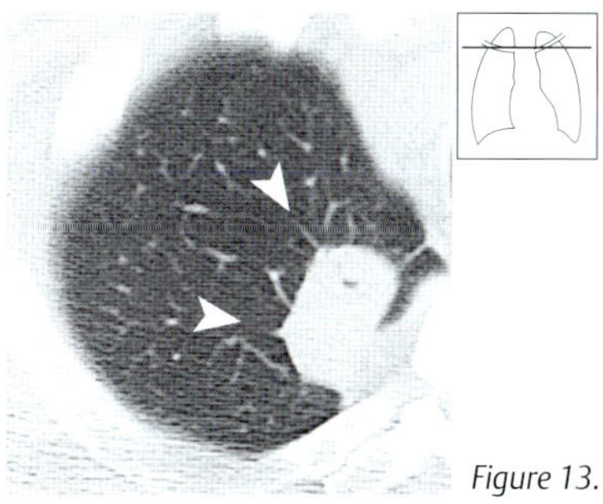

Figure 13. **Chest CT: Tuberculoma**

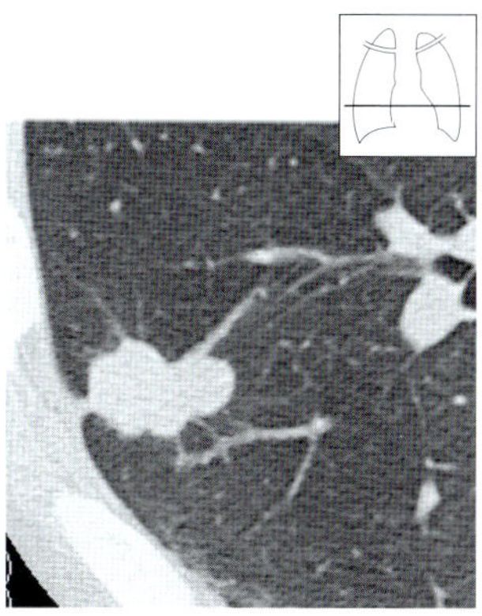

Figure 14. **Chest CT: Notch formation**

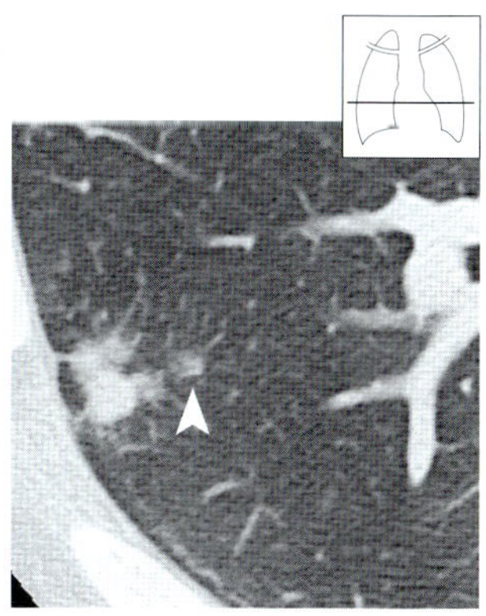

Figure 15. **Chest CT at the cranial level 4 mm higher than in Figure 14**

Case 3 Localized scattered tuberculosis

24-year-old female

Asymptomatic, found on regular checkup.

A plain chest radiograph (*Fig. 16*) shows granular shadows aggregating over an area of 4 x 4 cm in the right upper lung field. Compare this with the images taken 2 years previously (*Fig. 17*) which are essentially normal.

Chest CT (*Fig. 18*): Aggregation of minute nodules is found in the right upper lobe S^2. These are acinar foci, the smallest tuberculous lesions in the lung. Each individual focus is a tuberculous nodule formed in the bronchioles or surrounding alveolar areas. Their arrangement is irregular, making it difficult to recognize as centrilobular distribution. It is said that tubercular nodules are frequently located centrilobularly, but there are many cases to which this principle does not apply, most of which are chronic cases. In another level (*Fig. 19*), you can see branching shadows at the bronchiole level with minute nodules adhering at the tips of them (→) (tree-in-bud appearance). Areas where nodules have fused can also be seen (➤). Each of these findings is a characteristic of tuberculosis.

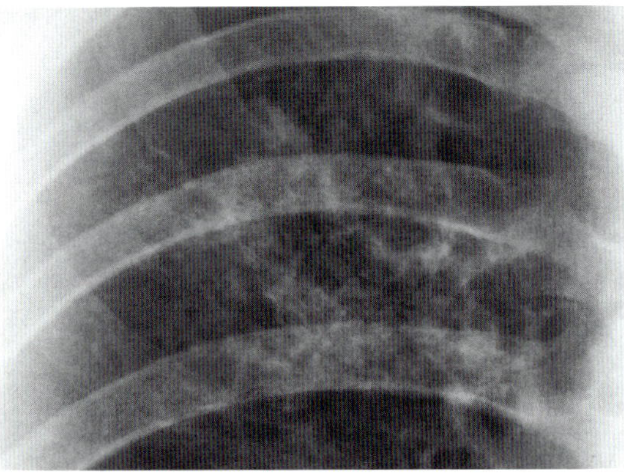

Figure 16. **Chest radiograph: Granular aggregation**

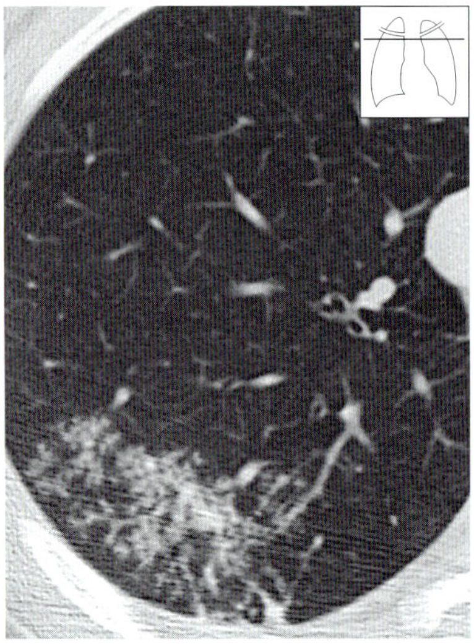

Figure 18. **Chest CT**

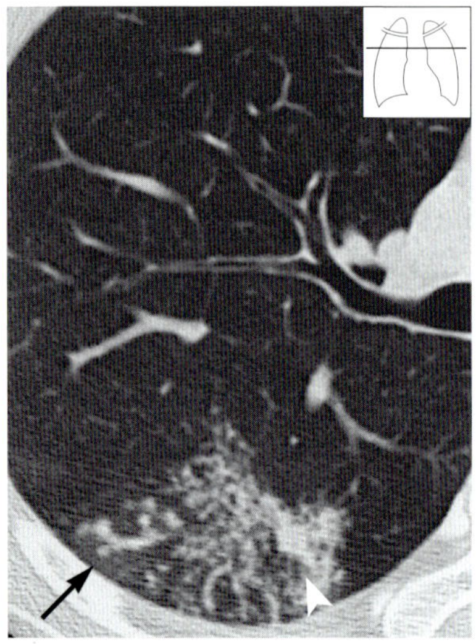

Figure 19. **Chest CT: Tree-in-bud appearance, a specific feature of pulmonary tuberculosis**

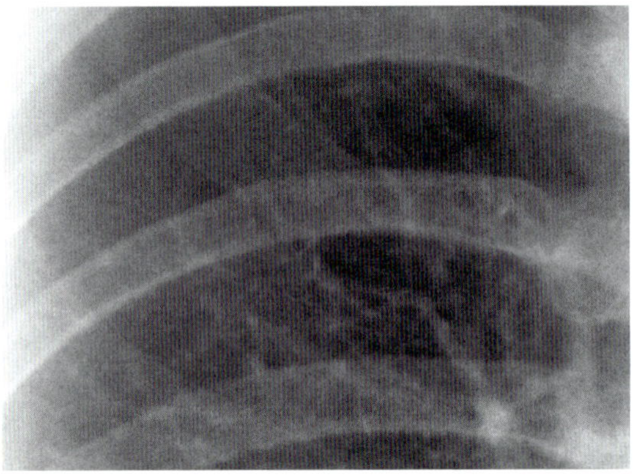

Figure 17. **Chest radiograph: taken 2 years previously (normal)**

Case 4 Localized organizing pneumonia

31-year-old male

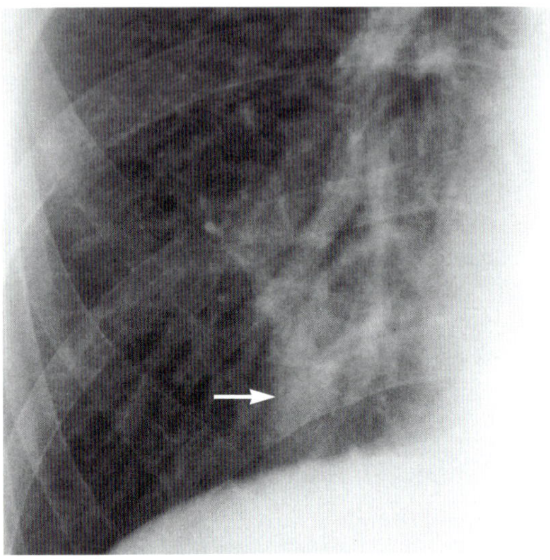

Figure 20. **Chest radiograph**

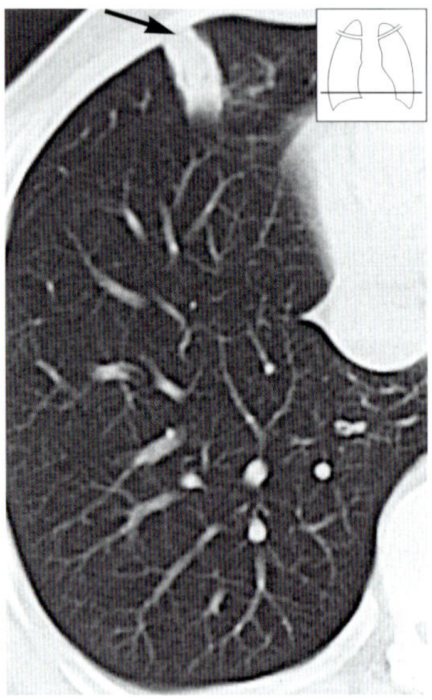

Figure 21. **Chest CT**

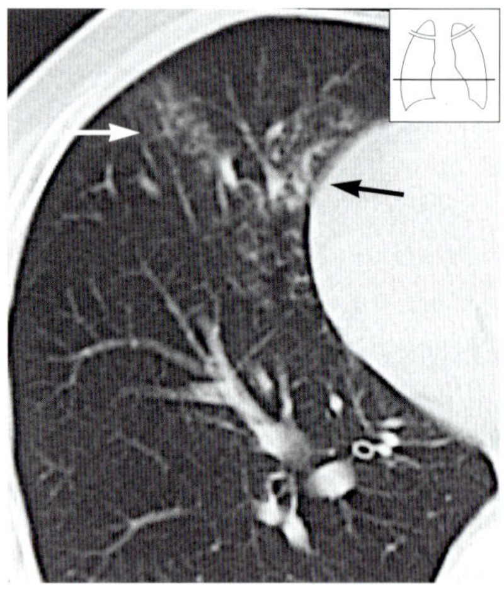

Figure 22. **Chest CT at the cranial level 3 cm higher than in Figure 21**

The disease was discovered on regular checkup but in fact the patient had a slight fever, cough and other cold-like symptoms for 2 to 3 days, 1 month previously.

Chest radiograph: A 2 x 1.5 cm nodular shadow (→) can be seen in the right lower lung field.

Chest CT: An enclosed lesion (→) with linear border can be observed at the periphery of the S^5 area. It is touching the parietal pleura and the interlobar pleura. Inside, an air bronchogram can be observed. It could comprise one lobular lesion. CT at the cranial level 3 cm higher (*Fig. 22*) shows scattered granular shadows (→), suggesting inflammatory origin. Localized organizing pneumonia was diagnosed, an antibiotic agent was administered and the shadows disappeared.

Case 5 Chronic lung abscess

51-year-old female

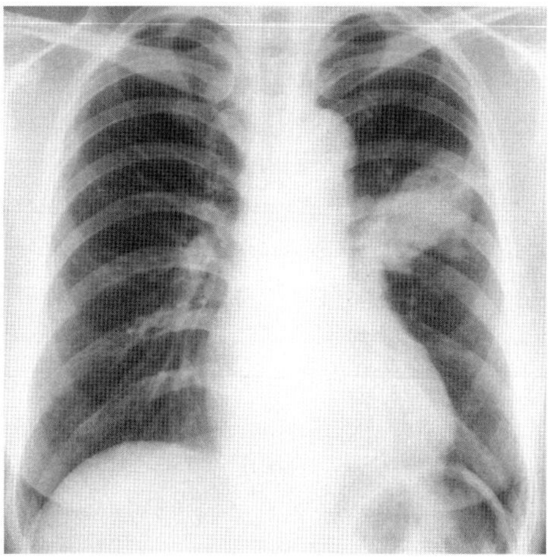

Figure 23. **Chest radiograph**

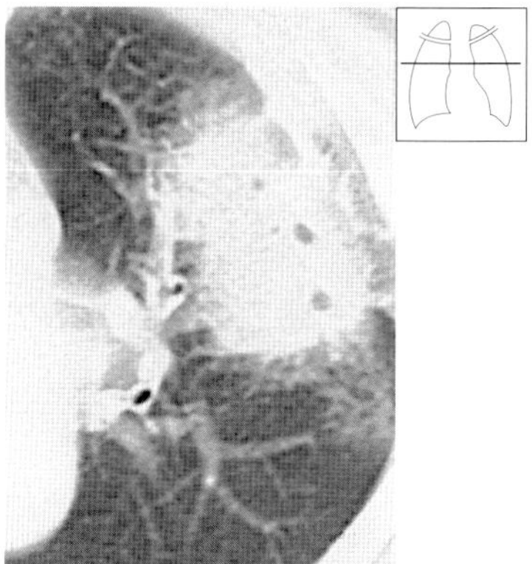

Figure 24. **Chest CT**

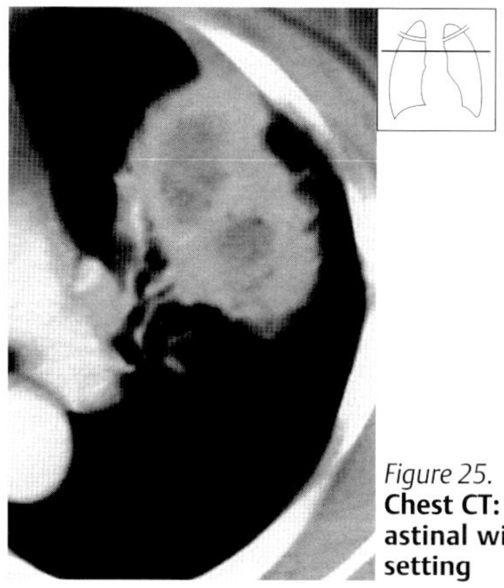

Figure 25. **Chest CT: Mediastinal window setting**

Since 3 months ago the patient had mild cold symptoms and a chest radiograph examination indicated an abnormality but it was left untreated. For the detailed examination the patient was referred to our hospital. The result of laboratory tests were WBC 8,700/μL, CRP 0.3 mg/dL and ESR 85/h. A bronchoscopy revealed floridity, edema and yellow sputum in the bronchial mucosa. Cytologic examination yielded Class II in atypism, and a large number of neutrophils. No proof of the presence of bacteria. Chronic lung abscess was diagnosed and penicillin and clindamycin were administered over an extended period. After 3 months the shadow finally disappeared.

Chest radiograph: A solitary 5.5 x 3.5 cm mass lesion in the left upper lung field.

Chest CT: In the lung window setting, ground glass opacity surrounds the tumor, with a bubbly, radiolucent image inside. In the mediastinal window setting, there is a low attenuation area inside the tumor indicating necrosis. With these images alone it is not possible to eliminate the possibility of squamous cell carcinoma (peripheral type). Either way, it should be emphasized that among cases of lung abscess (pulmonary suppuration) it is not uncommon for the course of the disease to be surprisingly indolent with few subjective symptoms.

Case 6 Rounded atelectasis

73-year-old male

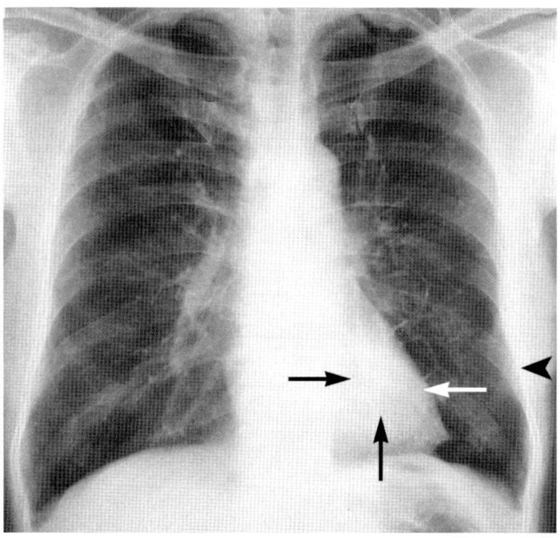

Figure 26. **Chest radiograph**

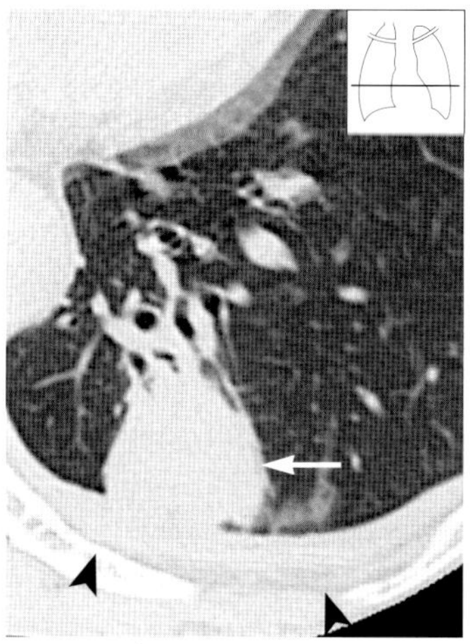

Figure 27. **Chest CT**

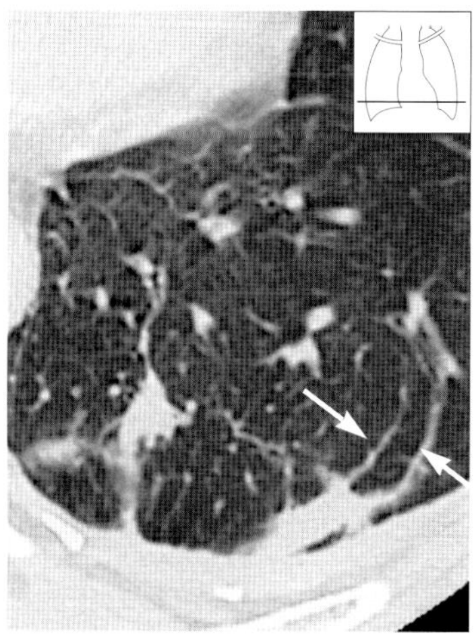

Figure 28. **Chest CT at the caudal level 2 cm lower than Figure 27**

Asymptomatic, found on regular checkup. Serology for inflammatory reaction and tumor markers are all negative.

Chest radiograph: A solitary 4 x 3 cm mass lesion (→) in the left lower lung field (behind the heart), accompanied by funicular shadows above and below. Thickening of the parietal pleura (➤) can be seen, and the existence of some kind of old pleural lesion is suspected.

Chest CT: There is a mass lesion (→) touching the pleura in the left lower lobe S^{10} area. B^9 and B^{10} bronchi appear to have converged and been drawn into the lesion. The pleura is considerably thickened (➤).

CT at the caudal level 2 cm lower (*Fig. 28*) shows marked pleural thickening with adjacent pulmonary structures drawn in and collapsed (→).

Rounded atelectasis readily occurs in cases of pleural thickening associated with pleurisy. It is considered to be related often to exposure to asbestos. Differentiating between cancer and tuberculosis may also be a problem. It was confirmed that this case was exposed to asbestos for 3 years and to glass fiber for 20 years in the past.

This section provided discussion of localized shadows in the lung field caused by inflammation. Most of the cases discussed are those of chronic infections whose pathological characteristics are reflected in imagings. Provided these characteristics are interpreted correctly, as may be seen, it is not difficult to arrive at the correct diagnosis.

Mycobacterium infection (pulmonary tuberculosis)

In this disease, the lesions may be as small as 1 cm or less in diameter or extend as far as the entire lung, and their extremely varied morphology can be anything from granular shadows and faint ground glass opacity to dense infiltrative shadows, nodular shadows and mass lesions. It is said to be difficult to make a diagnosis of infectious disease with imagings only, but pathologically, tuberculosis has characteristics that other infectious diseases do not have, and if these are taken into consideration diagnosis would be possible. These characteristics are 1) usually, the clinical course is extremely slow, 2) progression is mainly transbronchial, 3) individual lesions tend to be localized, and 4) there is a high incidence of peripheral airway disease.

The smallest of pulmonary tuberculous lesions are minute lesions called acinar lesions. Pathologically, due to the action of specific immunity, the lesions are encapsulated. Although these lesions often form in the respiratory bronchi and in surrounding pulmonary areas (in which case they appear to be centrilobular in CT), they can also extend into peripheral alveolar ducts (in which case it is difficult to recognize them as being centrilobular in CT). In either case, these minute lesions contain absolutely no air, and appear as high contrast granular shadows or branching shadows. This can be observed in CT of most cases of pulmonary tuberculosis, providing a key for the diagnosis of this disease.

Among infectious diseases, tuberculosis is also exceptional in that it causes strong pathological changes in airways. In addition to the central airway, this frequently occurs in peripheral airways. The combination of acinar nodular shadows and the bronchi-shaped branching shadows that seem to connect to them (tree-in-bud appearance) is often seen in CT but pathologically these are caseous bronchiolitis and peribronchiolitis, which provide valuable clues to diagnosing tuberculosis with CT.

Tubercles vary widely in size, ranging from a few millimeters to 2 to 3 cm in diameter. They are encapsulated, and inside caseous necrosis takes place. A solitary tubercle sized 1 to 3 cm is called a tuberculoma, which is difficult to differentiate from lung cancer. Important points in conducting imaging diagnosis are 1) in tuberculoma the border is distinct, and there are often scattered granular shadows in surrounding areas, 2) over time the lesion contracts and the border frequently exhibits a multi-cornered shape, with spicula at the corners, 3) contraction may be expressed as pleural indentation, 4) there may be notching, caused by fusion of multiple foci, and 5) inside density is uniform and calcification is often seen.

However, since some of these findings can also be seen with lung cancer, they are not necessarily absolute points for differentiation. It is often necessary to conduct some kind of invasive test to confirm diagnosis.

Organizing pneumonia

Although organizing pneumonia is the histopathological term, clinically, the term is actually used to refer to the pathological condition when healing of a microbial infection is protracted, and a shadow remains in chest radiograph for an extended period. As important pointers for suspecting an infectious disease, there are changes in surrounding areas (adjacent accompanying shadows, wide pleural indentation), and borders tend to be straight (pathologically, this corresponds to the interlobular septal border). It is natural to assume that organizing pneumonia is preceded by bacterial pneumonia, but even on detailed inquiry many patients have no recollection of recent respiratory symptoms. For diagnosis it is more useful to observe patients over an extended period, when in most cases lesions contract or disappear after 1 to 2 months.

Pulmonary mycosis

Aspergillosis and pulmonary cryptococcosis are the most common types of mycosis that form localized lesions in the lungs of healthy individuals. Here we have discussed fungus ball type (aspergilloma), but because of its frequency, pulmonary cryptococcosis is also important. In many cases of cryptococcosis, there are multiple nodular shadows in a single lobe. This is covered in the next section.

Chapter 4

Radiographs of intrapulmonary lesions with decreased radiolucency

9. Nodular shadow:

Multiple nodular shadows
[Pattern classification IV-D-2]

●Author — Jiro Fujita

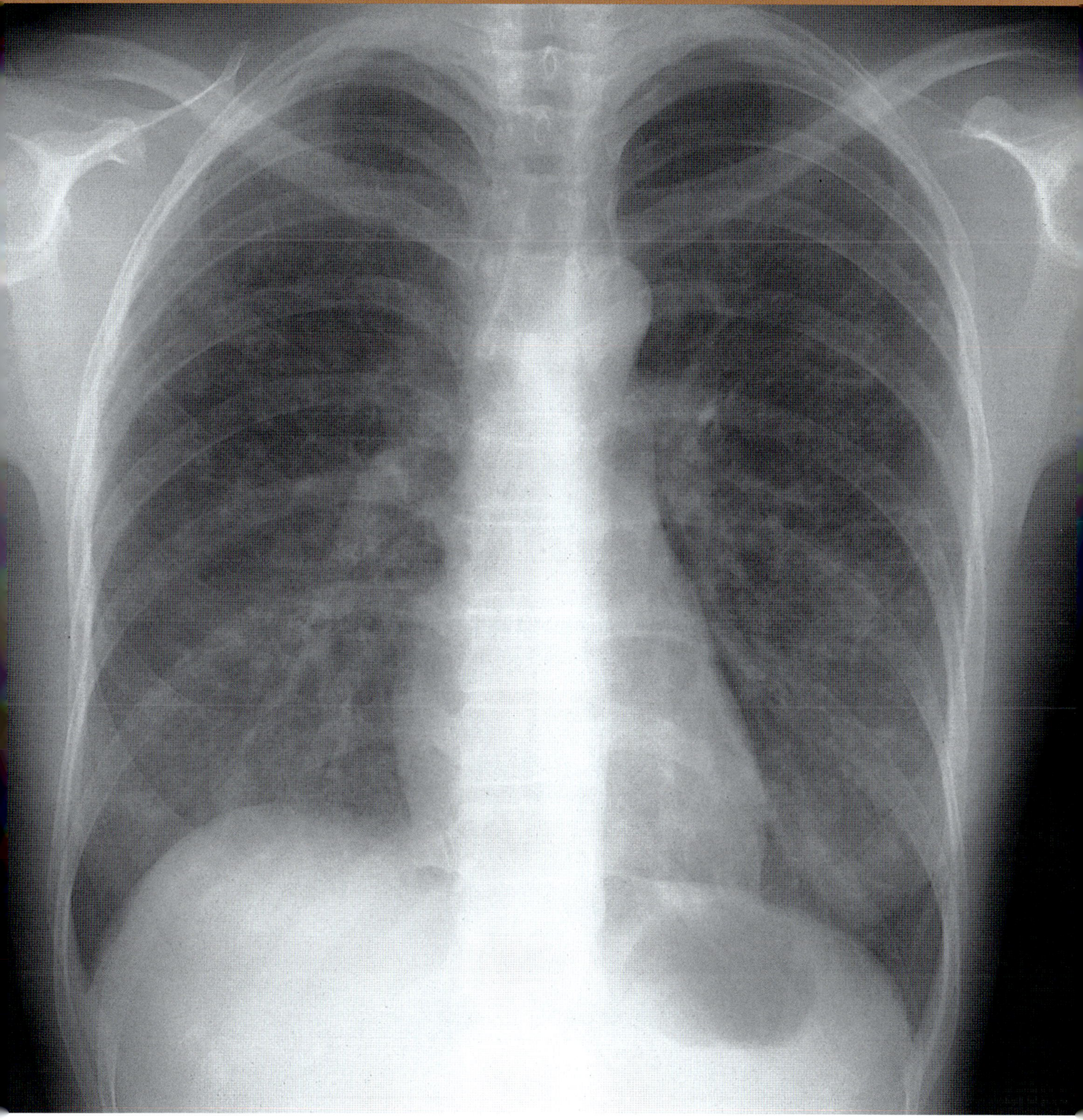

Keywords of this section

Adenocarcinoma
Pulmonary cryptococcosis
Pulmonary nocardiosis
Metastatic lung cancer
Alveolar cell carcinoma
Malignant lymphoma
Pulmonary hamartoma
Pulmonary plasmacytoma
Pulmonary amyloidosis
Pulmonary tuberculosis
Atypical (nontuberculous) mycobacteriosis
Bacterial pneumonia
Aspergillus
Sarcoidosis
Wegener's granulomatosis
Pulmonary eosinophilic granuloma
Pulmonary arterio-venous fistula

Multiple nodular shadows

Jiro Fujita
Department of Medicine and Therapeutics Control and Prevention of Infectious Diseases (1st Department of Internal Medicine), Faculty Of Medicine, University of the Ryukyus, Okinawa, Japan

A huge number of diseases show as multiple nodular shadows in chest radiographs. The definition of a node generally refers to something with a diameter of 8 mm or more. Nevertheless, there are frequently cavities in nodular shadows, and they sometimes change to small nodular shadows. In other words, chest radiographs show a wide range of patterns, combinations and changes. This section focuses on diseases in which multiple nodules with a diameter of 5 to 8 mm or larger are observed (including those which also show cavities, nodular shadows and patchy shadows). Case 1 is a typical example.

Case 1 35-year-old female

Chief complaint: Abnormal chest shadow observed during detailed examination

Medical history/Family history: Nothing of particular note

Smoking history: 15/day for 10 years

Present illness:

An abnormal chest shadow was indicated at a health examination. To examine this in detail, the patient received an examination at the Department of Internal Medicine, Kagawa Medical University. At the time of the first examination the patient had no subjective symptoms, and no physical abnormalities were observed.

A chest radiograph showed bilateral diffuse reticular shadows and nodular shadows.

Physical findings on admission:

Palpebral conjunctiva was slightly anemic, no superficial lymph nodes were palpable. Mild enlargement of the thyroid gland was observed. No cardiac, pulmonary or abdominal abnormalities were observed.

Laboratory data on admission:

Blood sedimentation rate increased to 65 mm/hour, but results were normal for CRP at 1.0 mg/dL and leukocyte count at 7,600/µL. Biochemical tests showed no abnormal findings. Pulmonary function tests indicated a high residual volume ratio of 62.7%, but arterial gas analysis showed no abnormalities.

In a chest radiograph at the time of admission (P. 109), pulmonary overinflation was observed, with bilateral reticular and nodular shadows throughout the lung fields.

Chest CT (*Figs. 1, 2*) showed multiple 5 to 8 mm nodules (→) distributed along bronchi in both lungs. Cavities were also observed in some nodules (➤). The nodules were distributed mainly in respiratory bronchioles and bronchiole areas.

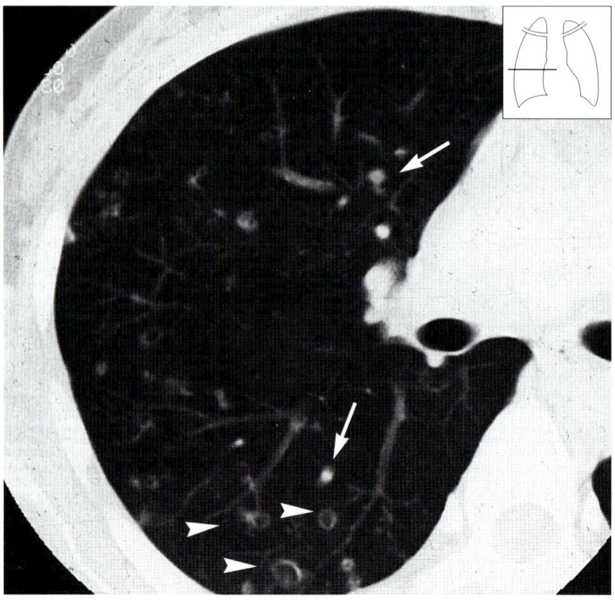

Figure 1. **Chest CT**

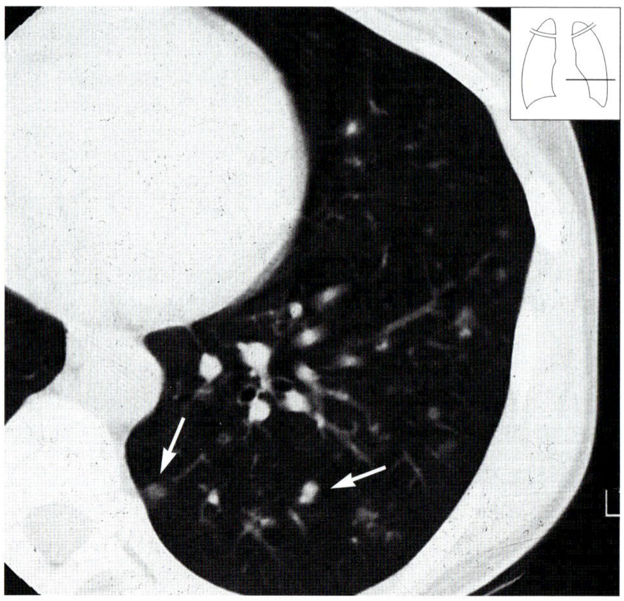

Figure 2. **Chest CT**

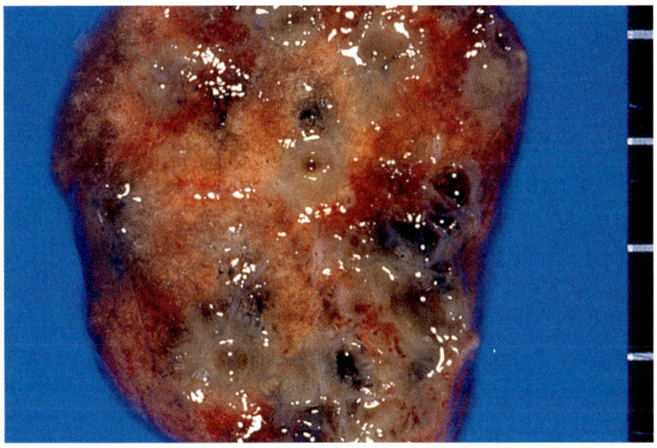

Figure 3. **Macroscopic picture**

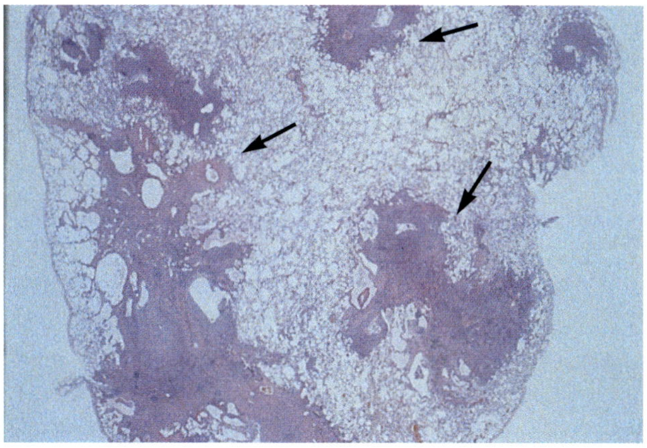

Figure 4. **Pathological findings: HE stain**

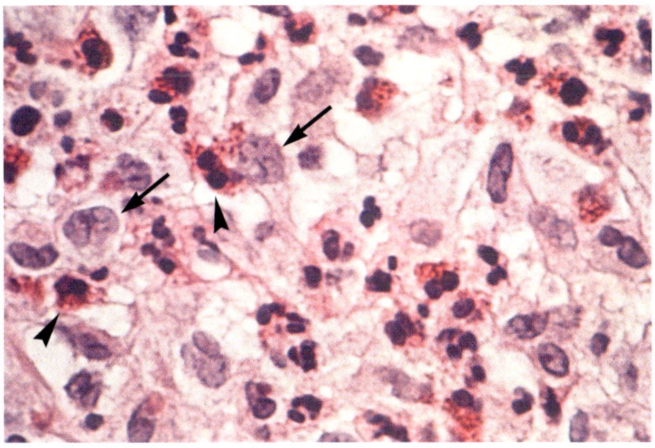

Figure 5. **Pathological findings: HE stain**

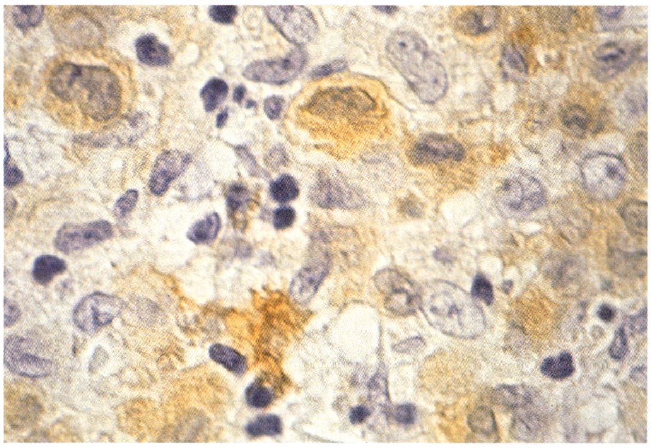

Figure 6. **Pathological findings: Anti S-100 protein stain**

Diagnosis

To arrive at a definite diagnosis, an open lung biopsy was performed immediately after admission. In a sample obtained from the biopsy, 8 mm nodules (→) could be observed surrounding bronchioles as indicated in the macroscopic picture (*Fig. 3*) and the pathological findings (HE stain) (*Fig. 4*). The cytological examination with hematoxylin and eosin stain (*Fig. 5*) indicates a large number of acidophilic vesicular bodies and proliferation of cells with large, irregular nuclei containing little chromatin (→), and formation of granuloma at the periphery due to eosinophil infiltration (➤). Large cells indicated positive findings with anti S-100 protein stain (*Fig. 6*). Examination with an electron microscope revealed indented nuclei in many of these cells, with little nuclear chromatin clumping, distinct nucleoli, and vesicle bodies with numerous large protrusions. From the above cytological and electron microscopic findings, a diagnosis of pulmonary eosinophilic granuloma was reached.

Because subjective symptoms were minimal, after arriving at a definite diagnosis the patient was told to stop smoking and was observed over an extended period as an outpatient, during which time reticular and nodular shadows in bilateral lung fields decreased markedly.

Conclusions of this case: Pulmonary eosinophilic granuloma

Pulmonary eosinophilic granuloma is a disease characterized by proliferation of Langerhans' cells and peripheral infiltration of inflammatory cells, including eosinophils. In chest radiograph, the shadows are mainly reticular and nodular, which develop into honeycomb lung if they progress. Shadows are densely distributed in the upper and middle lung fields, and in many cases there are no lesions in the costophrenic angle.

In chest CT, few lesions are observed directly below the pleura, but there are large changes in areas slightly further inside. On the bronchiole level, it is thought that nodular shadows and ring shadows are extremely specific findings for this disease. To arrive at a definite diagnosis, it is necessary to conduct cytological examinations on a sample obtained from an open lung biopsy to verify the presence of Langerhans' cells and peripheral infiltration of eosinophils. The cause of this disease is unclear but over 90% of patients are smokers. It is thought that smoking plays a role in the proliferation of Langerhans' cells.

Multiple nodular shadows and their differentiation

What are multiple nodules?

The nodular shadows that can be observed in chest radiographs are of many different sizes. When two or more nodules of at least 8 mm in diameter are observed, they are defined as multiple nodules. They are often accompanied by cavities and calcification. Nodular shadows are spherical with a distinct border with surrounding lung. Characteristics that must be differentiated are whether the nodules are multiple noncircumscribed lesions with indistinct border or irregular shape, or diffuse interstitial pattern nodules observed as 2 to 5 mm miliary shadows. It is difficult to draw a clear line between these two types, and in many cases two or more patterns are combined. The following explains how to differentiate multiple nodules in cases of metastasized cancer.

First, a case of metastasized cancer of the thyroid. In chest radiograph (*Fig. 7*), nodular shadows can be observed predominantly in bilateral lower lung fields. In chest CT (*Fig. 8*), diffuse nodular shadows (→) and scattered nodular shadows (➤) are observed in the lung field. This is an example of multiple nodular shadows coexisting with miliary shadows (diffuse interstitial pattern). Examples of the nodules indicating metastasized lung tumor are with metastasis from uterine smooth muscle tumor (*Fig. 9*) (large nodules, distinct borders), colorectal cancer (*Fig. 10*) (large nodules, comparatively distinct borders), biliary canal cancer (*Fig. 11*) (small nodules, slightly indistinct borders), and gastric cancer (*Fig. 12*) (nodules and cancerous lymphangitis). Those with a distinct border could be sarcomas, and those with an indistinct border could be adenocarcinomas. Differentiating multiple noncircumscribed lesions is particularly difficult in cases of metastasized gastric cancer.

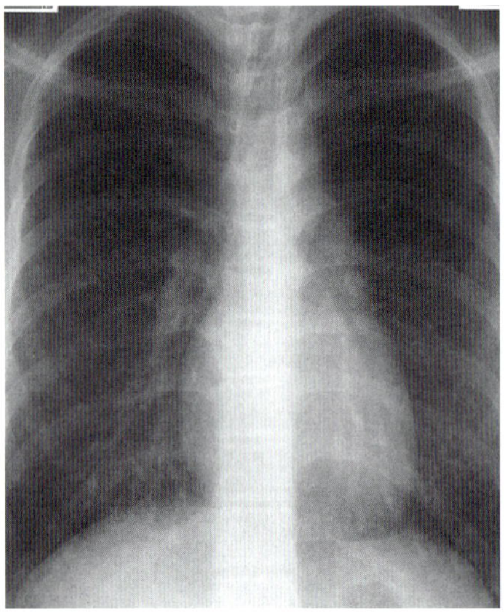

Figure 7. **Chest radiograph: Nodular shadows**

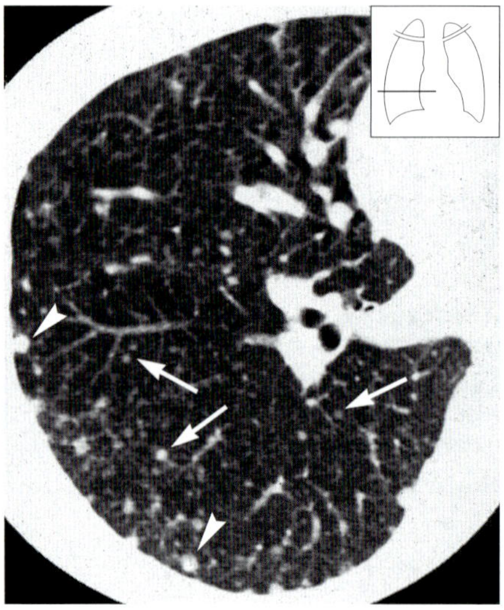

Figure 8. **Chest CT**

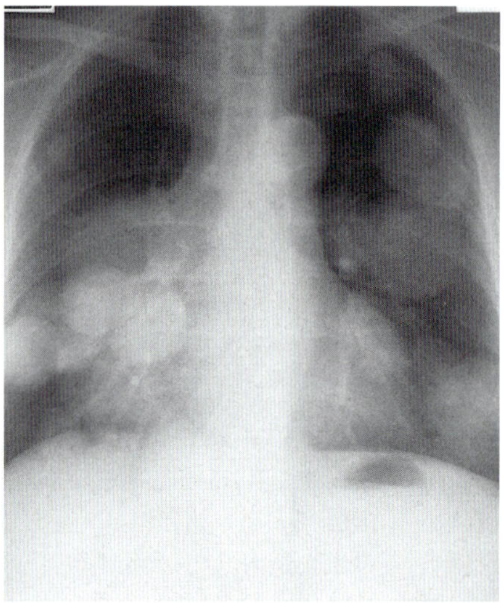

Figure 9. **Chest radiograph: Uterine smooth muscle tumor**

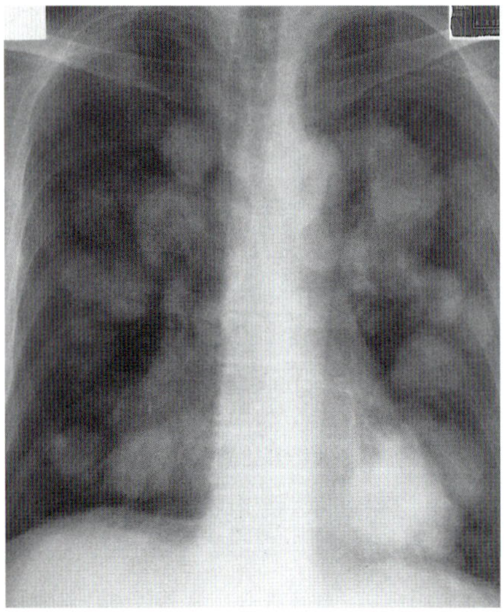

Figure 10. **Chest radiograph: Colorectal cancer**

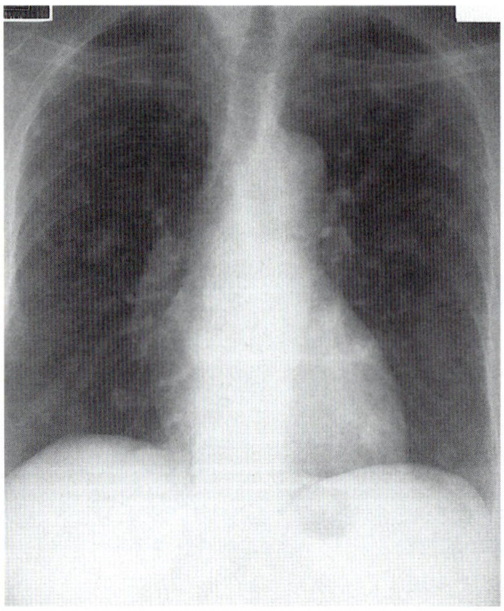

Figure 11. **Chest radiograph: Biliary canal cancer**

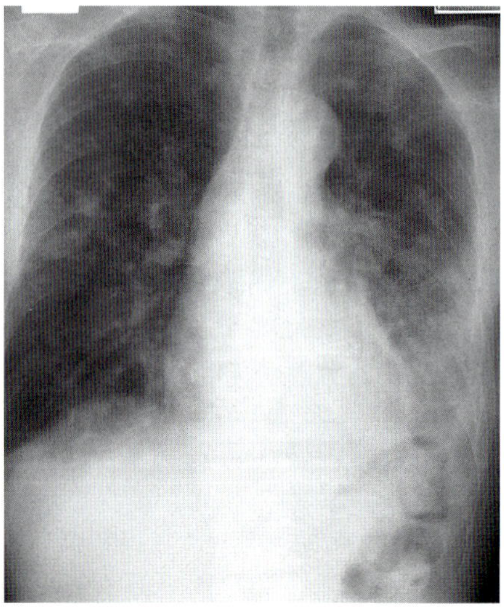

Figure 12. **Chest radiograph: Gastric cancer**

Case 2 Adenocarcinoma and atypical adenomatous hyperplasia

69-year-old female

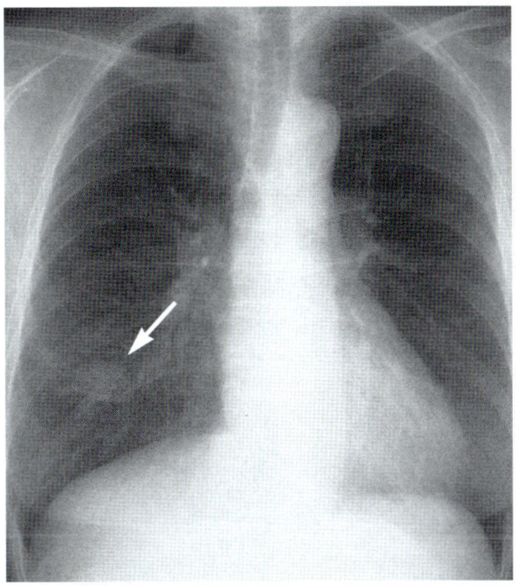

Figure 13. **Chest radiograph**

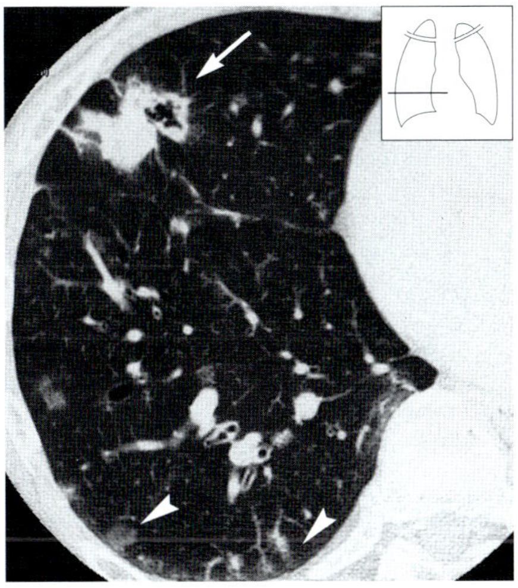

Figure 14. **Chest CT**

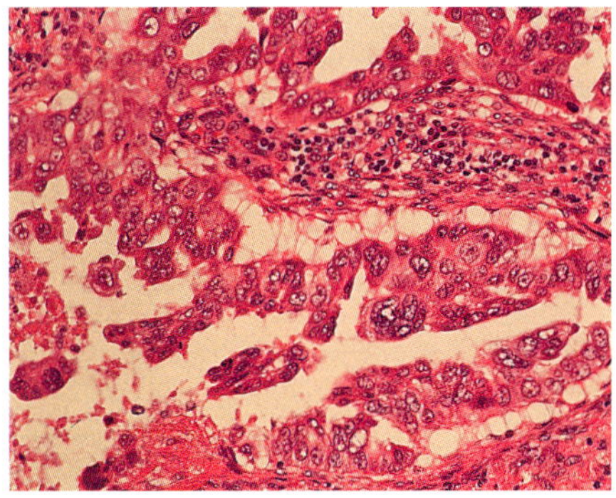

Figure 15. **Pathological findings: Adenocarcinoma originating in the right middle lobe**

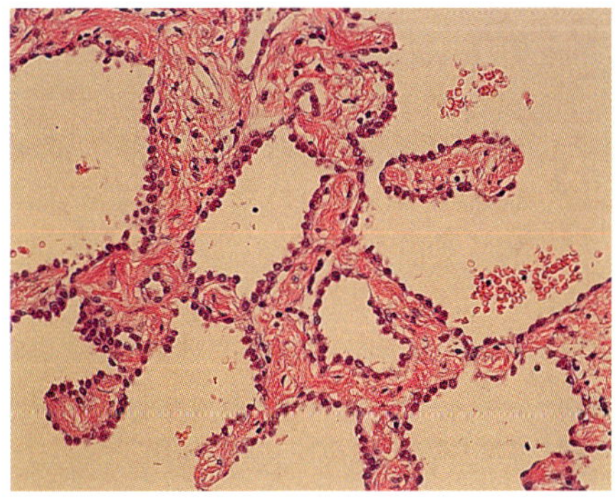

Figure 16. **Pathological findings: Atypical adenomatous hyperplasia**

Received an examination as an outpatient after complaining of cough. No smoking history observed but has a history of dust inhalation.

Chest radiograph shows a nodular shadow in the right lower lung field (→).

Chest CT shows a shadow (→) in the right middle lobe that could indicate adenocarcinoma, but multiple nodular shadows and patchy shadows (➤) are observed in the inferior lobe. Surgery clarified the existence of adenocarcinoma originating in the right middle lobe and multiple atypical adenomatous hyperplasia.

Case 3 Two cases of atypical (nontuberculous) mycobacteriosis

50-year-old female (*Fig. 17*) and 53-year-old female (*Fig. 18*)

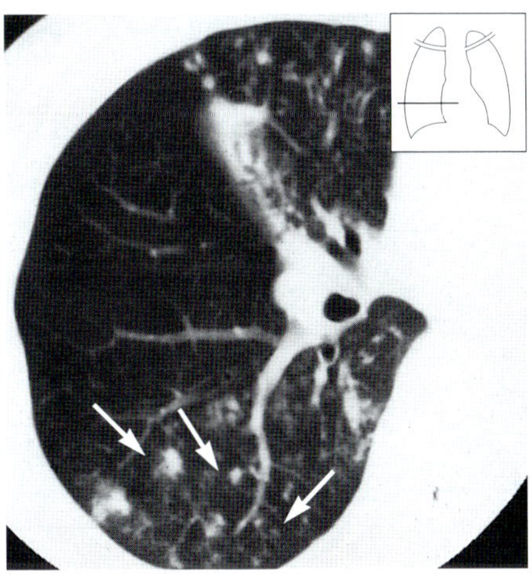

Figure 17. **Chest CT**

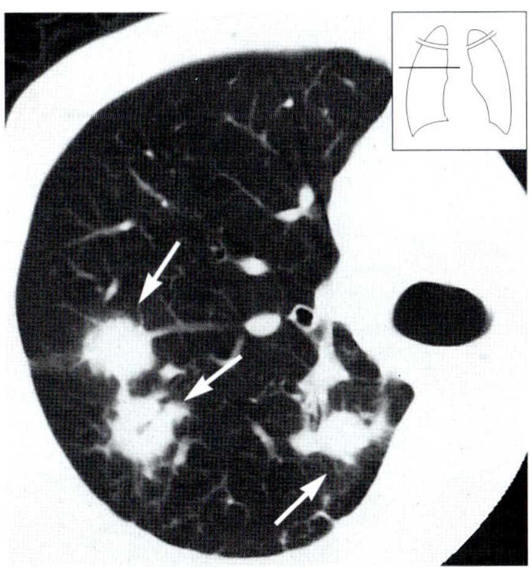

Figure 18. **Chest CT**

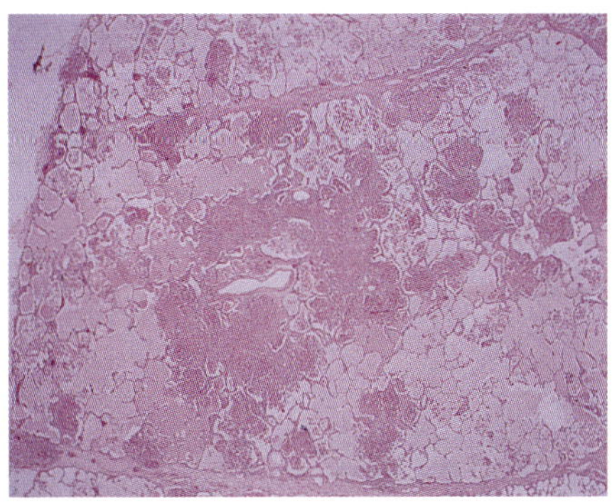

Figure 19. **Pathological findings: Granuloma**

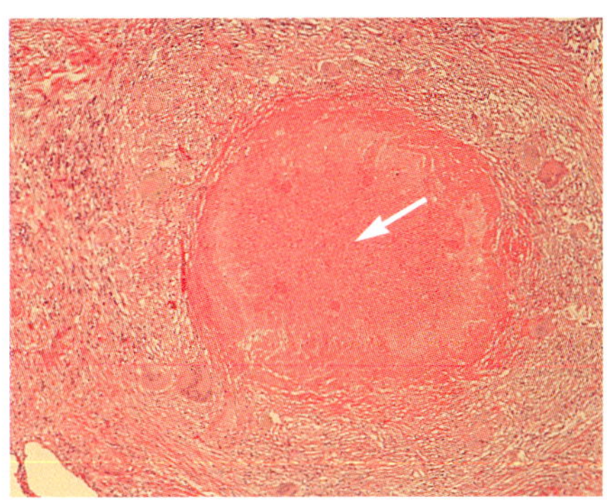

Figure 20. **Pathological findings: Granuloma**

The chest CT findings are typical for pulmonary atypical mycobacteriosis. With atypical mycobacteriosis, an extremely high incidence of bronchial expansion and centrilobular nodules (→) are observed (*Fig. 17*). Nodules of 1.5 to 2 cm in diameter (→) are also sometimes observed (*Fig. 18*).

With surgical specimens obtained from another case, pathological findings corresponding to the same pattern were examined and it was verified that there were also clear granulomas in the centrilobular lesions (*Fig. 19*), and that in the center of large lesions necrosis was occurring (→) (*Fig. 20*).

Case 4 Pulmonary cryptococcosis

40-year-old male

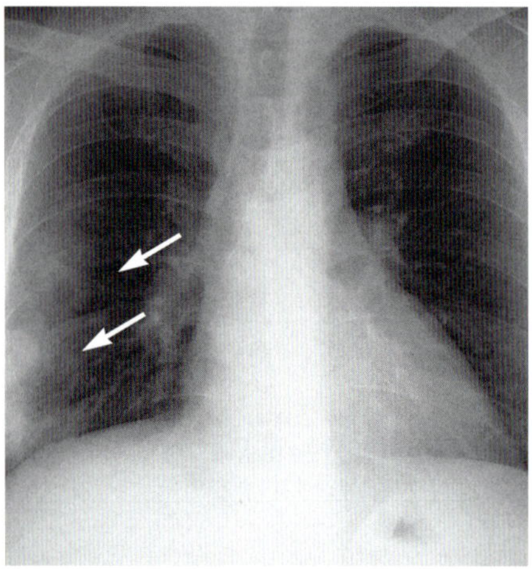

Figure21. **Chest radiograph**

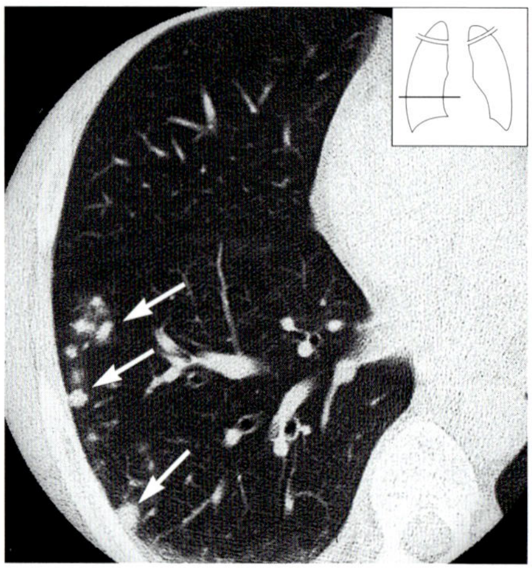

Figure 22. **Chest CT: on admission**

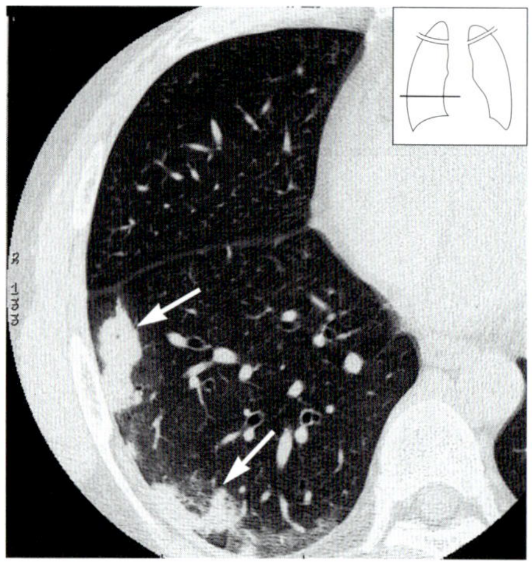

Figure 23. **Chest CT: 3 weeks after admission**

Received an examination as an outpatient after complaining of a cough. No fever observed.

A chest radiograph showed infiltrative shadow (→) in the right lower lung field. Nodules (→) indicating transbronchial scattering were observed in a chest CT before admission, but a chest CT 3 weeks later showed enlarged nodular shadows and adhesion (→).

A transbronchial lung biopsy verified the presence of granulomas and spherical bacterial bodies inside giant cells, and cryptococcosis was diagnosed. A Grocott stain clearly indicated the presence of *Cryptococcus*.

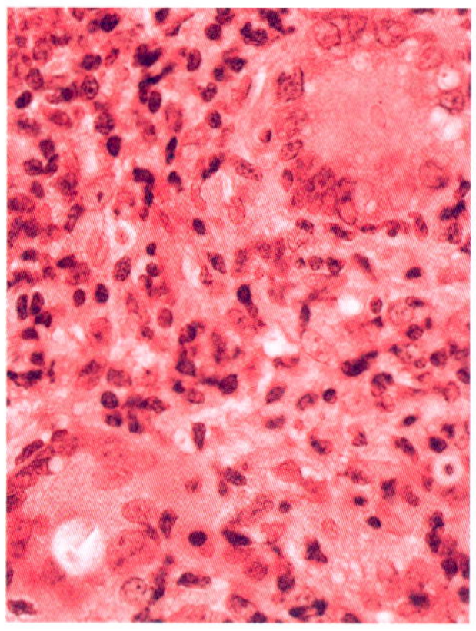

Figure 24. **Pathological findings: Transbronchial lung biopsy**

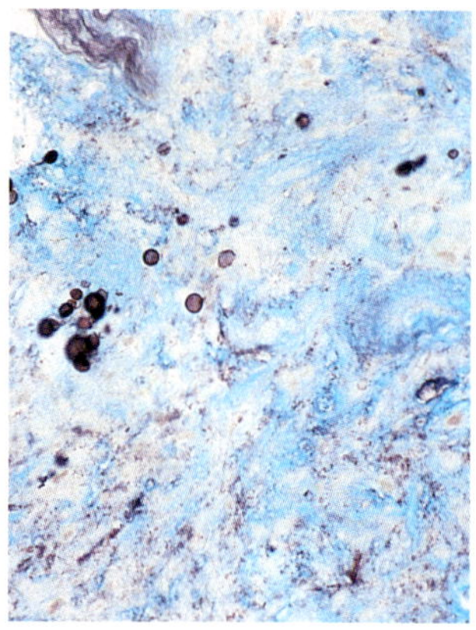

Figure 25. **Pathological findings: Grocott stain**

Case 5 Pulmonary nocardiosis

64-year-old male

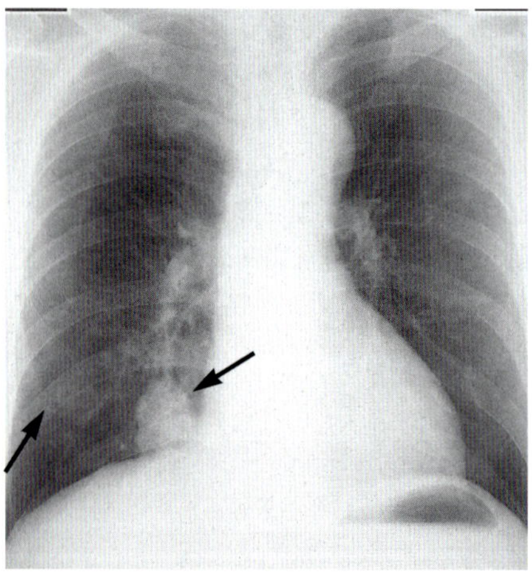

Figure 26. **Chest radiograph**

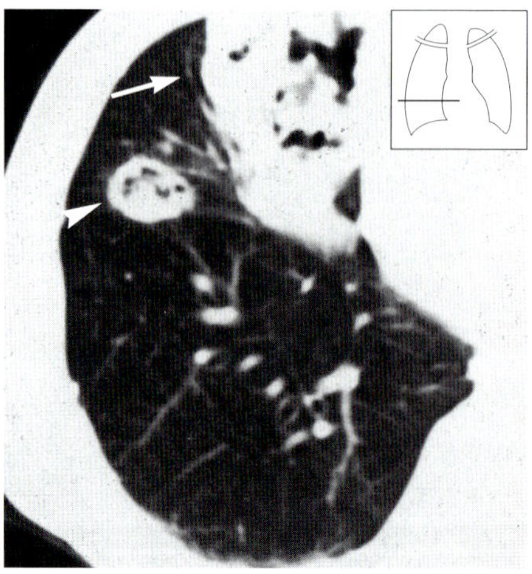

Figure 27. **Chest CT**

A patient diagnosed with nephrotic syndrome undergoing treatment with steroids.

A plain frontal chest radiograph shows multiple nodu-

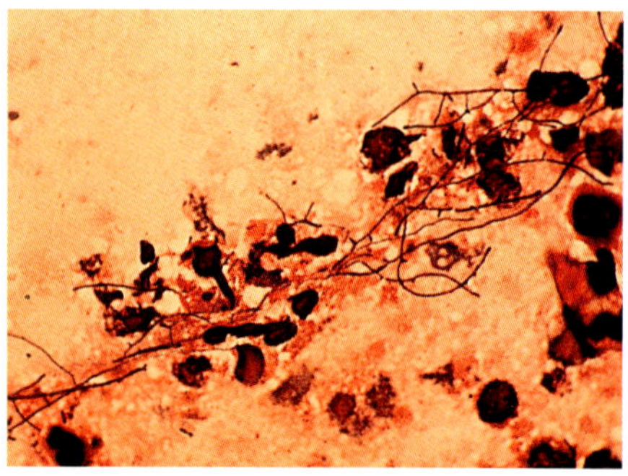

Figure 28. **Nocardia**

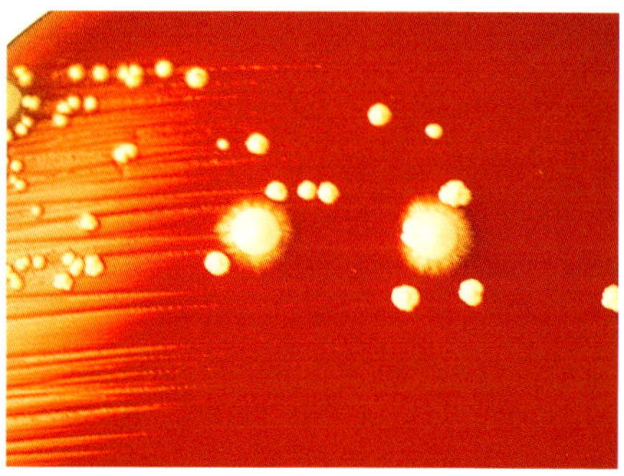

Figure 29. **Nocardia colonies on blood agar**

lar shadows (→) accompanied by cavities in the right lung field.

A chest CT shows tumor-like consolidation (→) in the center of right S^5, with multiple cavity formation inside. A 2.5 cm nodular shadow (➤) can also be seen in right S^4. *Nocardia* was detected in both sputum and bronchoalveolar lavage fluid. In addition, *Nocardia* colonies were seen to grow on blood agar.

Case 6 Pulmonary amyloidosis

68-year-old female

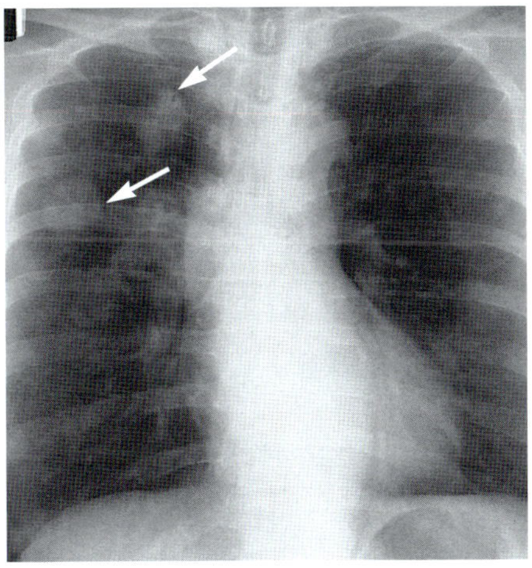

Figure 30. **Chest radiograph**

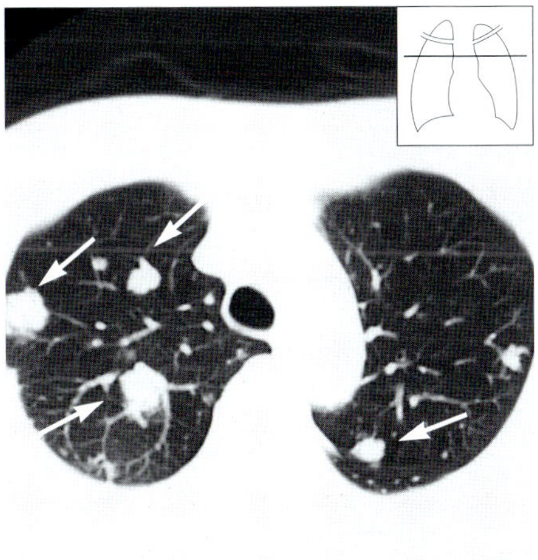

Figure 31. **Chest CT**

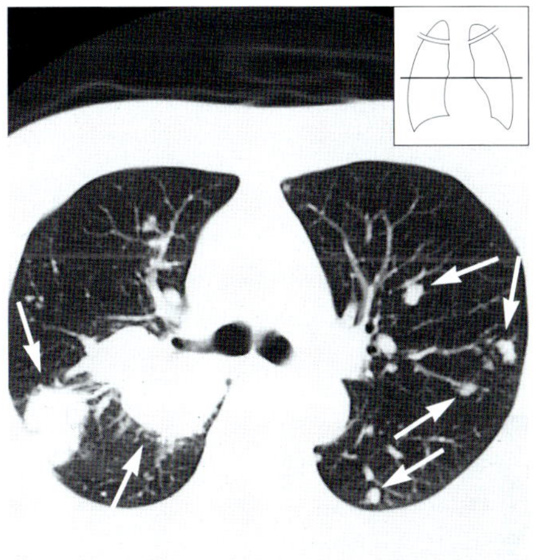

Figure 32. **Chest CT**

Asymptomatic, but abnormal chest shadow was indicated.

Multiple nodular shadows (→) are observed in chest radiograph and chest CT.

After a transbronchial lung biopsy, pulmonary amyloidosis was diagnosed. No complications of multiple myeloma or collagen disease were observed.

Case 7 Pneumoconiosis (silicosis)

57-year-old male

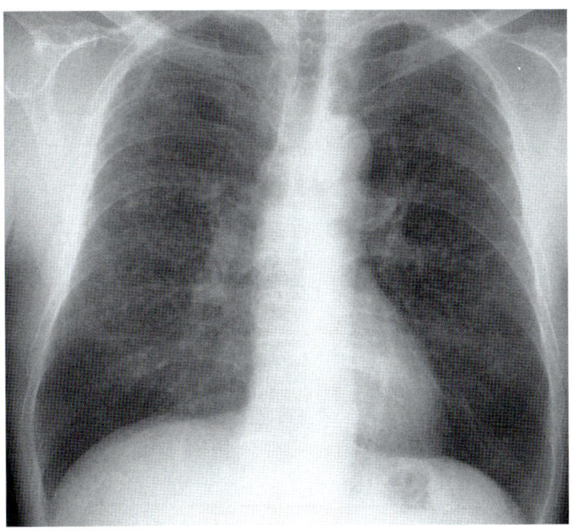

Figure 33. **Chest radiograph**

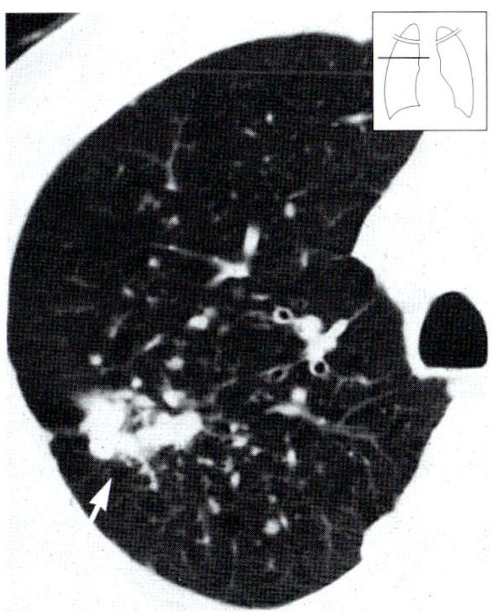

Figure 34. **Chest CT**

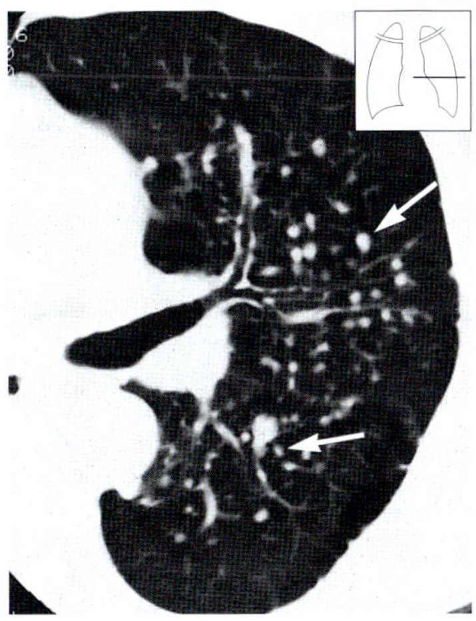

Figure 35. **Chest CT**

A patient with a long history of tunnel construction work, with the chief complaints of dyspnea on exertion, cough and sputum.

A chest radiograph shows bilateral diffuse nodular shadows.

In a chest CT, nodular shadows (→) can be observed in the bronchioles and bronchiole area, a typical indication of silicosis.

Conclusion

Nodular shadows are generally 8 mm or larger in size, but as mentioned earlier, they can occur together with smaller nodular shadows. They are also often accompanied by cavities. The following is an outline of typical diseases that show multiple nodular shadows.

Metastatic lung cancer

This is the most frequently encountered disease showing multiple nodular shadows. The nodules are spherical with either distinct or indistinct borders. Cavity formation is observed in roughly 5% of cases. It is sometimes possible to infer the primary site of origin by the size and border characteristics of nodules. For example, with a miliary metastatic pattern, consider metastasis from thyroid cancer or lung cancer. If the nodules are large, metastasis could have occurred from testicular cancer or sarcoma.

In the primary stage, the nodules may be only unilateral but they are generally bilateral. Calcification may be seen in cases of metastasis from ovarian cancer, mammary cancer, testicular cancer, osteosarcoma and chondrosarcoma.

Alveolar cell carcinoma

There are cases of bilateral multiple nodules but it is unclear whether they are multiple due to metastasis from the primary focus or scattered.

Malignant lymphoma

This is often accompanied by hilar and mediastinal lymph node enlargement, and in many cases borders are indistinct.

Other benign lung tumors

With pulmonary hamartoma nodules are generally solitary but on rare occasions they can be multiple. Borders are distinct, with popcorn-like calcification. They often occur as a complication of multiple myeloma, and are observed with pulmonary plasmacytoma. With pulmonary amyloidosis, they are accompanied by calcification and cavities. Multiple nodules are also seen with pulmonary chondroma. The borders are distinct and calcification is sometimes observed. Consider Kaposi's sarcoma with AIDS patients.

Pulmonary tuberculosis and atypical mycobacteriosis

These diseases progress transbronchially, forming centrolobular and acinar nodules (5 to 7 mm), and lobular nodules (1.5 to 2.0 cm). In general, many cases of tuberculosis involve the apex of the lung (S^1, S^2 and S^6), but in many cases of atypical mycobacteriosis it is centrilobular and lingular.

Bacterial pneumonia

Multiple nodules are formed by hematogenous pneumonia involving *Staphylococcus*.

Opportunistic infection

Patients undergoing immunosuppression show multiple nodular shadows due to a variety of infectious diseases (*Staphylococcus*, *Cryptococcus*, *Nocardia*, *Aspergillus*, *Candida* and *Pneumocystis carinii*).

Aspergillus

Multiple nodular shadows are sometimes seen with *Aspergillus* pneumonia. In many cases they are accompanied by cavities. Nodular shadows are also seen with the mucoid impaction observed in allergic bronchial pulmonary aspergillosis.

Sarcoidosis

Although rare, 0.5 to 3 cm nodules are sometimes observed.

Granulomas not caused by infection

Examples include pulmonary rheumatoid nodules (often accompanied by cavities), Wegener's granulomatosis, pneumoconiosis, pulmonary eosinophilic granuloma, lymphomatoid granulomatosis, bronchocentric granulomatosis and allergic granulomatosis (Churg-Strauss syndrome).

Parasites

Although rare, multiple nodules are seen with some parasitic diseases.

Pulmonary arterio-venous fistula

The nodules are spherical and lobed, with distinct borders and uniform internal density.

Pseudonodules due to extrapulmonary causes

Nodular-like shadows are sometimes seen in chest radiographs due to pleural plaque, papillary and skin tumors, subcutaneous nodules and localized hydrothorax.

Two or more diseases

Take into consideration that multiple nodules may be seen in the presence of two or more diseases that cause nodules.

When differentiating these nodules, important points to consider are whether the nodules are broadly classified as being bilaterally distributed, distributed along lymph ducts, or distributed hematogenously. Clarification in the case of lesions enable the pathology to be inferred, and, it should also be stressed, enable the breadth of differential diagnosis to be narrowed down.

References

- Felson, B.: Chest roentgenology. Saunders, Philadelphia, 1973
- Fraser, R. S. et al.: Diagnosis of diseases of the chest (4th ed.), Saunders, Philadelphia, 1999
- Lillington, G. A.: A diagnostic approach to chest diseases (3rd ed.), Williams & Wilkins, Baltimore, 1987
- Fujita, J. et al.: Pathological and immunohistochemical findings of resected lung specimens obtained from patients with *Mycobacterium avium intracellulare* complex. Eur. Respir. J. 13: 535–540, 1999

10. Ring shadow:
Cavity
[Pattern classification IV-E-1]

●Author — Yasuji Terada

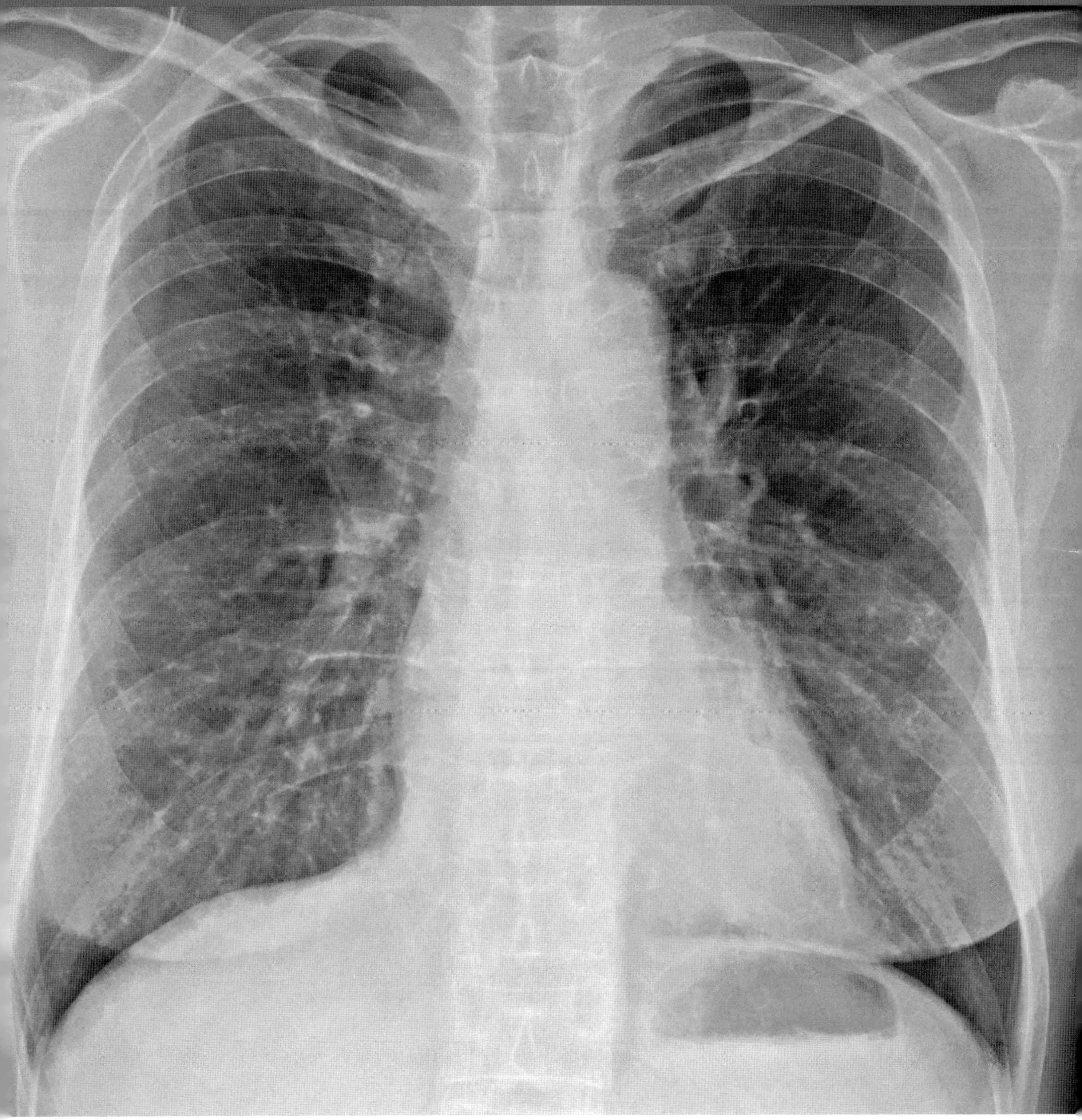

Keywords of this section

Cavity
Pleural indentation
Adenocarcinoma
Central necrosis
Wegener's granulomatosis
Staphylococcus aureus abscess
Pulmonary tuberculosis
Squamous cell carcinoma
Air-fluid level
Pulmonary aspergillosis
Fungus ball
Infectious bulla
Bronchogenic cyst
Echinococcus cyst
Metastatic lung cancer
Water lily sign

Cavity

Yasuji Terada
Department of Thoracic Surgery, Nagahama City Hospital, Nagahama, Shiga, Japan

In chest radiographs, lesions that have changed due to air in the center of the focus, which shows as increased density, are called cavities. They do not necessarily have an air-fluid level, and there is no limit to their size and wall thickness. Diagnosis of cavities using chest radiographs is difficult, but some can be easily identified with CT. Case 1 is an example of this.

Case 1 60-year-old female

Chief complaint: Abnormal shadow in chest radiograph
Medical history: Nothing of particular note
Family history: Nothing of particular note
Smoking history: None
Present illness:
Since a medical checkup in the spring of 1999 revealed an abnormal shadow in a chest radiograph and a mass shadow accompanied by a cavity in left S^6 in chest CT, the patient was referred to a local hospital for examination. No excretion of tubercle bacilli was observed but since the patient showed a strongly positive tuberculin reaction she was diagnosed as tuberculosis, admitted to hospital for 6 months and treated with antitubercular agents. However, although no excretion of bacilli was observed while in hospital, and despite the administration of antitubercular agents, no change was observed in CT. As a result, the patient was referred to this hospital for examination early the following year.

Although cytological examination of sputum and bronchoscopic examination revealed no malignant findings, lung cancer could not be ruled out and the patient was admitted for surgery.

Physical findings and laboratory data revealed no abnormalities, and about 3 weeks later an exploratory thoracotomy was performed.

In a chest radiograph (P. 117), a mass shadow roughly 2 cm in diameter with indistinct border can be observed on the outer side of the left central lung field. A cavity (→) can be observed in a close-up view (*Fig. 1*).

A chest CT (*Fig. 2*) shows a tumor shadow (→) with irregular border and cavity in left S^6. As wall thickness and density are nonuniform, no scattered image is observed.

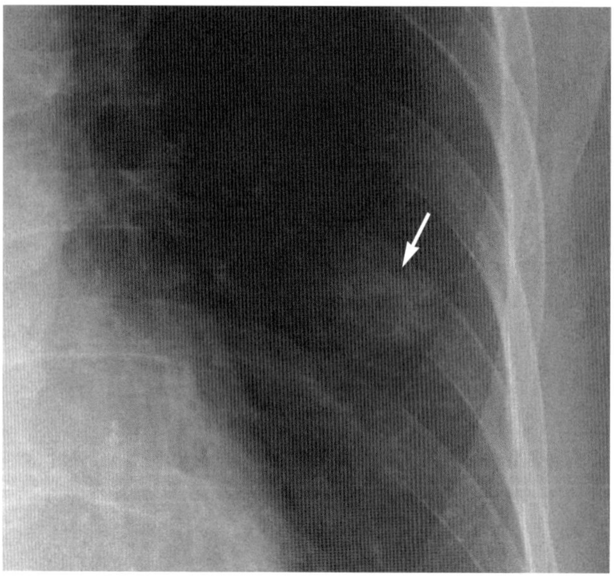

Figure 1. **Chest radiograph: Close-up view**

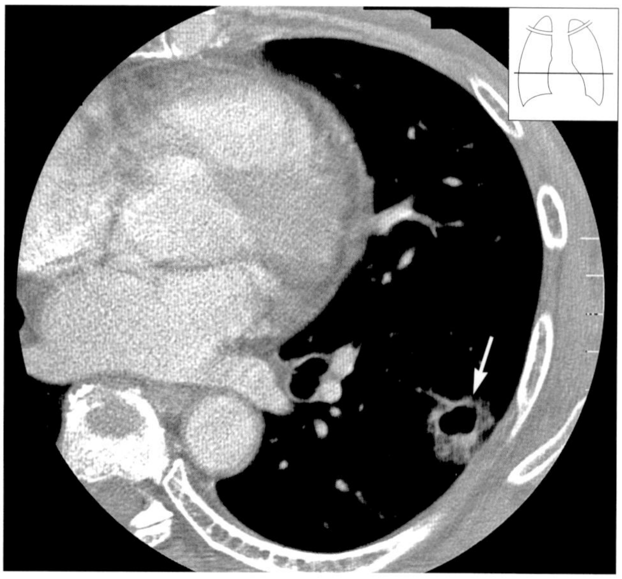

Figure 2. **Chest CT**

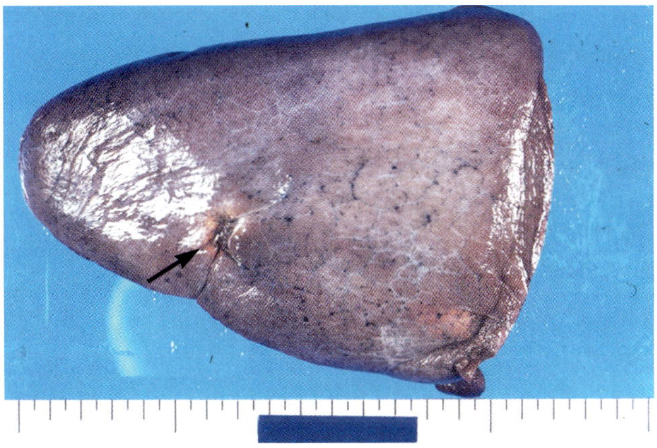

Figure 3. **Macroscopic specimen: Left side is cranial**

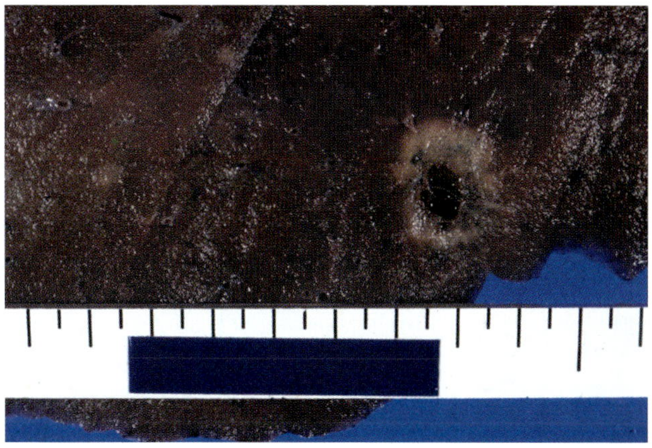

Figure 4. **Macroscopic specimen: Close-up view of a cut**

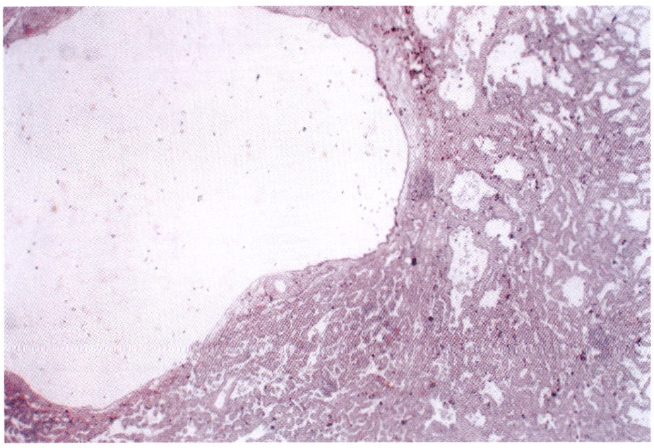

Figure 5. **Histological findings: HE stain, x 10**

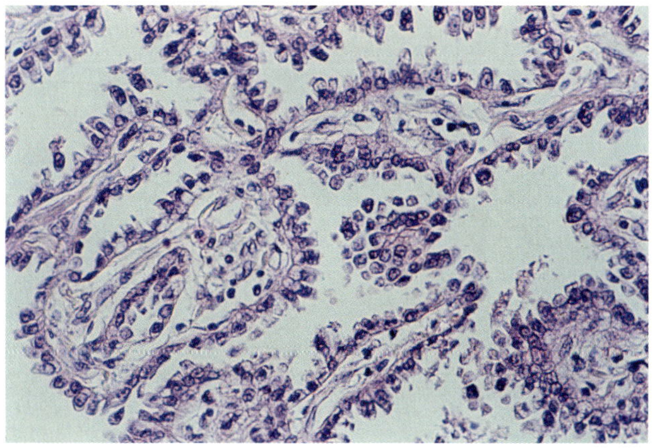

Figure 6. **Histological findings: HE stain, x 200**

Diagnosis

At the operation, an elastic hard mass with pleural indentation was palpable in S^{6}b. After intraoperative aspiration cytology, a diagnosis of adenocarcinoma was obtained. There was no lymph node metastasis to the hilum or mediastinum, and resection of the left lower lobe was performed.

A fixed macroscopic specimen (*Fig. 3*) shows pleural indentation, and as indicated by a CT, a close-up view of the cut surface (*Fig. 4*) shows a cavity accompanying a tumorous lesion.

In low magnification histopathological findings (HE stain, x 10, *Fig. 5*), no necrotic changes can be observed in the area surrounding the cavity. A high magnification (HE stain, x 200, *Fig. 6*) image shows idioblasts with distinct nucleoli with nuclear inclusion bodies, and nuclear groove indicating glandular cavity and papillary structures, which are findings of papillary type adenocarcinoma.

Conclusion of this case: Adenocarcinoma

Diagnosis is easy when a chest radiograph shows a cavity accompanied by air-fluid level, but for small cavities with nonuniform, nonpermeable areas (opacity) and cavities located near the mediastinum that are hard to diagnose analytically, diagnosis using chest radiograph alone is difficult. It was also difficult to verify the presence of a cavity in this case using radiographs, but clear verification was possible with CT. When tumorous or cavity lesions are suspected, tomography was previously useful for confirming diagnoses, but recently with the increasing use of CT, the location and size of cavities, and cavity wall and surrounding tissue characteristics are now clearly shown. There are even cases that can be verified by CT, and the use of CT is recommended as much as possible when an indistinct image is observed. It is thought that the cause of malignant neoplasm cavities is necrosis in the central areas resulting from insufficient blood flow, with many cases being seen with comparatively large squamous cell carcinomas. Nevertheless, as with this case, cavities are also sometimes exhibited with small adenocarcinomas. The view is that this is simply due to ischemia and cavity formation by another mechanism. From the above, even if a small tumorous shadow is accompanied by a cavity, malignant diseases must be included in the differential diagnosis.

Differentiation of cavities

Pulmonary ring shadows are caused either by cavities resulting from nodule tissue necrosis or by cysts covering airway epithelium. In many cases of cysts there are enlarged air spaces with an extremely thin wall showing as a spherical ring shadow and a typical example is bulla. In contrast to this, cavities are caused by necrosis of pulmonary tissue or tumors, with necrotic debris being expelled and replaced with intrabronchial gas. In radiographs, cavities are usually seen as an air space enclosed by a thick wall. There are also cavities with thin walls, so wall thickness alone is not sufficient to clearly differentiate between cavities and cysts.

The characteristics of the inside and outside surfaces of cavities vary widely depending on the disease and disease stage. Some cavities can be clearly seen in plain chest radiographs but if they are accompanied by nonuniform opacity or high-density infiltrative shadow, in many cases diagnosis is only possible by CT.

For differentiation, cavity characteristics include 1) cavity wall thickness, 2) cavity wall inner surface characteristics (smooth, uneven and irregular), 3) presence or absence of an air-fluid level, 4) presence or absence of a mass shadow inside the cavity (meniscus sign), and 5) infiltration shadow surrounding the cavity.

One disease other than cyst diseases that cavities should be differentiated from is sliding hernia. In chest radiographs, a sliding hernia appears dorsal to the heart with a wall that is not particularly thick, but depending on the volume of air it can be spherical or irregularly shaped. In some cases it also shows air-fluid level formation. An esophagram enables easy differential diagnosis of sliding hernia.

Case 2 Wegener's granulomatosis

54-year-old male

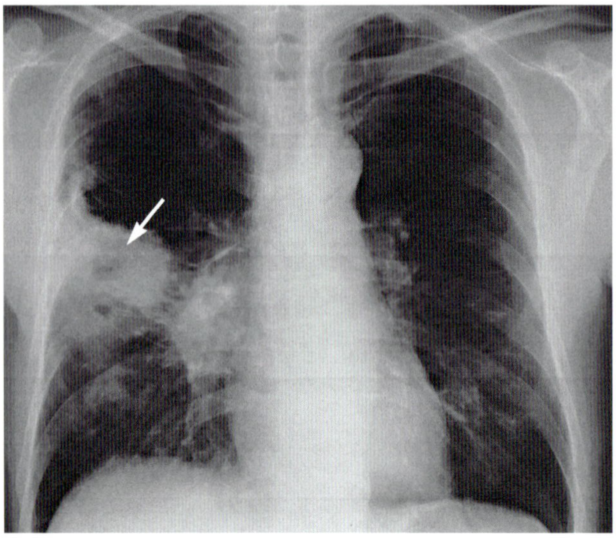

Figure 7. **Chest radiograph**

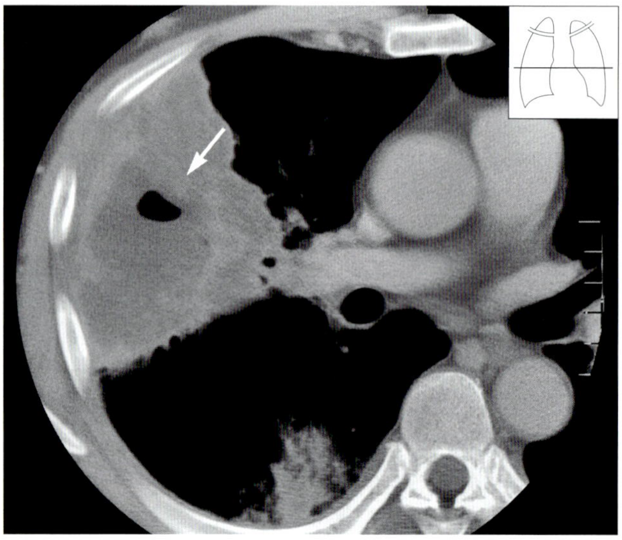

Figure 8. **Chest CT**

The patient received an examination at a local hospital for the major complaints of cough, fever and nasal pain. A chest radiograph showed infiltrative shadow in the right upper lung field, and he was referred to this hospital.

A chest radiograph shows a mass lesion with accompanying cavity in the right upper lobe, and infiltrative shadow in the right hilar area (→).

A chest CT shows a nonuniformly contrasted mass lesion with irregular border and accompanying cavity (→), with a noncontrasted part thought to be necrosis. In images other than this chest CT, a small tumor shadow was also observed on the left side, with tumors on both sides showing a tendency to enlarge.

An open lung biopsy was performed and Wegener's granulomatosis was diagnosed.

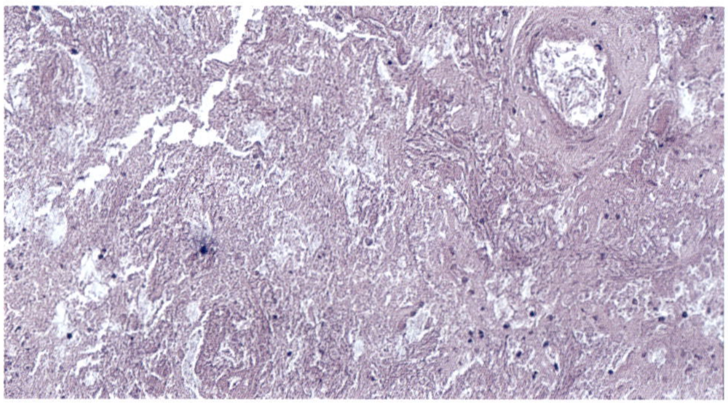

Figure 9. **Histological findings: HE stain, x 40**

Regarding pathological findings, perivascular inflammation can be observed. After the diagnosis, steroid treatment was started with prednisolone 60 mg/day, the symptoms disappeared and the patient stabilized.

Case 3 *Staphylococcus aureus* abscess

58-year-old male

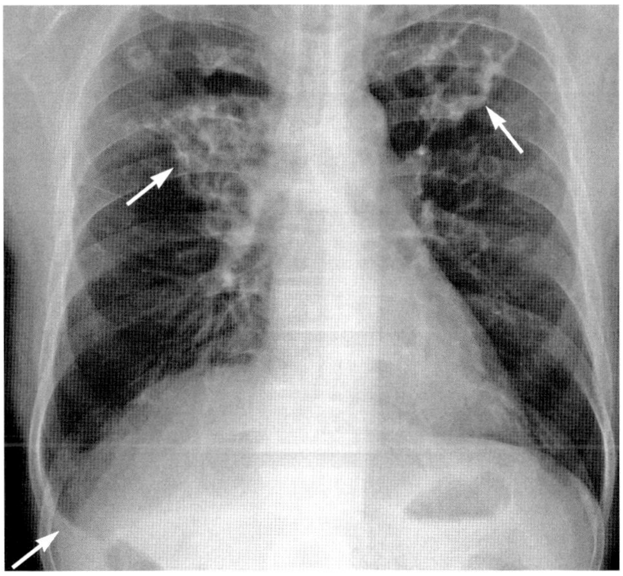

Figure 10. **Chest radiograph**

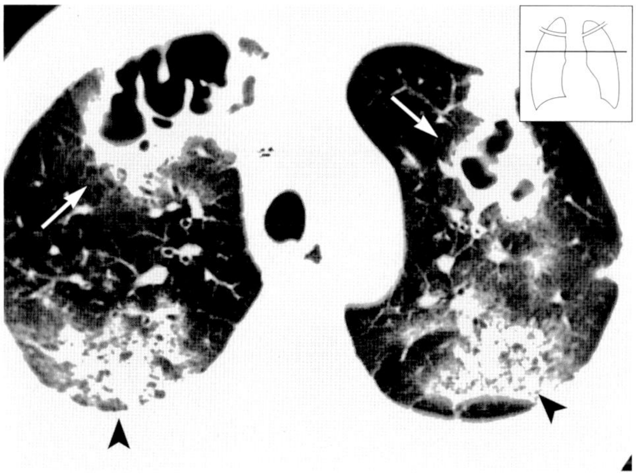

Figure 11. **Chest CT**

During hospitalization for another disease the patient developed a cough and fever, and a chest radiograph revealed an infiltrative shadow. Later, the infiltrative shadow spread throughout both lungs and was accompanied by cavities. *Staphylococcus aureus* was observed in sputum, and *Staphylococcus aureus* abscess was diagnosed.

A chest radiograph shows reactive pleural effusion retention on the right side (lower right →), and cavities with comparatively thin walls at the cranial side of the right hilar area and in the left lung field (→ in both upper lung fields).

A chest CT shows that cavity walls are irregular regardless of size (→), and the bilateral infiltration shadow (➤) is not accompanied by cavities.

Case 4 Pulmonary tuberculosis

48-year-old female

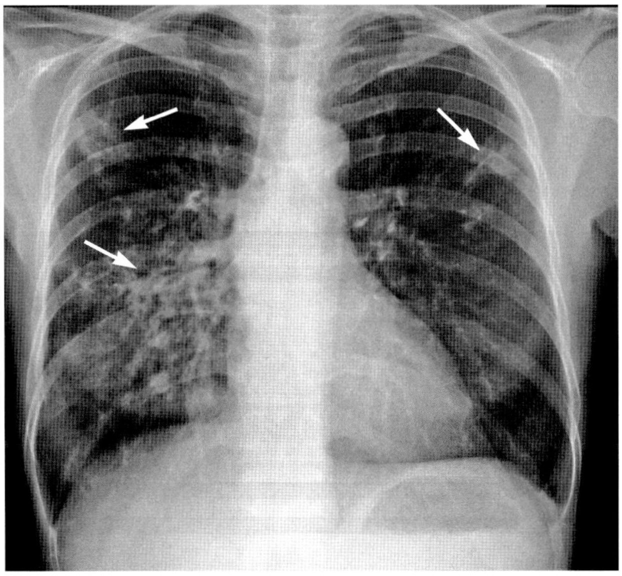

Figure 12. **Chest radiograph**

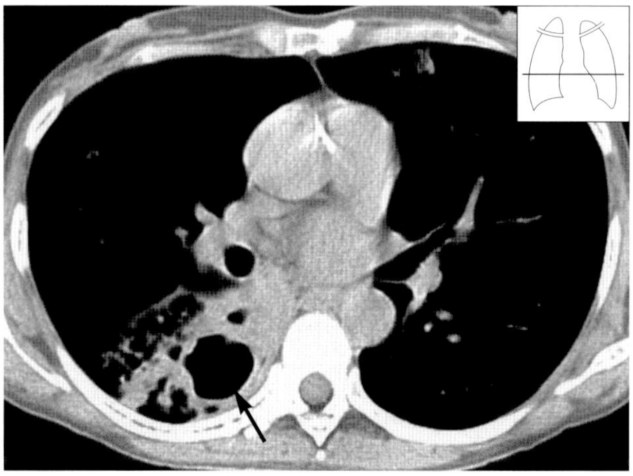

Figure 13. **Chest CT**

The patient was examined at a local hospital for continuous cough and fever. An infiltrative shadow was indicated in the right lower lung field, and the patient was referred to this department.

A chest radiograph shows a scattered infiltrative shadow in right S^6 (→), and additional infiltrative shadows in bilateral lung fields.

A chest CT shows a cavity with a comparatively smooth wall in right S^6 (→) surrounded by infiltrative shadow. After admission, Gaffky 7 tuberculosis bacilli were detected in sputum, and the patient was treated with antitubercular agents.

Case 5 Squamous cell carcinoma

78-year-old male

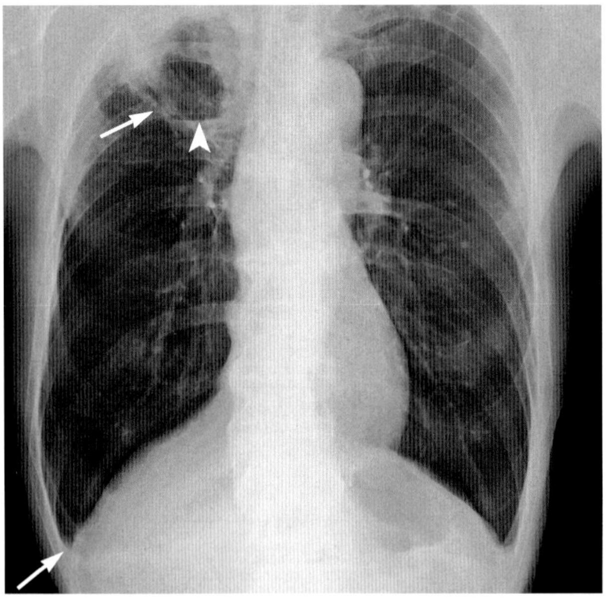

Figure 14. **Chest radiograph**

The patient received a medical examination for right back pain. A chest radiograph showed a cavity in the right upper lung field, and he was referred to this department. A bronchoscopy confirmed a tumor apparently completely obstructing B^1, and after a biopsy squamous cell carcinoma was diagnosed.

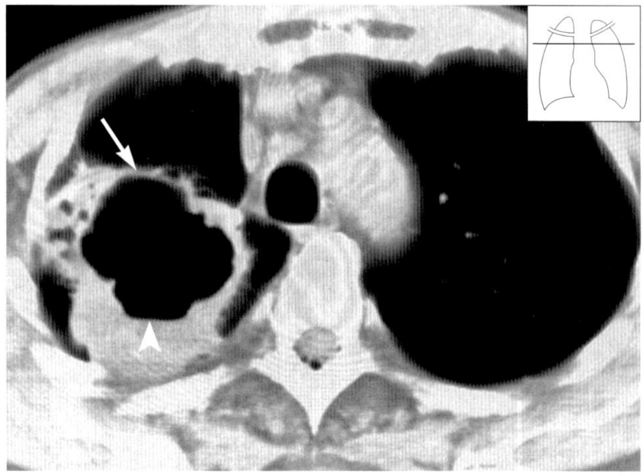

Figure 15. **Chest CT**

A chest radiograph shows that on the right side the costophrenic angle is a little blunt (bottom →), there is mild pleural effusion retention, and a cavity in the right apex (top→) with air-fluid level formation at the lower border (➤).

A chest CT shows a cavity in the right upper lobe with irregular wall of nonuniform thickness (→), with air-fluid level formation at the lower border of the cavity (➤).

Case 6 Pulmonary aspergillosis

78-year-old male

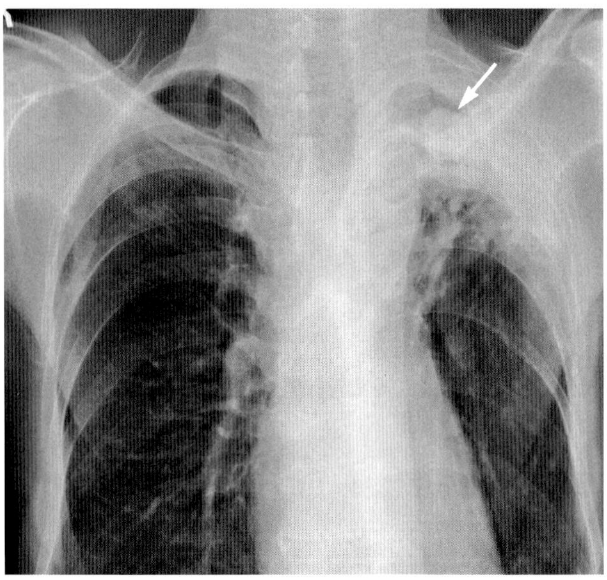

Figure 16. **Chest radiograph**

The patient visited hospital with the chief complaint of coughing. He had a past medical history of pulmonary tuberculosis and a cavity was observed in the left pulmonary apex on chest radiograph. An antitussive and antibiotics were administered but no improvement in symptoms was observed.

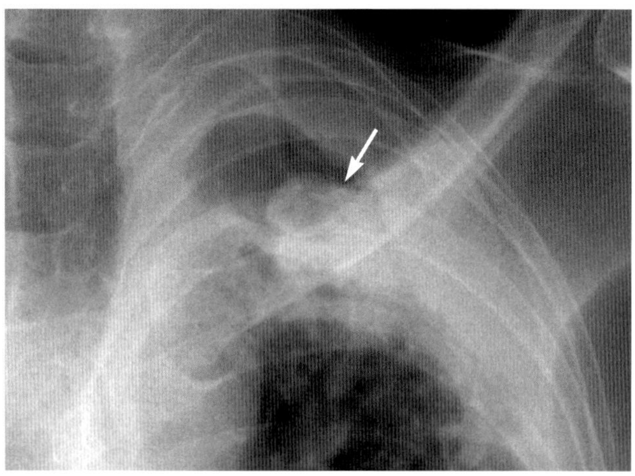

Figure 17. **Chest radiograph: Close-up view**

During observation over an extended period, the inside of the cavity tended to enlarge, a fungus ball appeared (*Fig. 16*), and pulmonary aspergillosis was diagnosed.

Symptoms improved with administration of antifungal agents. Since the patient has no symptoms at present, he is under extended observation as an outpatient.

A chest radiograph shows a cavity in the left pulmonary apex (→), with a spherical fungus ball inside.

A close-up view enables clear verification (→).

A chest CT also enables verification of the fungus ball (→). In most cases of fungus ball, it is seen in old pulmonary tuberculosis cavities, but in rare cases it can also occur in enlarged bronchi. It usually touches the wall but it may have mobility, changing location depending on posture.

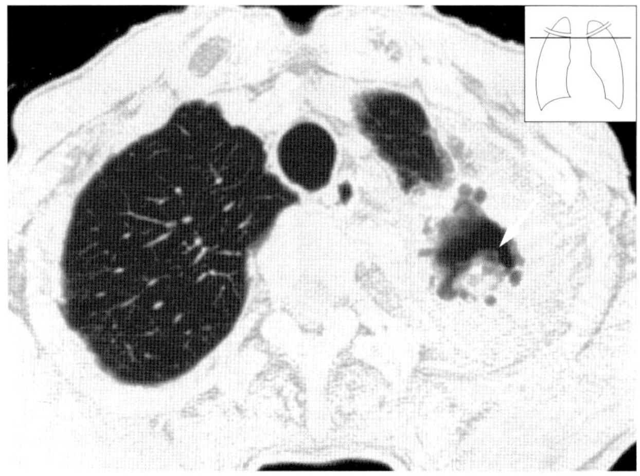

Figure 18. **Chest CT**

Case 7 Infectious bulla

73-year-old male

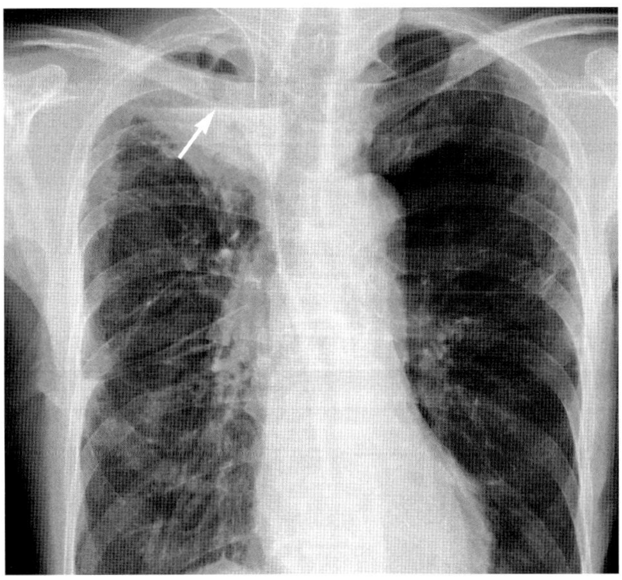

Figure 19. **Chest radiograph**

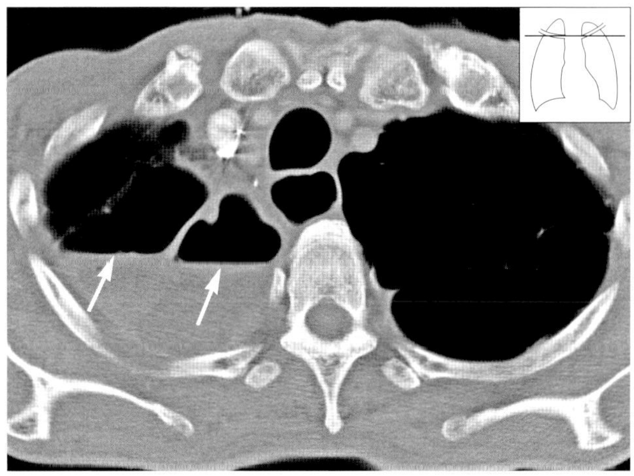

Figure 20. **Chest CT**

Patient had continuous high fever following subtotal esophagectomy by right thoracotomy for esophageal cancer.

A chest radiograph showed bullae in bilateral pulmonary apexes but air-fluid level formation (→) was observed in the bulla on the right side, and it was diagnosed as infectious bulla.

A chest CT also showed fluid retention in two bullae in the right pulmonary apex (→), with slightly different fluid level heights, and walls comparatively thicker than those of ordinary bullae. An Aspiration kit® was inserted into each of the infectious bullae from the axilla and back, and debridement and irrigation were continued until the cysts healed.

In chest radiographs, a cavity is defined either as an area of increased density, in which the center has been replaced with air, regardless of size or wall characteristics,[1] or as a ring shadow with a thick, irregular wall 2 mm or more thick,[2] When differentiating from bullae, if the wall is thick there is no problem calling it a bulla but it is difficult if the wall is thin. The following is a list of cases generally called cavities.

Most pulmonary cavities are due to tissue necrosis followed by discharge of necrotic debris into the airway. Causes other than this are extremely rare, and examples are rupture of bronchogenic cyst and Echinococcus cyst, and infection to cystic space-like bullae.

The mechanism behind necrosis differs depending on the underlying disease. During the course of acute *Staphylococcus* infection, tissue dies due to the toxin of the bacilli. With pulmonary embolism due to sepsis, it is believed that both insufficient blood flow and inflammation play a role. It is thought that insufficient blood flow is involved in more than a few malignant neoplasm cavities. However, since even extremely small malignant tumors (diameter of 1 cm or less) exhibit cavities, another mechanism is thought to be involved.

In specific diseases the characteristics of cavity formation differ widely, but in most cases with ordinary patients there are findings that suggest an underlying disease. Regardless of the case, factors that must be considered when viewing radiographs of pulmonary cavities include cavity wall thickness, whether the line of the inside wall of the cavity is regular or not, whether the cavity contains anything, and if it does, the characteristics of the contents, whether the lesions are solitary or multiple, and the number of cavities in the case of multiple lesions. Several patterns will be presented as follows, but there are frequent exceptions.

Cavity wall

Usually, a thick wall indicates diseases such as acute pulmonary abscess, primary or metastatic lung cancer or Wegener's granulomatosis. A thin wall points to diseases such as infectious bulla or posttraumatic cyst.

Cavity wall internal line characteristics

In many cases, there is fluid in the center of a cavity but there are no clear characteristics. There are almost no exceptions, and the air-fluid level in the cavity is distinct. With some diseases, cavity contents have sufficient characteristics to be used as diagnostic material. For example, if a mobile fungus ball (mycetoma: aspergilloma) is observed inside a cavity, it is possible to arrive at a diagnosis of pulmonary aspergillosis. Furthermore, the collapsed membrane of a ruptured Echinococcus cyst floats on the fluid surface to exhibit as a characteristic water lily sign. Although rare, a large amount of pulmonary tissue necrosis results in pulmonary gangrene, showing as a characteristic mass shadow inside the cavity.

Multiple lesions

In many cases of disease such as primary lung cancer, acute pulmonary abscess and posttraumatic cyst, lesions are solitary. Multiple lesions can occur with many diseases such as metastatic lung cancer, Wegener's granulomatosis, acute coccidoidomycosis and acute pulmonary abscess.

References

1) Fraser, R. G., Pare, J. A. P.: Diagnosis of diseases of the chest. Saunders, Philadelphia, 1973, p.443
2) Felson, B. : Chest roentgenology. Saunders, Philadelphia, 1973, p.314

Chapter 4

Radiographs of intrapulmonary lesions with decreased radiolucency

11. Ring shadow:

Cystic shadow

[Pattern classification IV-E-2]

●Author — Toshiharu Matsushima

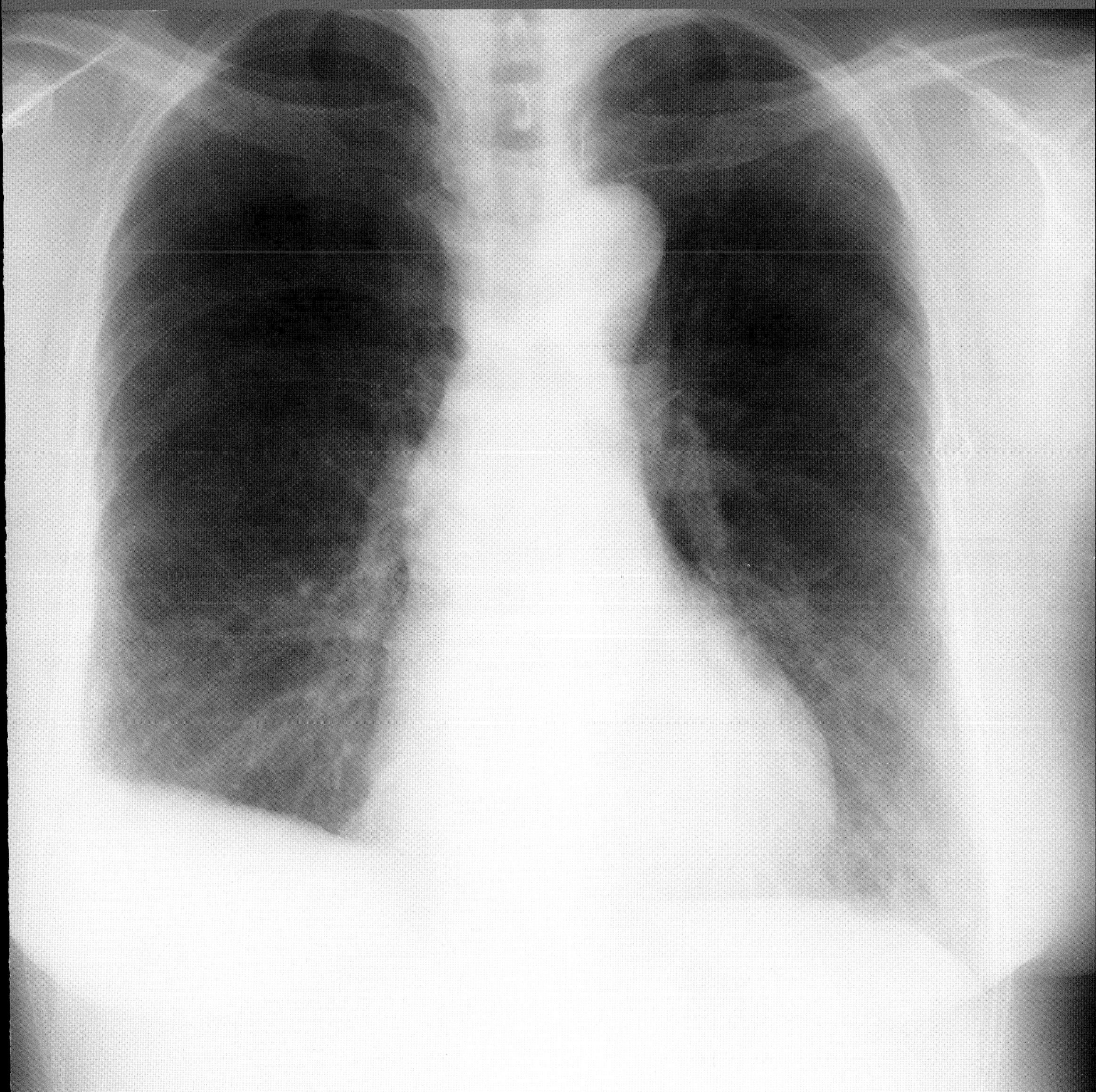

Keywords of this section

Cystic shadow
Pulmonary lymphangiomyomatosis
Tuberous sclerosis
Pulmonary cyst
Pulmonary eosinophilic granuloma
Metastatic lung cancer
Cystic bronchiectasis
Hermansky–Pudlak syndrome
Panlobular emphysema
Centrilobular emphysema

Cystic shadow

Toshiharu Matsushima
Respiratory Center, Kurashiki Daiichi Hospital, Junpukai Foundation, Okayama, Japan

Cystic lesions show on chest radiographs as a hyperlucent shadow surrounded by a thin wall with increased radiolucency. Frequently they are accompanied by ring shadows. Ring shadows with a thin wall are called cysts. Cysts are divided into solitary and multiple types. This section mainly deals with the multiple type with typical cases. Chest CT is also excellent for detecting cystic lesions.

Case 1 38-year-old female

Chief complaint: Dyspnea on exertion (H-J III degree)
Medical history: Epilepsy attacks and facial steatocystoma at school age, and vascular steatocystoma of bilateral kidneys at 21 years of age
Family history: Eldest daughter afflicted with epilepsy, mental retardation and facial steatocystoma (tuberous sclerosis)
Smoking history: None
Occupational history: No work in a dusty environment
Present illness:
Dry cough and dyspnea on exertion since 4–5 years ago, the patient was admitted to a hospital in April 1985 with right-side pneumothorax, and an abnormal shadow was found in a chest radiograph. In October of the same year, she came to our hospital for examination of a lung lesion.
Physical findings on admission:
Steatocystomas on bilateral face, molluscum pendulum on trunk, fibromas on fingers and toes about the nails (Koenen tumor). No fine crackles were audible on auscultation of thorax except slight attenuation of breathing sound.
Laboratory data on admission:
Slight reduction of PaO_2 in arterial blood gas analysis was recognized, but lung function test showed almost normal VC $FEV_{1.0}$ and slight reduction of diffusion capacity.

The spiral CT of a healthy control taken at the level of bilateral bifurcating B^6 (*Fig. 4*) shows the pulmonary

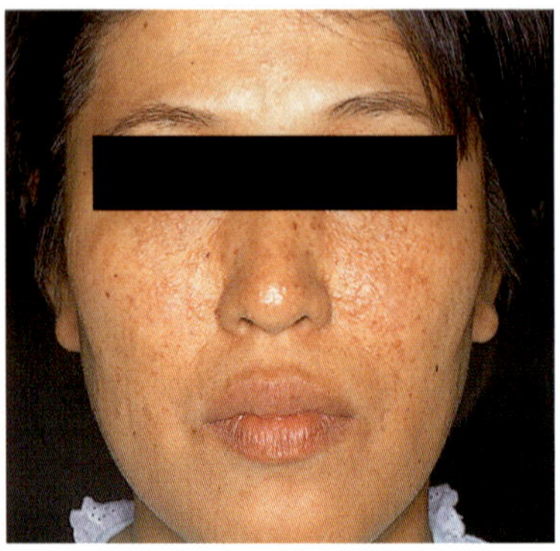

Figure 1. **Facial steatocystoma**

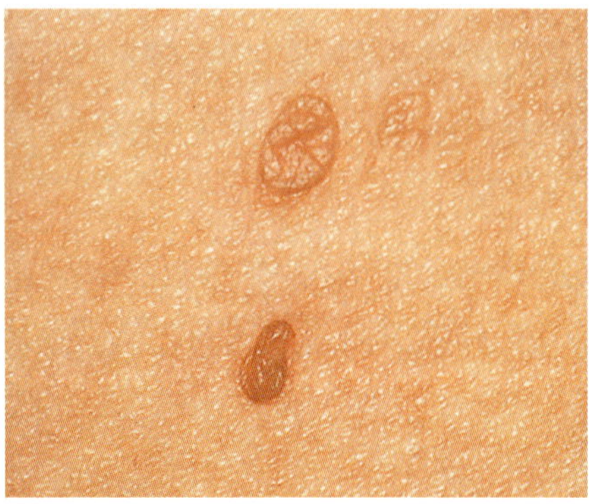

Figure 2. **Molluscum pendulum**

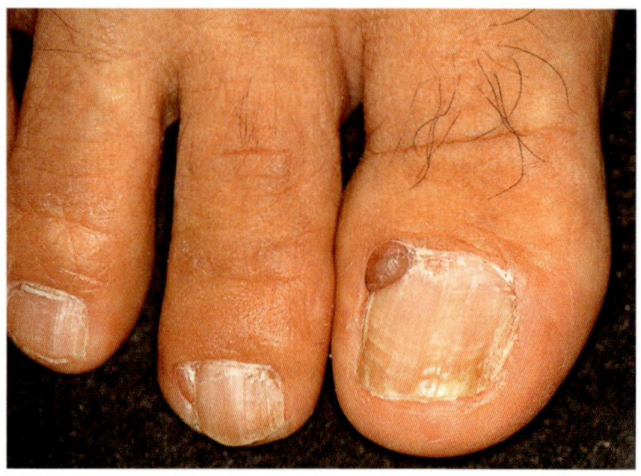

Figure 3. **Koenen tumor**

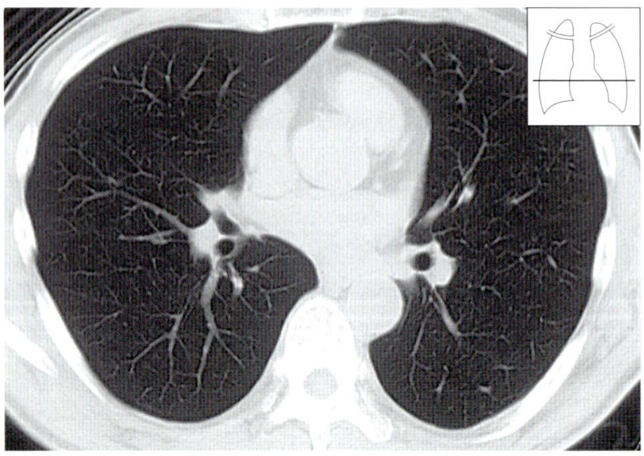

Figure 4. **Spiral CT of a healthy control person**

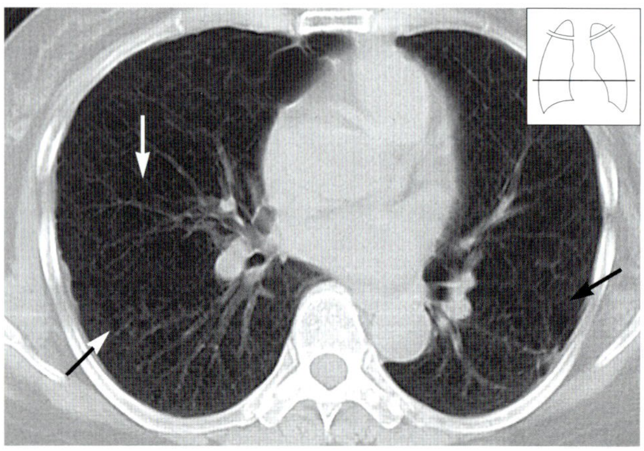

Figure 5. **Spiral CT of the patient, showing multiple cystic lesions**

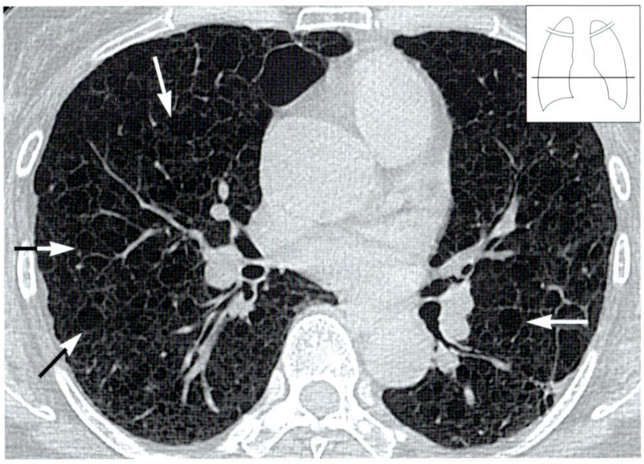

Figure 6. **HRCT of the patient**

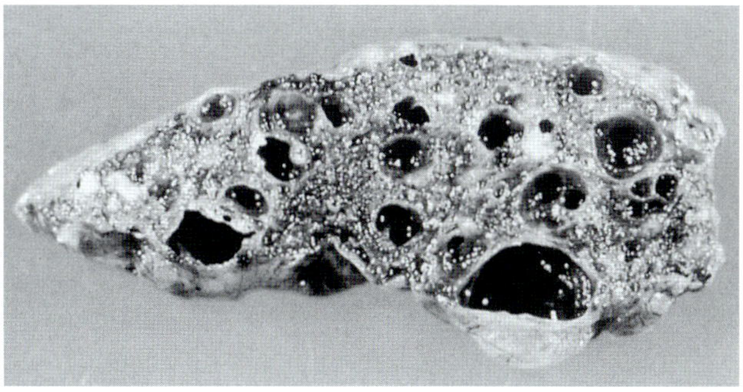

Figure 7. **Biopsy specimen**

artery and vein gradually branching and reaching the periphery. The bronchus of bilateral basal bronchus, left side B^6 and B^4 are visible. However, the CT of Case 1 (*Fig.* 5) taken at the same level showed only large to medium blood vessels, and a reticular pattern. HRCT (1-mm slices) (*Fig. 6*) of the same case reveals formation of numerous cysts, corresponding to the biopsy findings (*Fig.* 7).

CT is very convenient for showing ring shadows. In particular, HRCT is suitable for revealing cysts and bullae.

Diagnosis

The conventional chest radiograph (P.125) shows diffuse nodular and reticular shadows in bilateral lung fields, but volume reduction is less pronounced and radiolucency is rather enhanced in the upper lung fields. Numerous ring shadows on CT could indicate cystic lesions.

The lung biopsy showed numerous emphysematous cysts of 5–15 mm in diameter, the so-called "Ikura" (roe) shape as shown in *Figure 7*. Histologically, swelling and hyperplasia of smooth muscles affecting the pleura, bronchiole walls, alveolar septum and perivascular interstitium were observed. There were numerous intrapulmonary cysts of various sizes immediately beneath the pleural surface. These findings corresponded to diffuse pulmonary lymphangiomyomatosis.

Final diagnosis: Pulmonary lymphangiomyomatosis (LAM)

This woman was afflicted by facial steatocystoma, Koenen tumors and steatocystoma of renal blood vessels in her childhood. Although mental retardation was not observed, we could ascertain epilepsy attacks and cerebral calcification. Tuberous sclerosis (TS or Bourneville–Pringle disease) was suggested from family history and confirmed. We also considered that her pulmonary lesions were the result of the disease. TS is characterized by the three main symptoms of facial rash, mental retardation and epilepsy attacks. Lymphangiomyomatosis, believed to originate from mesenchymal and ectomorphic growth impairment, is a hereditary disease that can affect various organs including the skin, brain, eyeballs, retina, kidneys, lung and heart. On the other hand, the main symptoms of LAM are dyspnea, pneumothorax, hemoptysis and chylous hydrothorax. Pathological features are swelling and hyperplasia of smooth muscles in the alveolar and bronchial walls, pulmonary arteries, and lymph vessels. The disease occurs only in women of child-bearing age. Since TS and LAM have the same pathological symptoms, LAM is regarded as an incomplete type of TS, while other authors think they are separate entities.

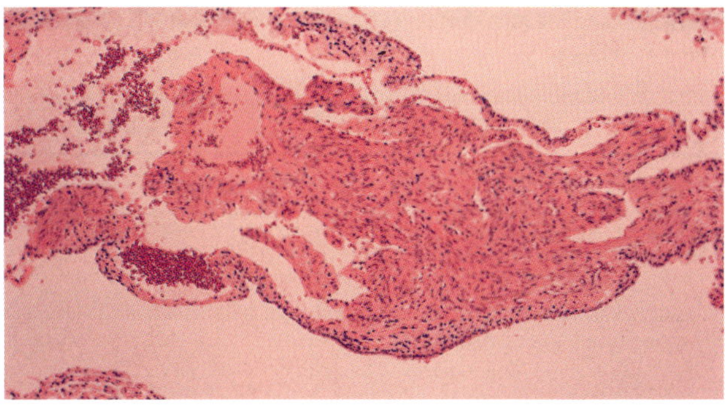

a

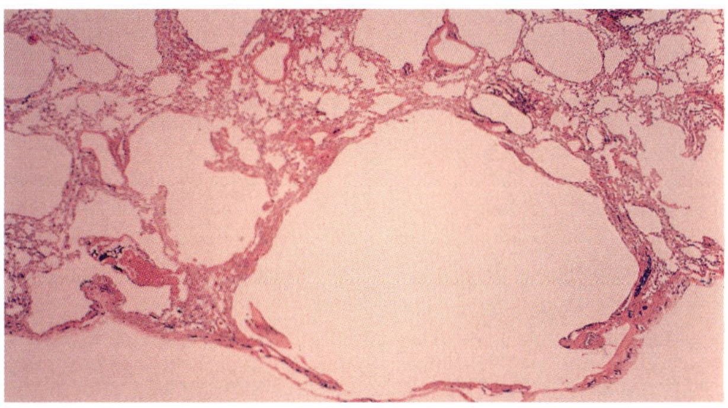

b

Figure 8 a–b. **Lung histology of biopsy**

Differential diagnosis based on cystic sign

What is a cyst?

An intrapulmonary ring shadow with over 2 mm of cavity wall indicates a cavity mainly caused by tissue necrosis of nodules. On the other hand a ring with under 1 mm of wall thickness is called a cyst that is usually covered by airway epithelium. The latter is divided into bronchial cyst covered by bronchial epithelium and alveolar cyst covered by alveolar epithelium. Furthermore, a cyst caused by fusion of the alveolar space, a typical alveolar cyst, is usually called a bulla. A cavity on a radiograph is characterized by ring shadows with thick and irregular walls (≥ 2 mm). A cyst has thin walls (1–2 mm) which can be traced distinctly.[1, 2] A lesion with thinner walls (≤1 mm) with an indistinct border is called a bulla. But these distinctions are sometimes blurred in imaging and clinics. In this section a cyst is defined as a bag-shaped (ring) shadow with thin walls and containing air.

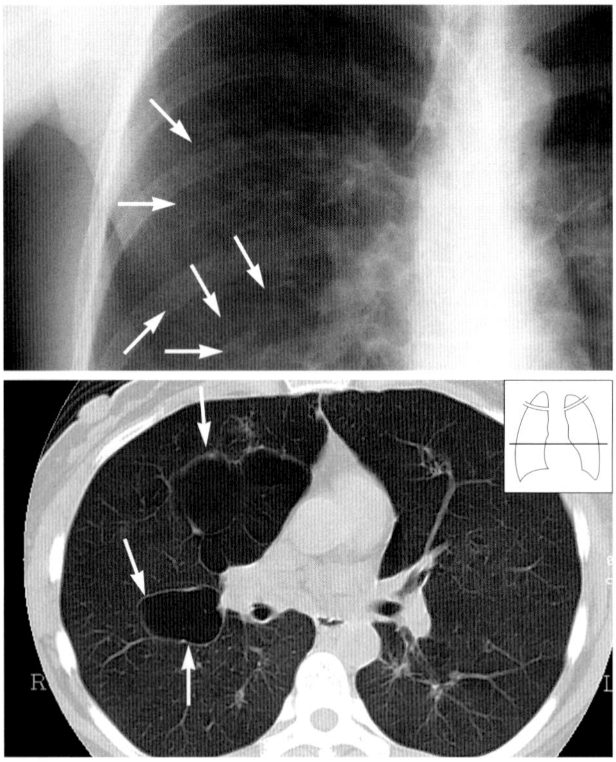

Figure 9 a–b. **Cyst**

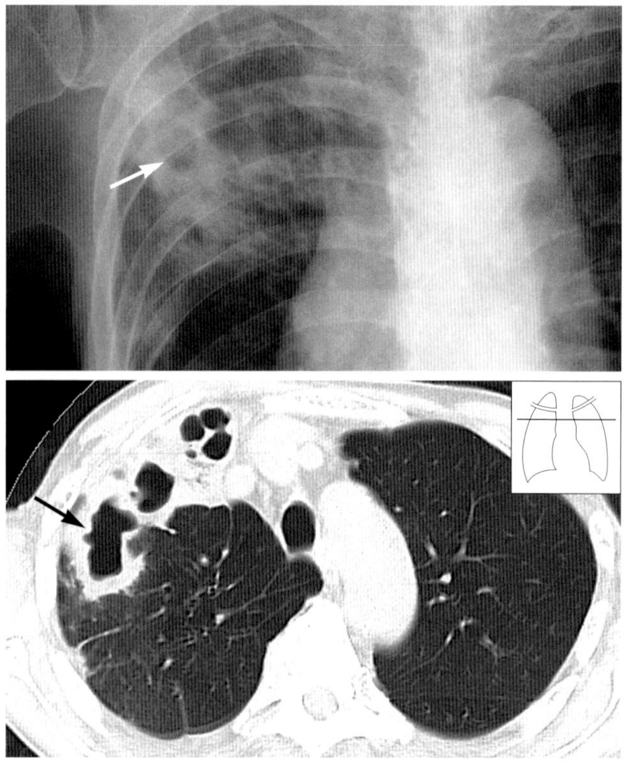

Figure 10 a–b. **Cavity**

Point of differentiation / Disease	Wall thickness		Number of ring shadows	
	Thin (cyst)	Thick (cavity)	Solitary	Multiple
Acidfast bacillus infections (tuberculosis, etc.)	○	◎	○	○ Hematogenic dissemination
Staphylococcus aureus abscess	○	◎	○	
Abscess caused by other pyrogenic bacteria		○	○	
Aspergillosis		○	○	
Cryptococcosis	◎	○	○	○
Carinii pneumonia (complicated with AIDS)	○			○
Lung cancer	○	◎	◎	
Metastatic lung cancer	◎	Mixed		◎
Bronchiectasis	◎	At time of infection		◎
Emphysematous cyst	○	At time of infection		◎
Cyst-forming diseases (EG, LAM, etc.)	◎			◎
Wegener's granuloma	(Mixed type) ○	○	○	○
Pulmonary embolism	○	○	○	
Trauma of lungs (including laceration)	○		○	○

◎ type is common

Table. **Differential diagnosis of ring shadows by wall and number**

(Original concept of the author)

Case 2 Eosinophilic granuloma
39-year-old male

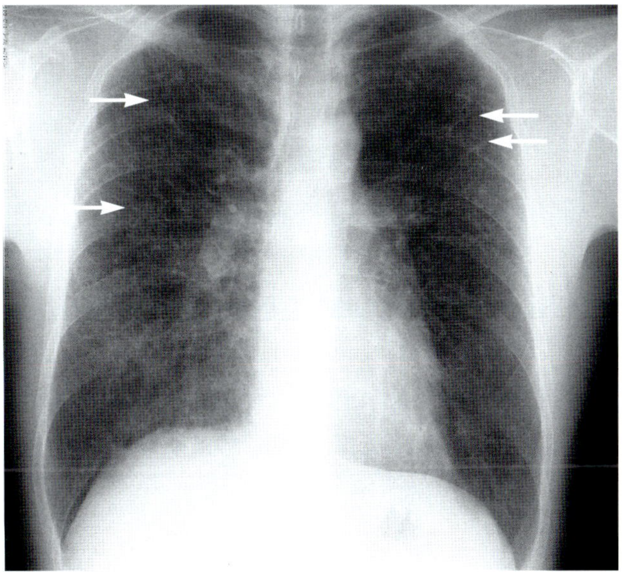

Figure 11. **Chest radiograph**

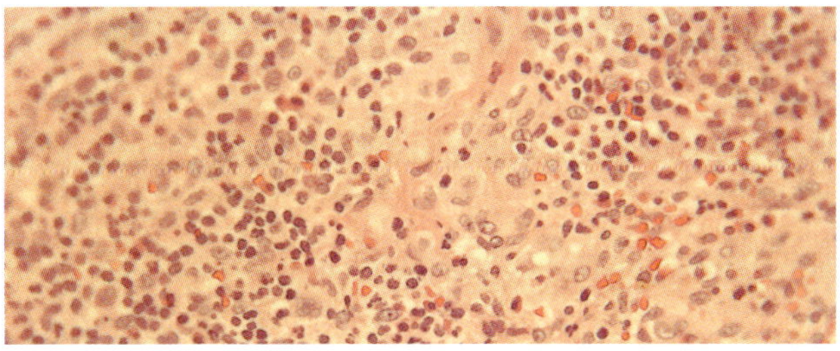

Figure 12. **Histology of biopsy**

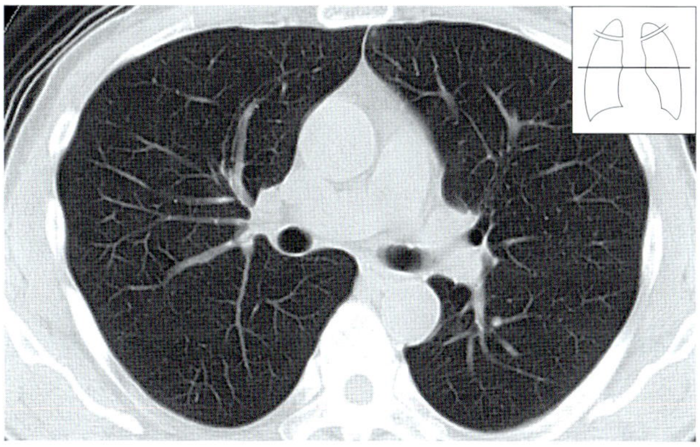

Figure 13. **Chest CT of healthy control**

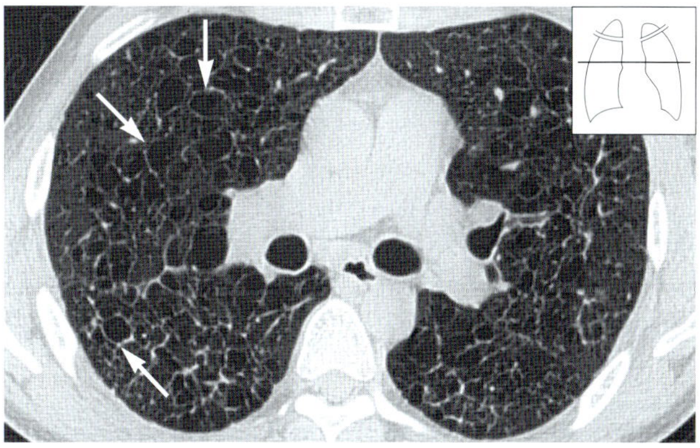

Figure 14. **HRCT of the patient**

Normal lung markings have disappeared from the conventional plain chest radiograph, replaced by striated, reticular, honeycomb-like and large cystic shadows. Lesions are most pronounced in the upper lung fields and less so in the basal lung. The HRCT (1 mm) shows numerous cysts still more clearly. A comparison of the CT with the healthy control at the same level emphasizes the distinction.

Case 3 Metastatic lung cancer (adenocarcinoma of the primary lung cancer)
39-year-old female

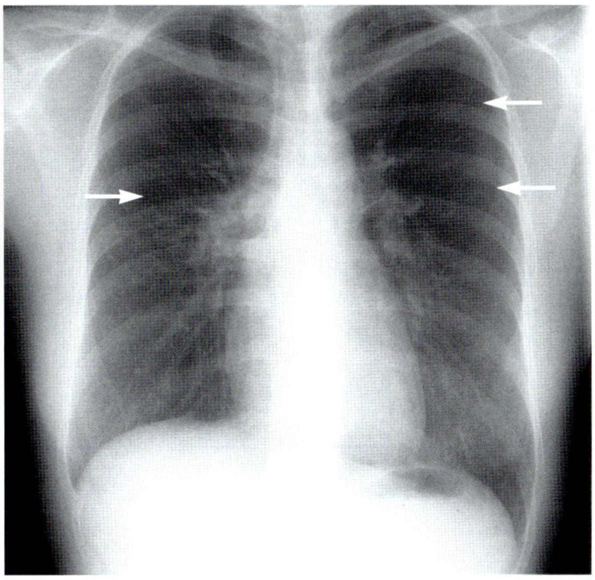

Figure 15. **Chest radiograph**

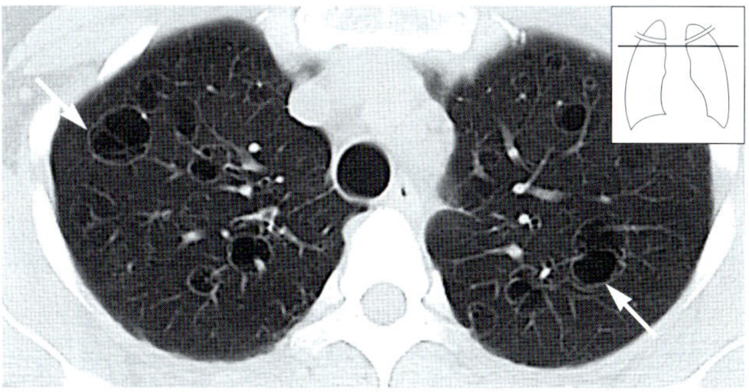

Figure 16. **Chest CT**

The patient was afflicted with a slight fever and cough. The first radiograph did not reveal abnormal findings but cysts appeared gradually.

CT (5 mm slices) distinctly showed numerous cysts of various sizes. LAM was suspected by chest imaging at first, but adenocarcinoma was confirmed by sputum cytology later.

Case 4 Cystic bronchiectasis

28-year-old female

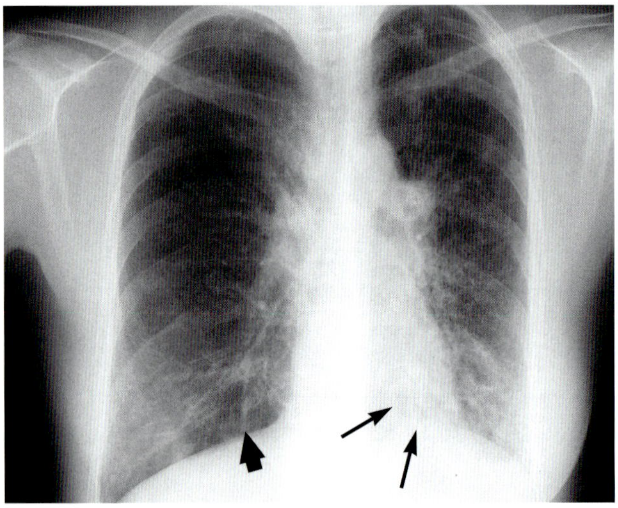

Figure 17. **Chest radiograph**

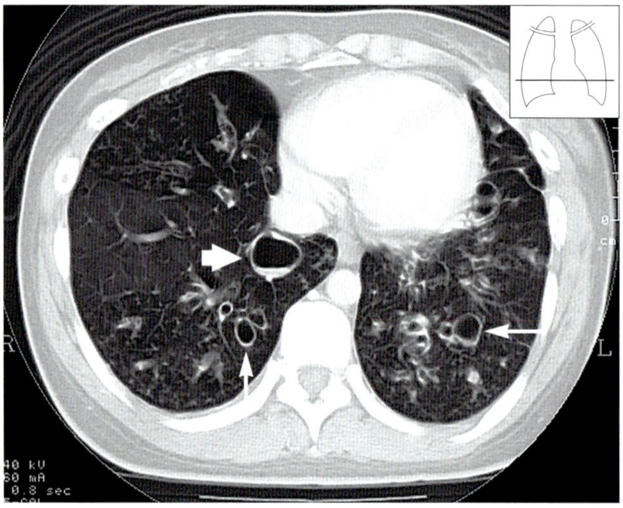

Figure 18. **Chest CT**

The patient suffered from recurrent pneumonias and had been hospitalized frequently since the age of 20.

A frontal chest radiograph showed bronchiectasis with thickened walls as well as numerous cysts (especially in the right lower lung field) indicated by the long arrows. A bulla was observed in the left apex, while a shadow in the left lower lung field suggested cysts with consolidation. Some of the cysts had thickened walls and niveau (indicated by the short arrow).

A CT showed these findings more clearly.

Case 5 Hermansky–Pudlak syndrome

43-year-old female

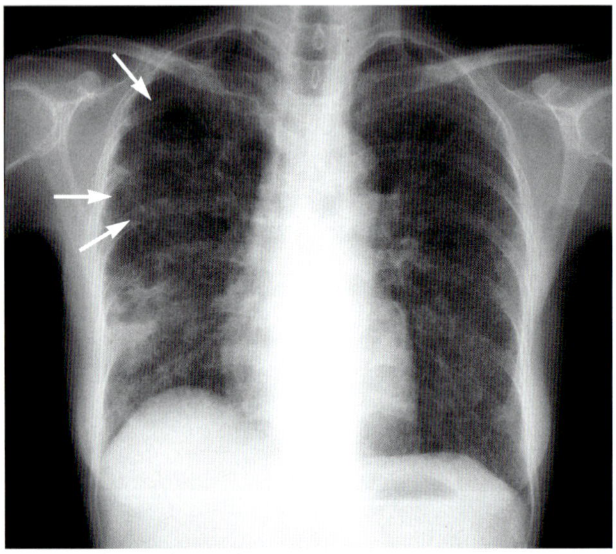

Figure 19. **Chest radiograph**

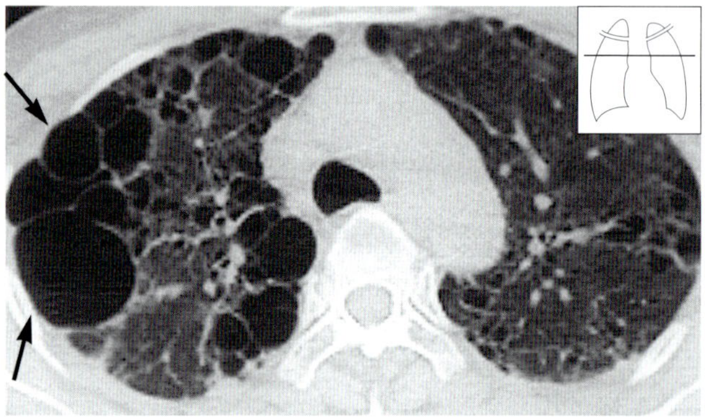

Figure 20. **Chest CT**

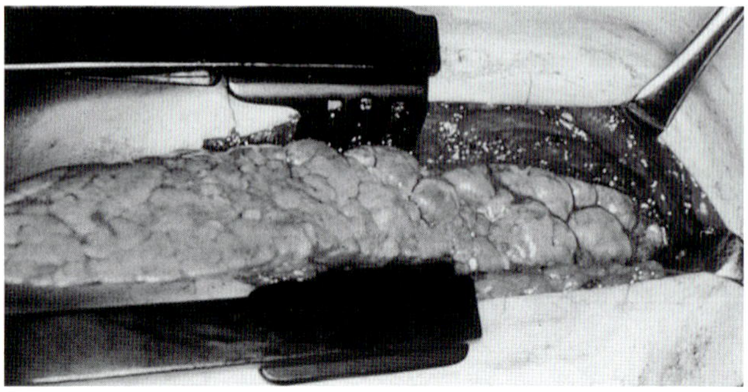

Figure 21. **Macroscopic findings at biopsy**

The patient visited the hospital with dyspnea on exertion. Skin and ocular albinism were noticeable.

A frontal chest radiograph revealed numerous cystic lesions, which were confirmed as being mainly subpleural bullae by CT. Interstitial pneumonia and fibrosis formation accompanying Hermansky–Pudlak syndrome were observed by autopsy.

Case 6 Panlobular emphysema

82-year-old male

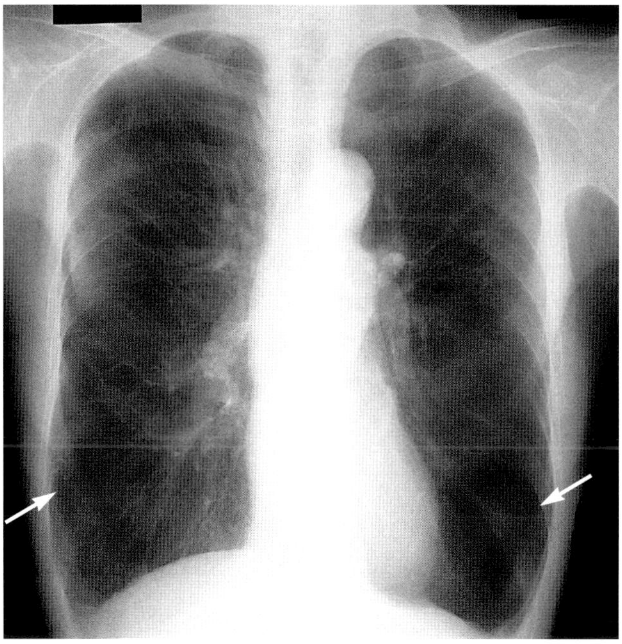

Figure 22. **Chest radiograph**

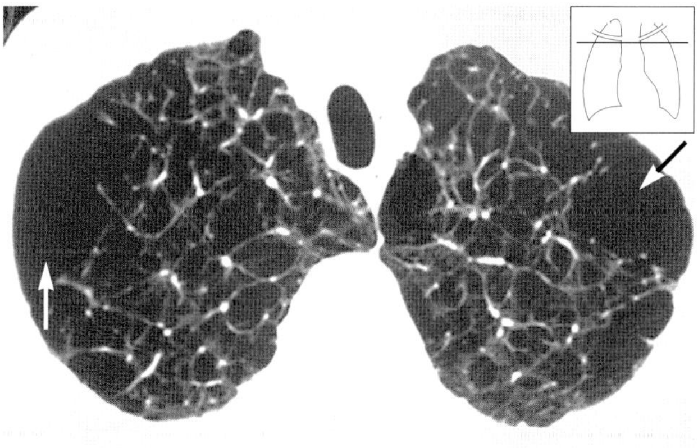

Figure 23. **Chest CT**

Case 7 Centrilobular emphysema

74-year-old female

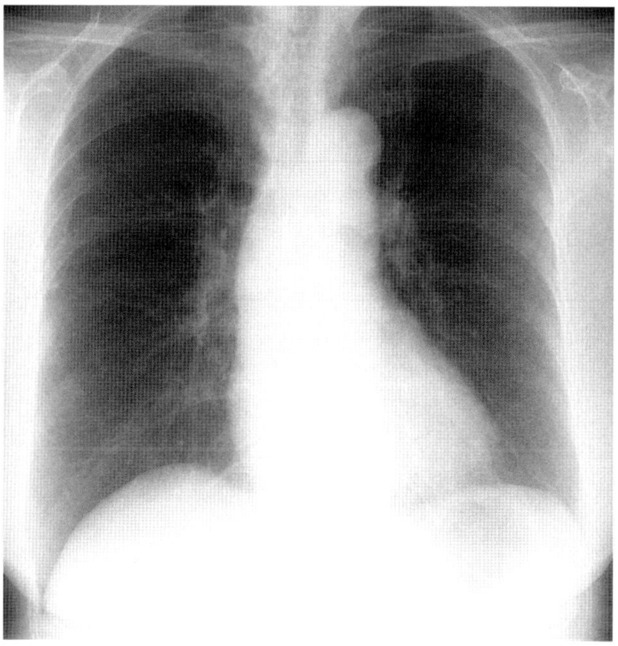

Figure 24. **Chest radiograph**

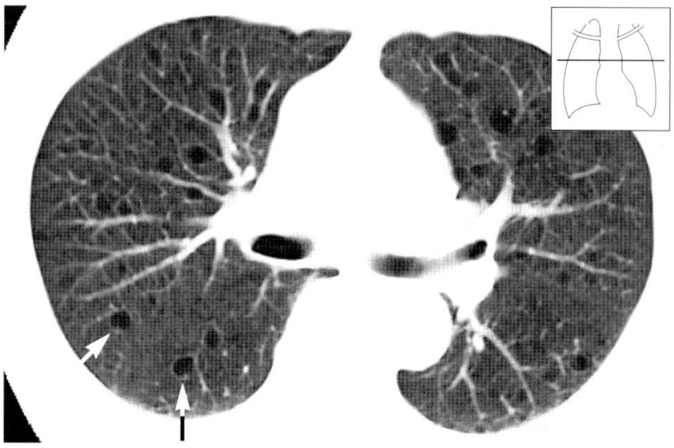

Figure 25. **Chest CT**

Case 6 *(Figs. 22, 23)*: Dyspnea on exertion was the main symptom. The diaphragm was low and flattened with pronounced loss of pulmonary markings in the frontal chest radiograph. CT revealed loss of vascular markings and normal alveolar tissues replaced by emphysematous bulla.

Case 7 *(Figs. 24, 25)*: The patient had no subjective symptoms and there were no abnormalities in lung function tests.

A frontal chest radiograph showed no abnormal shadow, but CT (10 mm slices) revealed numerous cysts of unknown origin. Biopsy confirmed the diagnosis of centrilobular pulmonary emphysema. Emphysema is known to destroy normal alveolar tissues and form numerous bullae. Lung tissues disappear in wide regions in typical cases of panlobular emphysema. Bullae are formed sporadically in centrilobular pulmonary emphysema. The distinction between cystic shadow and bulla is that the septum is clear in the former and indistinct in the latter. However, bullae in Case 7 were clearly visible as cysts.

Conclusion

When a ring shadow is recognized inside the lungs, the hyperlucent ring formed through necrosis or defoliation is called a cavity, while the ring expanded through pressure or fusion of the alveolar space is called a cyst. Cysts are divided into bronchial cysts (in which the inner surface is covered by bronchial epithelium) and alveolar cysts (covered by alveolar epithelium). However, it is impossible to confirm this difference by chest radiograph in clinical practice. Hence, we sometimes classify ring shadows into cavities with thick walls and cysts with thin walls. Cysts are classified further into two types. One type are cysts when the walls of their pneumatic space can be traced distinctly in all their circumference as shadows, and the other are bullae and emphysematous cysts when the walls are indistinct. Chest CT is suitable for observing tiny or indistinct abnormalities. Also, cysts are more readily observed through CT than through conventional chest radiograph. Details of the cyst wall are also obtained. In particular, CT is excellent for the detection and observation of bullae and emphysematous cysts, and is indispensable for their detailed differentiation.

Cysts are either solitary or multiple. The latter are more numerous and clinically more important in pulmonary lesions, and often require differential diagnosis.

Main cyst-forming pulmonary diseases are listed in the previous table. The prevalence of solitary or multiple cysts is marked with circles. Their importance is different depending on the country and hospital. There are also diseases not covered by this table. Only illnesses of interest causing multiple cysts are listed. Owing to limited space, only a few typical clinical cases are included in this section. Hence, some other cyst-forming illnesses are omitted.

Numerous infectious diseases including abscess and tuberculosis form solitary or multiple cavities. Some cysts remain after healing. It is well known that hematogenic pulmonary abscesses, especially those caused by *S. aureus*, induce cystic lesions.

Lung cancers also produce cystic shadows. Various causal mechanisms have been proposed, including the formation of cysts by the so called "check-valve phenomenon" and infiltration of cancer cells to the cyst walls. Hematogenic metastasis cancers often form cystic and nodular lesions of various sizes.

Advanced pneumoconiosis and chronic interstitial pneumonias are almost always accompanied by cysts in characteristic locations. In these cases diagnosis of the underlying disease is essential.

Cysts are also characteristic of generalized or systemic diseases. Diagnosis of the cause is not always easy and depends on detection of the underlying disease or histological findings. Various diseases are responsible including Wegener's granuloma. In this section I have given eosinophilic granuloma and pulmonary lymphangiomyomatosis as examples.

Thoracic trauma and pulmonary embolism are also able to make cysts.

Airway lesions including bronchiectasis and DPB (diffuse panbronchiolitis) can cause cystic shadows. In particular, bronchiectasis is a typical disease causing cystic lesions. Sputum production and recurrent infections are characteristic of this illness.

Pulmonary emphysema tends to form large pneumatic bulla. Cysts can be explicitly visible, or can remain latent, simply assuming the form of disappearance or defect of the pulmonary substance.

The present section only dealt with cyst-forming diseases. But there are many other diseases with similar symptoms, which require careful differential diagnosis.

References

1) Felson B.: Chest roentgenology. Saunders, Philadelphia, 1973, p.314
2) Fraser R. S. et al.: Diagnosis of diseases of the chest (4th ed.), Saunders, Philadelphia, 1999, p.504, p.510
- Toshiharu Matsushima: Roentgenological diagnosis of disease of the chest (2nd ed.), Kinpodo, Kyoto, 1996 (In Japanese)
- Toshiharu Matsushima et al.: Interesting Cases of Pulmonary Disease as seen in Thoracic X-Ray Images, Makoto-printing Co, Kyoto, 1992 (In Japanese)
- Shah R. M.: High-resolution CT in the evaluation of obstructive lung disease: Structure-function correlation. Clin. Pulm. Med. 4: 247–253, 1997

Chapter 4

Radiographs of intrapulmonary lesions with decreased radiolucency

12. Lesions of trachea and bronchus

[Pattern classification IV-F-1]

●Authors — Tatsuji Enomoto, Shoji Kudoh

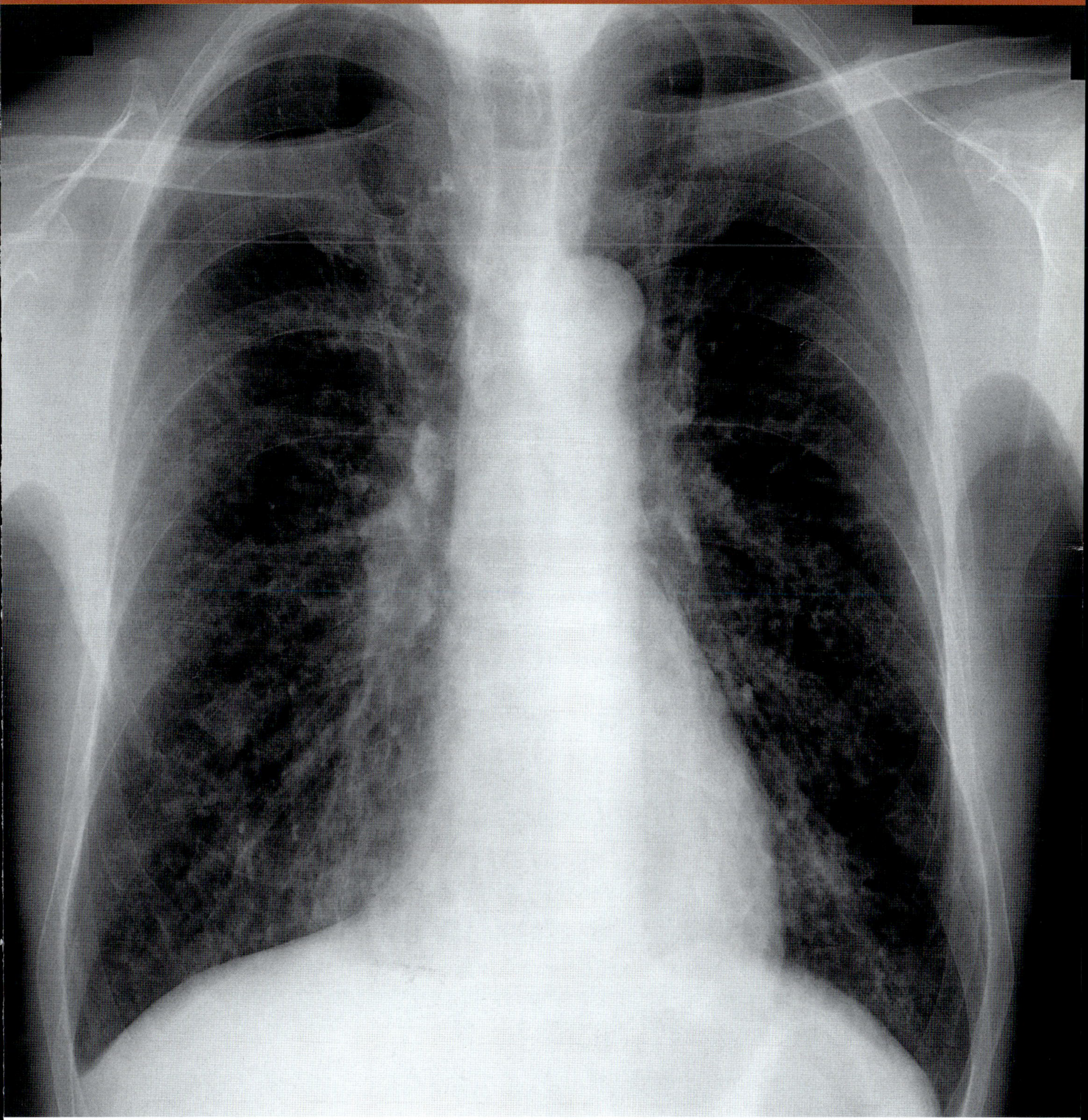

Keywords of this section

Diffuse panbronchiolitis
Centrilobular branching opacity
Centrilobular nodules
Bronchiectasis
Tram line
Signet ring sign
Diffuse aspiration bronchiolitis
Pulmonary tuberculosis
Tree-in-bud appearance
Endobronchial spread
Mycoplasma pneumonia
Allergic bronchopulmonary aspergillosis

Lesions of trachea and bronchus

Tatsuji Enomoto[1)], **Shoji Kudoh**[2)]
1) Department of Respiratory Medicine, Tokyo Metropolitan Hiroo General Hospital, Tokyo, Japan
2) Department of Pulmonary Medicine/Infection and Oncology, Nippon Medical School, Tokyo, Japan

Bronchial lesions include lesions in the central bronchi which can be observed in CT, and lesions in the bronchioles, which are not normally recognizable. However, with peripheral airway lesions, even if bronchi themselves cannot be identified, it is possible to infer the primary lesions from the findings of centrilobular nodular opacity and branching opacity. Case 1 is a typical example.

Case 1 60-year-old male

Chief complaints: Wet cough, nasal obstruction, dyspnea

Medical history: Chronic paranasal sinusitis at the age of 40, anxiety neurosis

Family history: Elder sister had bronchitis, younger sister had gastric cancer

Smoking history: 20/day for 27 years (18 to 45)

Present illness:

The patient has been receiving treatment at this hospital's Department of Otolaryngology for chronic sinusitis for 20 years. Subjective symptoms of nasal obstruction and wet cough. Exhibited dyspnea (Hugh-Jones II) from 4 to 5 years ago, and after having accompanying bloody sputum was referred to this department. He was admitted for detailed examination and treatment.

Physical findings on admission:

Height 165 cm, weight 48 kg, coarse crackles heard in bilateral lower lungs on the dorsal side, no other findings of note observed.

Laboratory data on admission:

WBC 7,000/μL, CRP 1.8 mg/dL, cold hemagglutinin titers 256 times, HTLV-antibody (-), arterial blood gas analysis pH 7.416, $PaCO_2$ 45.7 Torr, PaO_2 70.7 Torr, HCO_3^- 38.8 mmol/L.

Imaging findings:

Chest radiograph (P. 133): Pulmonary overinflation findings and diffuse nodular opacities can be observed in bilateral lower lung fields.

Chest CT (*Figs. 1, 2*): Diffuse centrilobular nodules and centrilobular branching opacities, so called tree-in-bud appearance (→) can be observed. Dilated bronchi and bronchioles can be seen (➤).

Diagnosis

In consideration of continuous cough and sputum, shortness of breath on exertion, chronic sinusitis, chest CT showing diffuse centrilobular nodules in bilateral lung fields, coarse crackles on auscultation of the chest, hypoxia and elevated serum cold hemagglutinin titers, diffuse panbronchiolitis was diagnosed.

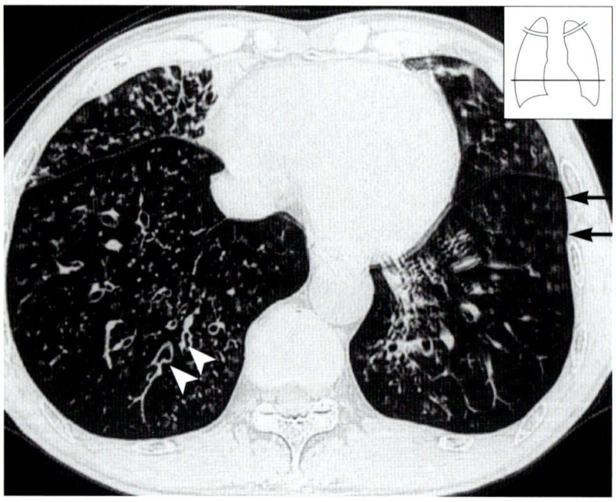

Figure 1. **Chest CT**

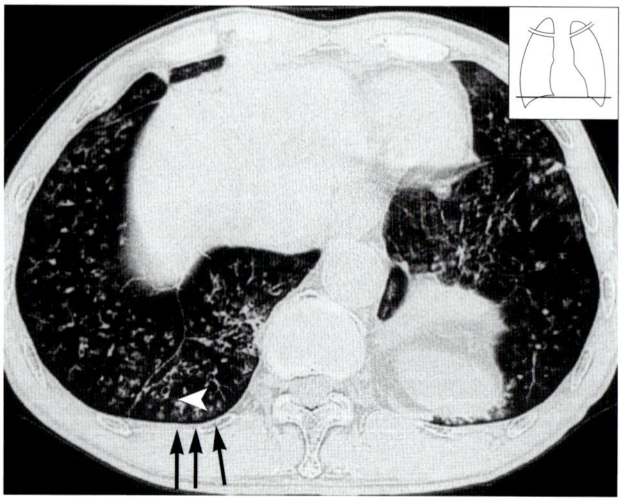

Figure 2. **Chest CT**

Conclusions of this case
Diffuse panbronchiolitis: DPB

DPB is characterized by diffuse bilateral chronic inflammation in the respiratory bronchiole area, and is a disease that impairs respiratory function.

For both males and females, the peak of onset is from 40 to 50 years of age, spanning a wide range of age groups. Major symptoms are chronic cough and sputum, and dyspnea on exertion, and it is frequently associated with chronic sinusitis and a history of chronic sinusitis. It has been suggested that hereditary factors may be involved.

Histopathologically, characteristic findings of this disease include bronchiolitis and peribronchiolitis, with round cell infiltration of lymphocytes and plasma cells and striking accumulation of foam cells, principally at the level of the respiratory bronchioles (*Fig. 3*). It is frequently accompanied by lymphoid follicle formation, with respiratory bronchiole obstruction due to granulation tissue and scars, leading to bronchiectasis as the disease progresses.

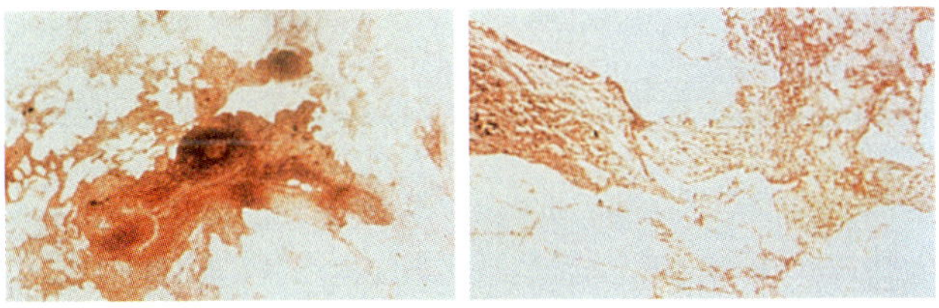

a *b*
Figure 3 a–b. **Histopathological findings: DPB**

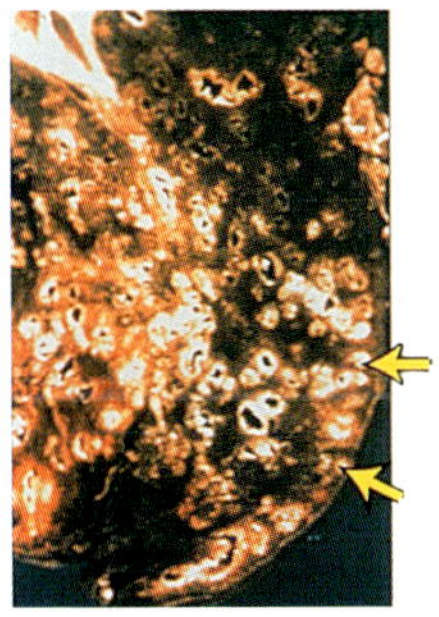

Figure 4. **Cross-section of lung: DPB**

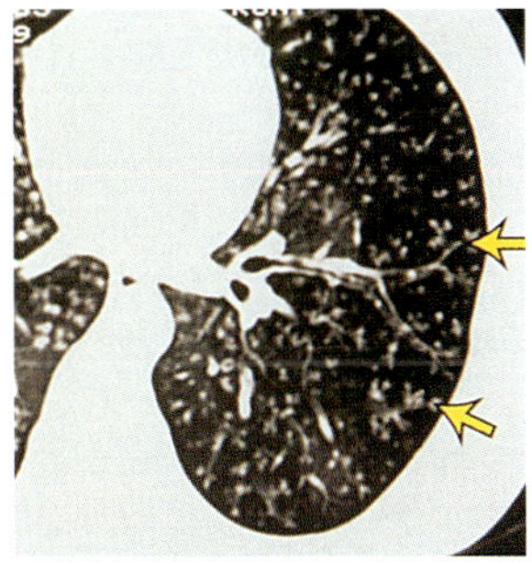

Figure 5. **Chest HRCT**

Guidelines for the diagnosis of diffuse panbronchiolitis
(Diffuse Panbronchiolitis Research Committee of the Ministry of Health, Labor and Welfare, revised on December 12, 1998)

1. Outline

Diffuse panbronchiolitis (DPB) is characterized by diffuse bilateral chronic inflammation in the respiratory bronchiole area, and is a disease that impairs respiratory function. Histopathologically, it is a disease mainly of the respiratory bronchioles, causing bronchiolitis and peribronchiolitis, with round cell infiltration of lymphocytes and plasma cells and foamy alveolar macrophage accumulation. It is frequently accompanied by lymphoid follicle formation, with respiratory bronchiole obstruction due to granulation tissue and scars, leading to bronchodilation as the disease progresses.

For both males and females, the peak of onset is from 40 to 50 years of age, spanning a wide range of age groups. Major symptoms are chronic cough and sputum, and dyspnea on exertion, and it is frequently associated with chronic paranasal sinusitis and a history of chronic paranasal sinusitis. Due to its relationship with human leukocyte antigen and other factors, it has been suggested that hereditary factors may be involved.[*1] Previously, due to respiratory failure occurring as chronic airway infection progressed, the prognosis was poor but treatment with erythromycin in recent years has improved the prognosis.

2. Chief clinical findings

(1) Mandatory
① Clinical symptoms: Continued cough and sputum, and shortness of breath on exertion
② Medical history or coexistence of chronic parasinusitis [*2]
③ Chest radiograph and CT findings:
Chest radiograph: Diffuse, scattered nodular opacities [*3] in bilateral lung fields and
Chest CT: Diffuse centrilobular nodular lesions in bilateral lung fields [*4]

(2) Reference
① Chest auscultation findings: Discontinuous rales [*5]
② Respiratory function and blood gas findings: $FEV_{1.0}$ reduction (70% or lower) and hypoxia (80 Torr or lower) [*6]
③ Blood findings: Elevated titers of cold hemagglutinin[*7]

3. Clinical diagnosis

(1) Diagnostic criteria

Definite	If all three of the above mandatory chief findings and two or more of the reference findings are satisfied.
Almost definite	If all three of the above mandatory chief findings are satisfied.
Possible	If items ① and ② of the above mandatory chief findings are satisfied.

(2) Differential diagnosis
Important diseases for differential diagnosis include chronic bronchitis, bronchiectasis, immotile cilia syndrome, bronchiolitis obliterans and cystic fibrosis. Histopathological examinations are useful for arriving at a definite diagnosis of this disease.

Notes
*1 There are high rates of carriers of HLA-B54 in Japanese cases and HLA-A11 in South Korean cases, and at present the disease shows a high degree of racial dependence in the South Asia region.
*2 Confirmation with radiographs.
*3 Frequently accompanied by findings of overinflation. If the disease progresses, findings of bilateral bronchodilation are seen, and occasionally focal pneumonia.
*4 Bronchiole dilation and wall thickening are frequently seen.
*5 Many cases are accompanied by coarse crackles, and occasionally wheezes, rhonchi or squawk.
*6 If the disease progresses, there is reduced vital capacity and increased residual volume (rate). No reduction of diffusing capacity is seen.
*7 64 times and more with human erythrocyte agglutination tests.

(Taken from reference literature 1. Colored text indicates changes made to diagnostic standards)

Comparing lung cross-section and HRCT, diffuse centrilobular nodules can be seen, reflecting peripheral lung tissue reaction (*Figs. 4, 5*).

Diagnosis is made following the guidelines (*Table*) of the Research Committee of the Ministry of Health, Labor and Welfare, revised in 1998. Medical history and CT play an important role in diagnosis. Histological decision is not necessary.

DPB was a disease with a poor prognosis, causing repeated airway infection that can lead to respiratory failure and even death. However, with the spread of extended treatment with low doses of erythromycin, the prognosis has improved markedly, and at present the 5-year survival rate is over 90%. It is a disease that can be cured if treated in its early stage, and one that points to the importance of imaging diagnosis in particular.

Bronchial lesion differentiation

Bronchial lesions include lesions in the bronchi which can be seen in CT as being comparatively central, and lesions in the bronchioles, which are not normally easy to ascertain. If the bronchi are thick-walled and appear larger than adjacent pulmonary arteries (signet ring sign), this can be taken to indicate bronchial dilatation. Peripheral airway lesions are observed as conspicuous bronchovascular bundles. It is important to identify the findings of distinctive bronchial lesions of centrilobular branching opacity and centrilobular nodules.

Case 2 Bronchiectasis

53-year-old female

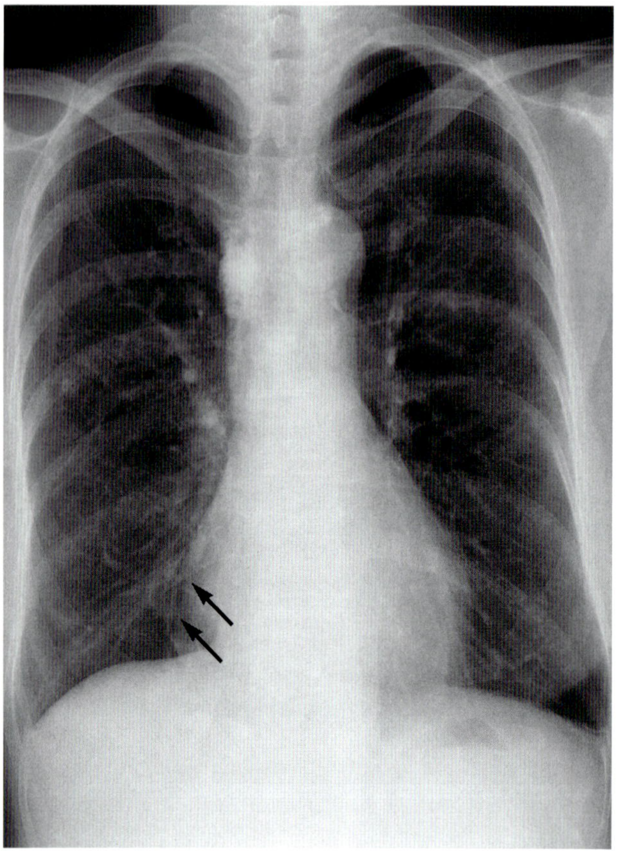

Figure 6. **Chest radiograph**

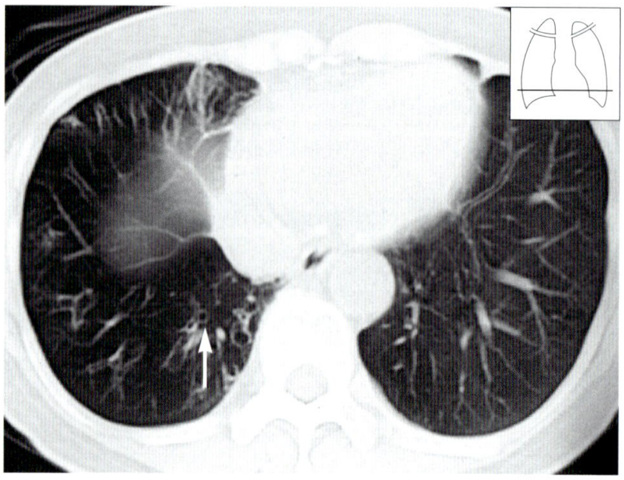

Figure 7. **Chest CT**

Chief complaint: Hemoptysis

Chest radiograph: Tram lines (→) can be observed in the right lower lung field.

Chest CT: A thick ring shadow can be observed in right S^{10}. This is the so-called signet ring sign (→). Unlike normal bronchi, there is no thinning with branching, and it can be clearly seen that the external diameter is larger than the adjacent pulmonary arteries. This is a finding of cylindrical bronchiectasis.

Case 3 Bronchiectasis

72-year-old female

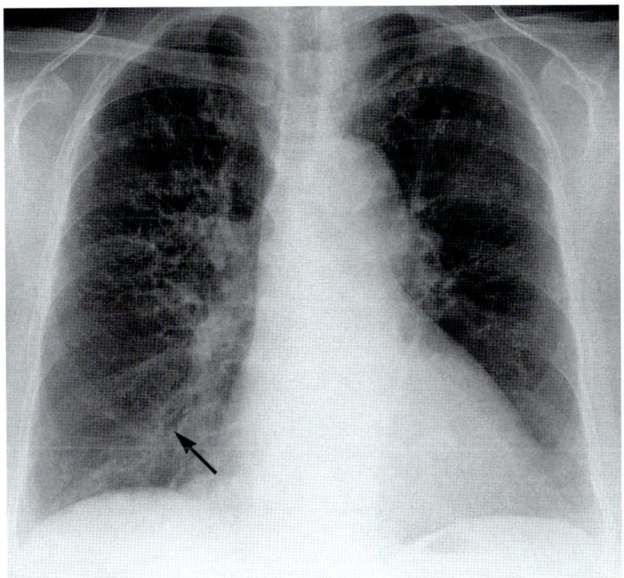

Figure 8. **Chest radiograph**

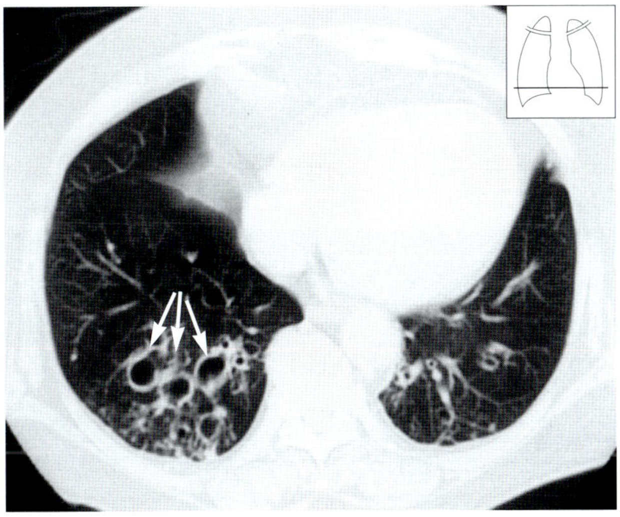

Figure 9. **Chest CT**

Chief complaints: Hemoptysis, dyspnea (Hugh-Jones III)
Chest radiograph: Tram lines (→) can be observed in the right lower lung field.

Chest CT: As with Case 2, the signet ring sign (→) is observed around S^{10}. Centrilobular nodules can also be observed at the periphery. Centrilobular nodules can be seen even if bronchiole lesions accompany usual bronchiectasis, but a finding that differentiates it from DPB is nonuniformity. With bronchiectasis, even in the same lobe normal parts exist together with bronchi that are dilated to varying degrees. Furthermore, even though DPB is accompanied by diffuse bronchial dilatation in cases where the disease progresses, in usual bronchiectasis cases the lesions are localized. Clinically, an important point for differentiation is to establish whether there is also the complication of chronic paranasal sinusitis.

Case 4 Diffuse aspiration bronchiolitis

68-year-old female

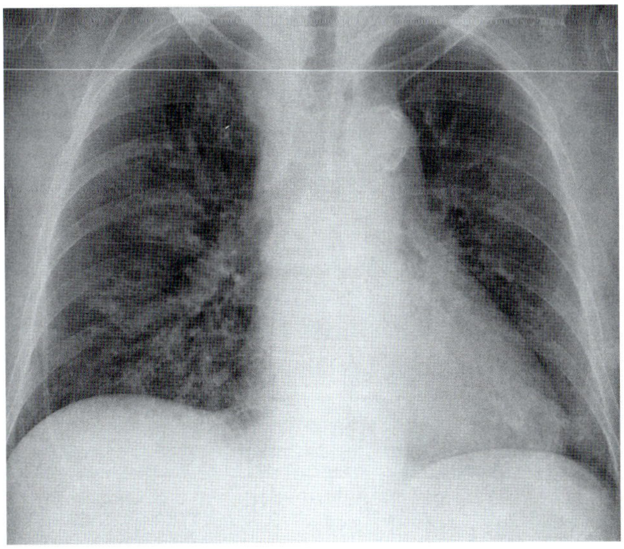

Figure 10. **Chest radiograph**

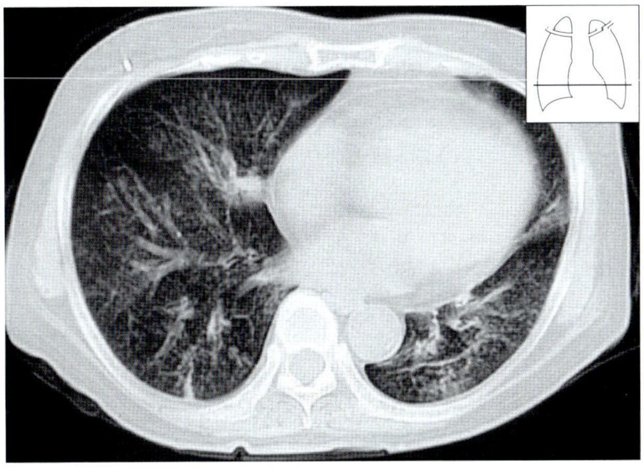

Figure 11. **Chest CT**

Chief complaint: Fever (Postoperative V-P shunt for hydrocephalus due to cerebellopontine angle tumor)
Chest radiograph: Diffuse nodular opacity can be observed from the bilateral upper lung field to the lower lung field. There is partial accumulation and patchy shadows can be seen.

Chest CT: Fine nodular opacity can be observed from the bilateral upper lung field to the lower lung field. This is with 10 mm-thick CT, but these nodular opacities can be observed at a distance from the pleura, and could be centrilobular. Unclear bronchial dilation and fewer findings of peripheral overinflation are points for differentiating the disease from DPB.[2)] Together with an underlying disease that can cause aspiration, these findings point to suspected diffuse aspiration bronchiolitis (DAB).

Case 5 Pulmonary tuberculosis

62-year-old male

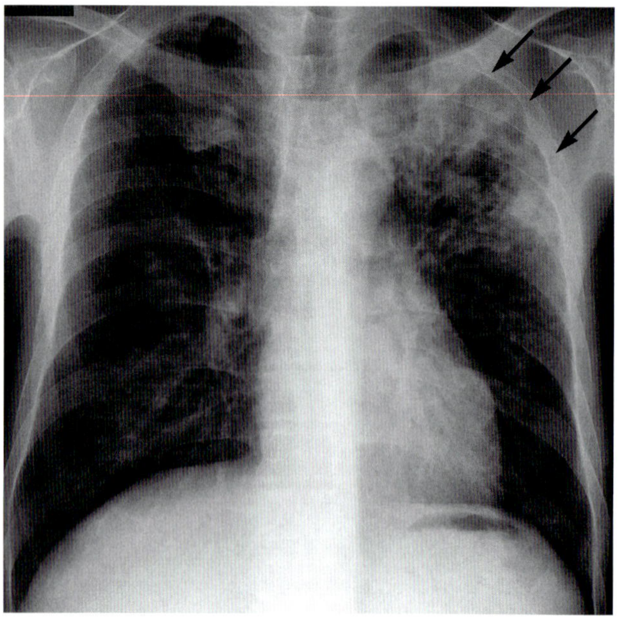

Figure 12. **Chest radiograph**

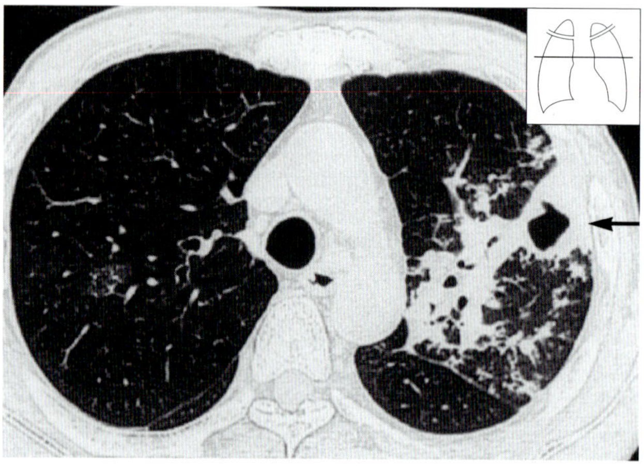

Figure 13. **Chest CT**

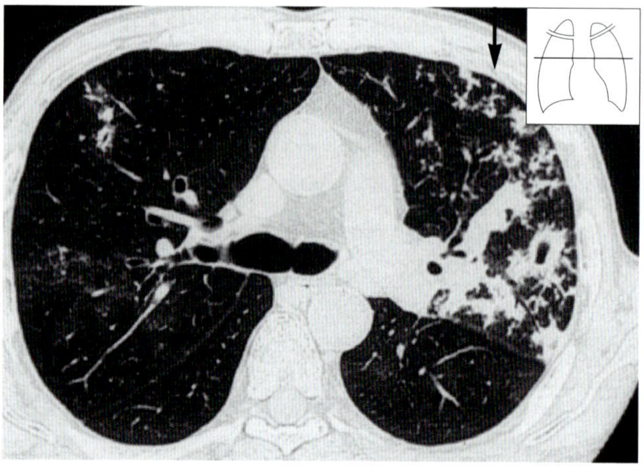

Figure 14. **Chest CT**

Chief complaint: Hemoptysis

Chest radiograph (*Fig. 12*): Consolidation (→) accompanied by air bronchogram can be observed in the left upper lung field. Nodular opacities can be seen in the surrounding area.

Chest CT (*Figs. 13, 14*): A thick-walled cavity, 2 cm in size (*Fig. 13*, →) can be seen in left S^3a. The accompanying bronchi are dilated, and the inside is filled. In addition to the dilated bronchi, there is centrilobular branching opacity with nodular tips, so-called tree-in-bud appearance (*Fig. 14*, →). These findings are typical of endobronchial spread of tuberculosis infection.

Case 6 *Mycoplasma* pneumonia

24-year-old male

Chief complaints: Wet cough, fever

Chest radiograph: Nonuniform consolidation (→) can be seen in the right lower lung field.

Chest CT: Centrilobular nodular opacities (→) centered in right S^{10} can be observed. There is accompanying surrounding ground glass opacity. The contrast of nodules is not distinct. This is a case of *Mycoplasma* pneumonia. Even with *Mycoplasma* pneumonia, centrilobular nodular opacity indicating bronchiole lesions can be seen, but since inflammatory cell infiltration spreads to the bronchioles, peribronchiole areas and alveolar spaces, it may not be possible to obtain nodular opacity contrast as good as in the previous cases.

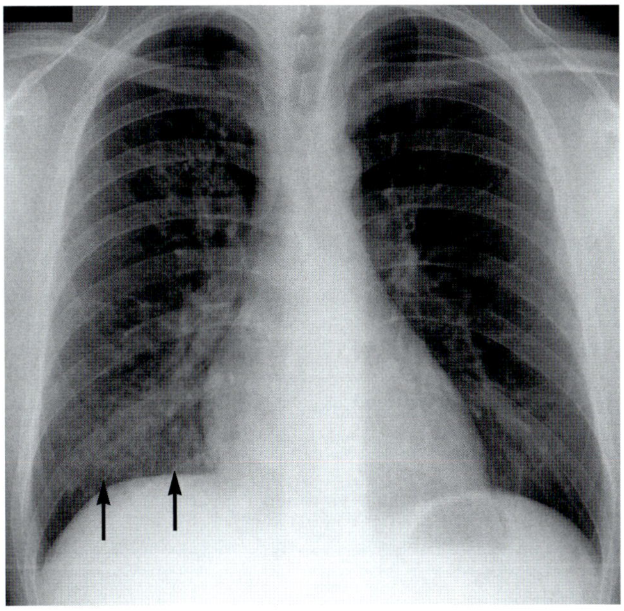

Figure 15. **Chest radiograph**

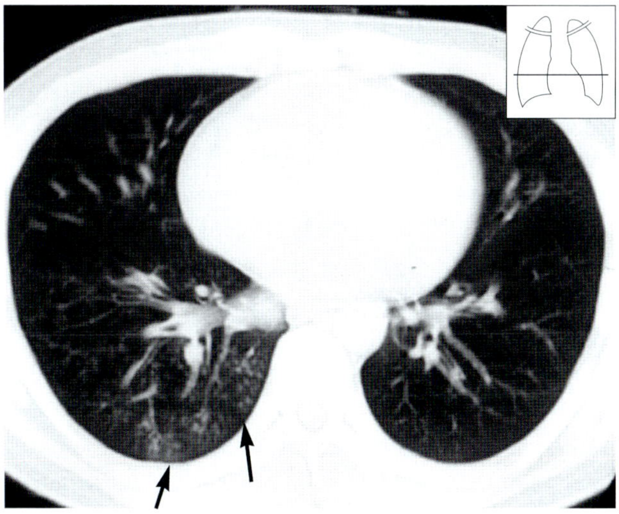

Figure 16. **Chest CT**

Case 7 Allergic bronchopulmonary aspergillosis

37-year-old male

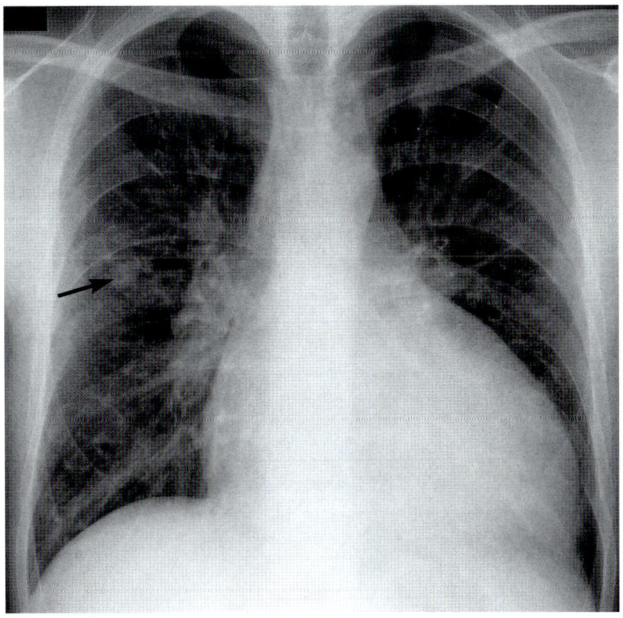

Figure 17. **Chest radiograph**

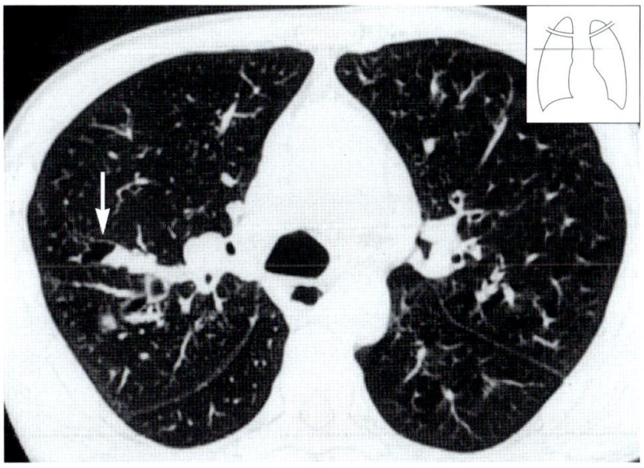

Figure 18. **Chest CT**

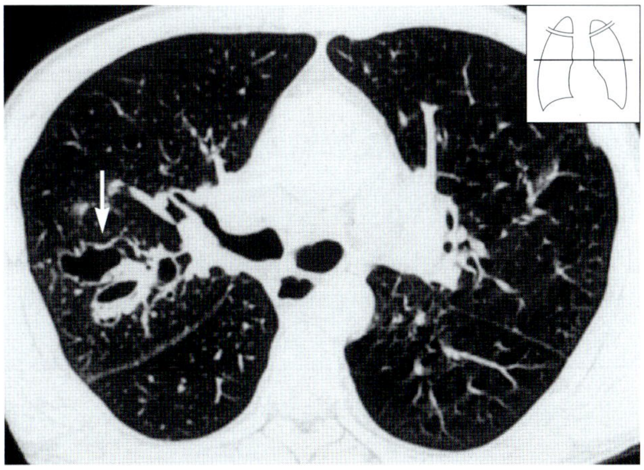

Figure 19. **Chest CT**

Chief complaints: Fever, wet cough (visiting hospital for bronchial asthma)

Chest radiograph (*Fig. 17*): An infiltrative shadow (→) is observed in the right middle zone (cardiomegaly is remarkable but it is not directly related to this disease).

Chest CT (*Figs. 18, 19*): Central bronchiectasis with mucoid impaction (→) in right S^2 can be observed. Unlike the dilated bronchi in the previous cases, these are central with mucus or fluid retention in the bronchial lumen (*Figs. 18* →) that could be mucus plug. Peripheral nodular and branching opacities can also be seen. This is a typical case of allergic bronchopulmonary aspergillosis (ABPA).

Conclusion

When talking about bronchial lesions, the interpretative methods for lesions of comparatively central bronchi that can be observed in CT, and lesions of peripheral airways which are not seen in normal subjects are different. In general, taking lung structure as consisting of an inner level, a middle level and an outer level, even with high resolution CT (HRCT), bronchi can be detected as far as the middle level in a normal lung. Up to this level, if vertical sections of bronchi are obtained, bronchiectasis is considered to be present when the internal diameter of a bronchus is greater than the diameter of the adjacent pulmonary artery branch.

Direct CT findings of bronchiolar disease in the outer level could include bronchiolar wall thickening, bronchiolar dilation or luminal impaction. That is to say, normal bronchioles with no wall thickening are 1 mm or less in diameter and are not depicted in CT (*Fig. 20 A*). When bronchiolar wall thickening occurs, CT can show abnormal bronchioles in profile or as ring shadows in the periphery where they are not normally visible (*Fig. 20 B*). If the external diameter of dilated bronchioles is 2 mm or more, they can be seen in CT (*Fig. 20 C*). Bronchioles whose secretions have become impacted show as centrilobular nodular opacities and centrilobular branching opacities (*Fig 20 D*). If bronchiolar impaction is severe, resulting in clubbing of distal bronchioles, this shows as tree-in-bud appearance (*Fig 20 E*).

To interpret centrilobular lesions, the following points must be understood. 1) Lungs consist of numerous secondary pulmonary lobules about 1 cm in diameter. 2) Bronchovascular bundles run through the center of these secondary lobules, and there are pulmonary veins and interlobular septa at the borders of the lobules. 3) The tips of bronchioles are almost uniformly located about 3 mm away from the borders of lobules.

Taking the above into consideration, regardless of whether there are findings of bronchodilation, wall thickening, bronchovascular bundle swelling in peripheral lung (centrilobular branching opacities) or centrilobular nodular opacities due to lesions becoming more severe, if there are no lesions on the lobular borders or lesions are mild, bronchial lesions should be suspected.

Frequently, central bronchiectasis resembles an overly pruned tree in images, peripheral bronchiolectasis and bronchiolar luminal impaction resemble a tree budding

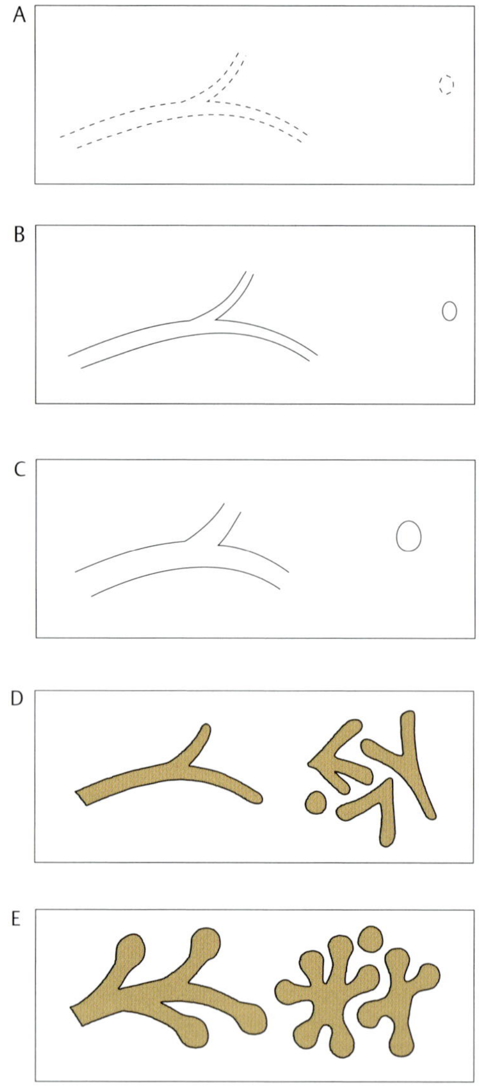

Figure 20. **Illustrations of direct findings: Normal bronchioles and bronchiole lesions** (taken from literature 3)

in springtime, and extensive airway and lung parenchyma lesions resemble a tree in full summer foliage. These should be kept in mind when interpreting images.

References

1) Respiratory System Disease Research Committee of the Ministry of Health, Labor and Welfare Diffuse Pulmonary Disease Subcommittee, Annual Research Report, 1998
2) Satoshi Noma et al.: HRCT Images of Diffuse Aspiration Bronchiolitis (DAB), Clinical Radiology, 41: 129–133, 1996
3) Janet Collins et al.: CT Patterns of Bronchiolar Disease: What Is "Tree-in-bud"? Am. J. Roentgenol. 171: 365–370, 1998

Chapter 4

Radiographs of intrapulmonary lesions with decreased radiolucency

13. Abnormal linear shadow

[Pattern classification IV-F-2]

●Author — Hitoshi Tokuda

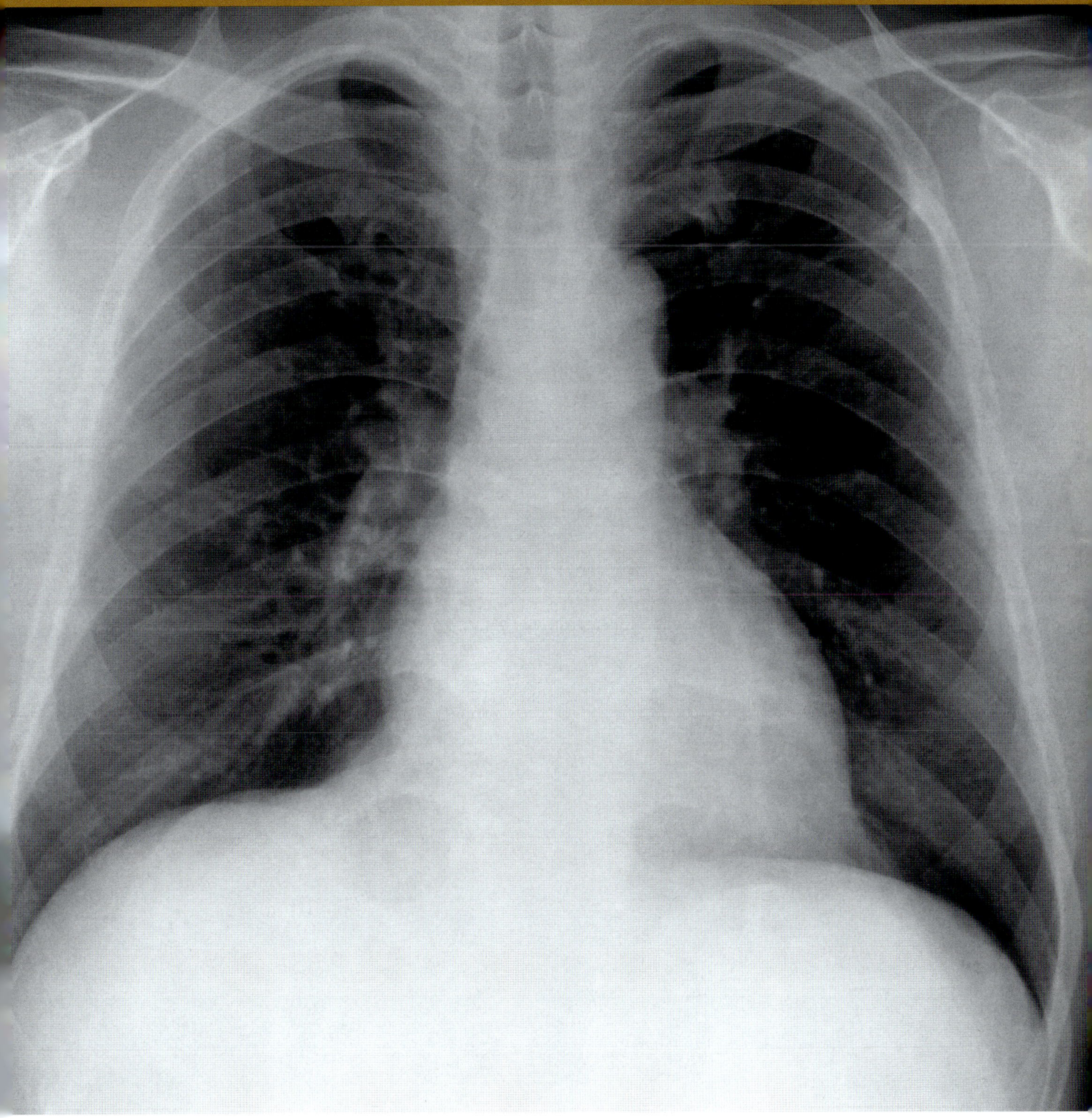

Keywords of this section

Well-differentiated adenocarcinoma
Pleural indentation
Pneumonia
Parenchymal band
Scar
Plate atelectasis
Discoid atelectasis
Linear atelectasis
Pulmonary infarction
Kerley's B lines
Cardiac failure
Lymphangitic carcinomatosis
Acute eosinophilic pneumonia
Giant bulla
Pneumomediastinum
Azygos fissure
Azygos lobe

Abnormal linear shadow

Hitoshi Tokuda
Department of Internal Medicine, Respiratory Medicine, Social Insurance Central General Hospital, Tokyo, Japan

In addition to those originating from bronchial walls (Chapter 4-*12*), abnormal linear shadows seen in plain chest radiographs can be caused by numerous factors such as 1) manifestation of the pleura due to leakage of air (pneumothorax, pneumomediastinum), 2) the borders of cystic change, 3) partial collapse of pulmonary tissue (inflammatory scars, atelectasis, occasionally in the vicinity of tumors), and 4) interstitial diseases in general, particularly thickening of interlobular connective tissue. Since diagnosis is comparatively easy in many cases and most of them are benign, chest imaging diagnosis is not considered important for this situation, but occasionally serious diseases might show as abnormal linear shadows. For this reason it is important to know about general variations.

Case 1 47-year-old male

Chief complaint: Abnormal chest shadow
Medical history: Nothing of particular note
Smoking history: 20/day for 27 years
Present illness:
On a health check a chest radiograph showed an abnormal shadow in the left upper lung field. A local doctor conducted a CT examination which indicated a small, faint shadow in left upper lobe S^{1+2}, and the patient was referred to this hospital.

Laboratory data showed no abnormality of note.

Chest radiograph (P. 141): There is a short linear shadow reaching the pleura in the left upper lung field. No abnormalities can be seen in any other areas of the lung field including the lung apex. It is a solitary abnormal shadow. There is no pleural effusion or lymph node swelling.

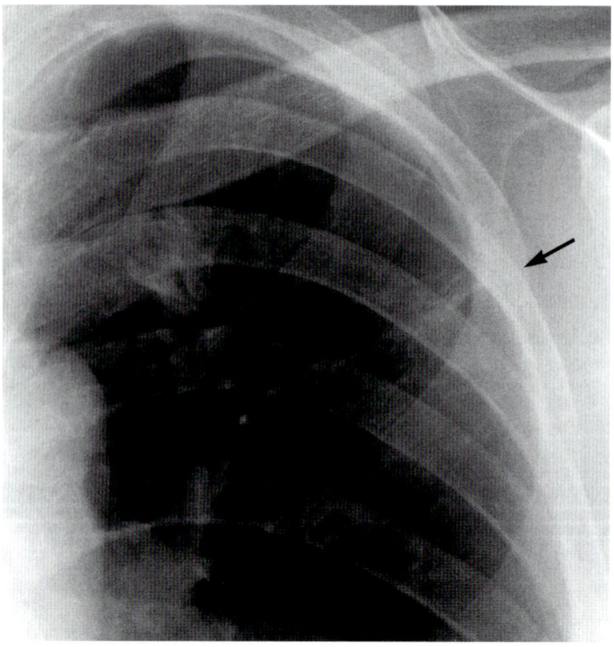

Figure 1. **Chest radiograph**: Slightly irregular linear shadow reaching the pleura, with no clear nodular shadows in the vicinity.

Chest radiograph (*Fig. 1*): The linear shadow is slightly irregular-shaped and composed of multiple lines (➞). In the vicinity no clear nodular shadows or consolidation can be seen. This shadow could be taken as a scar and left alone, but being a solitary shadow it raises doubts. A CT scan was then conducted.

Chest CT (*Fig. 2*): There is an irregularly-shaped faint shadow beneath the pleura in left S^{1+2}. Inside the shadow density is uneven, and there is also aeration that could be an air bronchogram. The pleura is pulled in toward the shadow.

Diagnosis

For this case diagnosis could not be reached with a bronchoscopy or CT-guided needle biopsy, so video-assisted thoracoscopy was conducted. A frozen section diagnosis indicated adenocarcinoma and a left upper lobe lobectomy was performed.

Micropathology of excised material (*Fig. 3*) indicated carcinoma extending in alveolar lining pattern, which is a typical finding of well-differentiated adenocarcinoma. However, a look at the indented part (Elastica van Gieson stain, *Figure 4*) shows marked elastosis which might have caused the contraction (Noguchi type C).

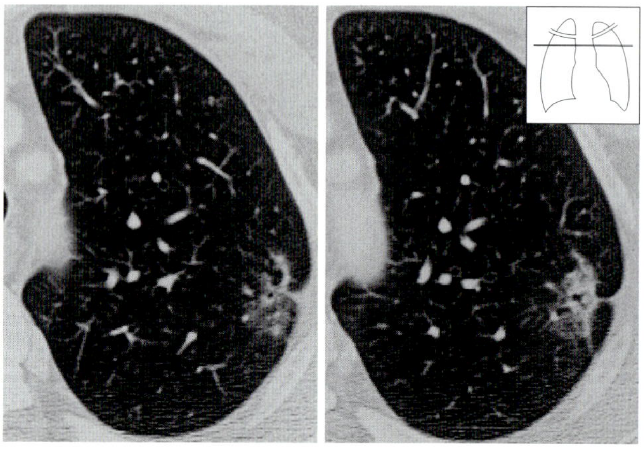

Figure 2. **Chest CT**: A small, faint, irregular-shaped shadow beneath the pleura in S^{1+2}, with uneven density inside the shadow, air bronchogram, pleural indentation and other typical findings of well-differentiated adenocarcinoma (Noguchi type C).

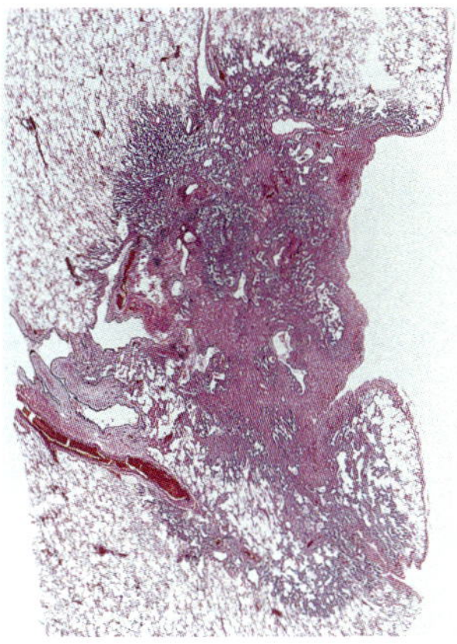

Figure 3. **Pathological findings**

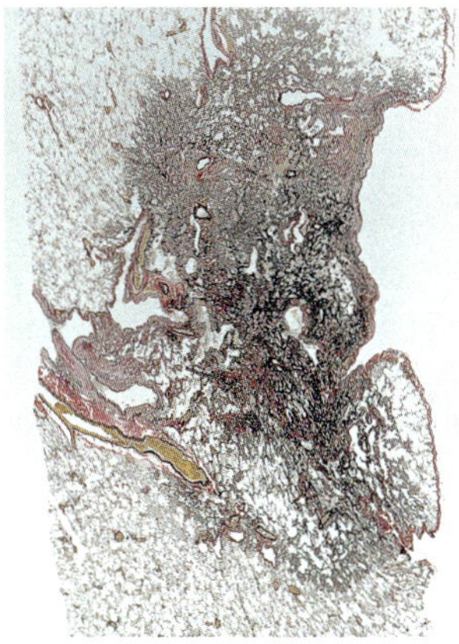

Figure 4. **Pathological findings: Elastica van Gieson stain**

Pleural indentation is a well-known finding of well-differentiated adenocarcinoma in chest imagings. In most cases of adenocarcinoma lesions can be found (nodular shadows or small consolidation) that are clearly visible in plain chest radiographs. When linear shadows are seen at the periphery of these nodular lesions, there is little need to hesitate making a diagnosis of adenocarcinoma, even with plain chest radiographs. As is well known, adenocarcinoma with central fibrosis causes pleural indentation when located near the pleura, which is displayed as a linear shadow, and such a type of adenocarcinoma itself is usually radiopaque and recognizable in plain chest radiographs.

This is an exceptional case, the tumor itself being extremely difficult to recognize in plain chest radiographs. The only conspicuous feature is pleural indentation. But such a phenomenon may occur depending on the ratio of the alveolar lining part and the fibrotic part, and so attention to this point is required.

Another point in this case is the patient's constitution. He was apparently obese. With this body type, the subpleural area of plain chest radiographs is obscured by thick soft tissue density, making it difficult to recognize faint lesions in that area.

Reference case

This is another case resembling the previous one (kindly provided by Dr. Masashi Sato, Assistant Professor, Department of Radiology, Nippon Medical School).

76-year-old male. Found at a health check. A plain chest radiograph shows a short linear shadow (→) extending to the pleura in the right upper lung field. Since the scapula interferes with the reading of this image, it seems that no apparent nodular shadow is observed in this area.

Chest CT findings show a faint, irregular-shaped shadow, with a linear shadow reaching the pleura which must be pleural indentation.

In this case no precise comparison between the pathology and chest radiograph was conducted, but a fibrotic focus was found in the tumor and it could cause the pleural indentation. Like the previous case, this is well-differentiated adenocarcinoma.

To avoid overlooking this kind of small lung cancer seen as a linear shadow in plain chest radiographs and mistaking it as scarring, one must carefully check the surrounding area and confirm that there are no abnormal shadows in the vicinity. When no scar shadows are found in the vicinity, that is, if it is determined to be a solitary linear shadow, lung cancer should be suspected. More thorough interpretation should be conducted, with CT scan desirable if there is even a hint of doubt.

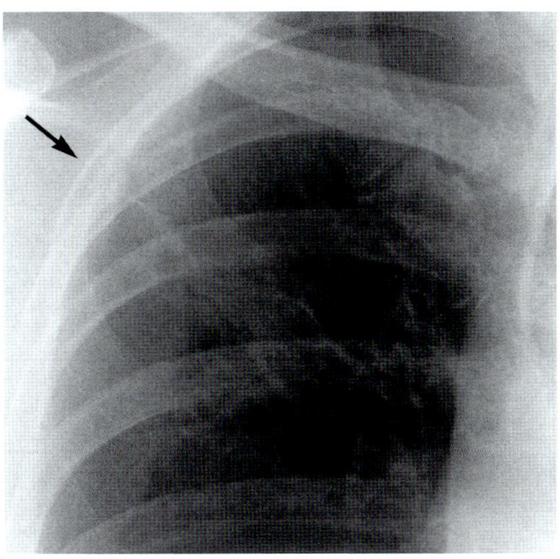

Figure 5. **Chest radiograph**: Short linear shadow reaching the pleura in the right upper lung field. There appears to be a very faint shadow nearby but it is not clear.

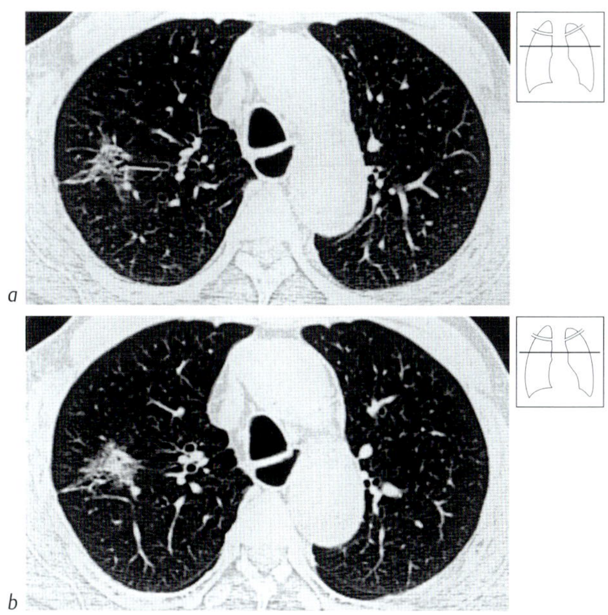

Figure 6 a–b. **Chest CT**: Faint, irregular shaped lesion in right upper lobe accompanied by linear shadow reaching the pleura, possibly pleural indentation. Well-differentiated adenocarcinoma.

Case 2 Pneumonia scar

72-year-old male

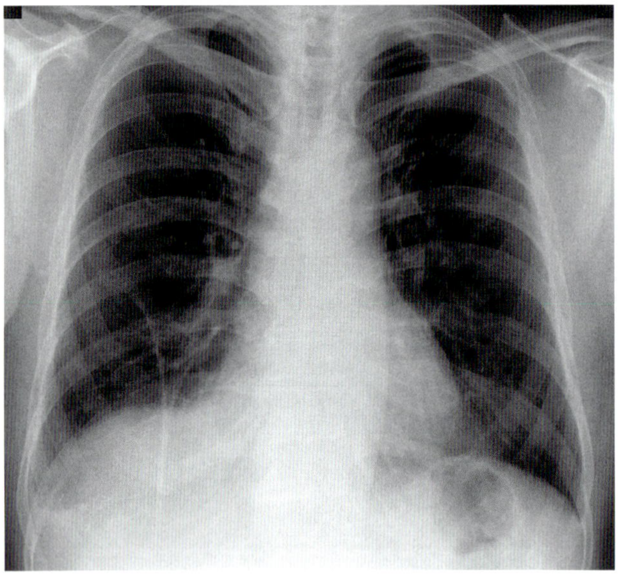

Figure 7. **Chest radiograph**

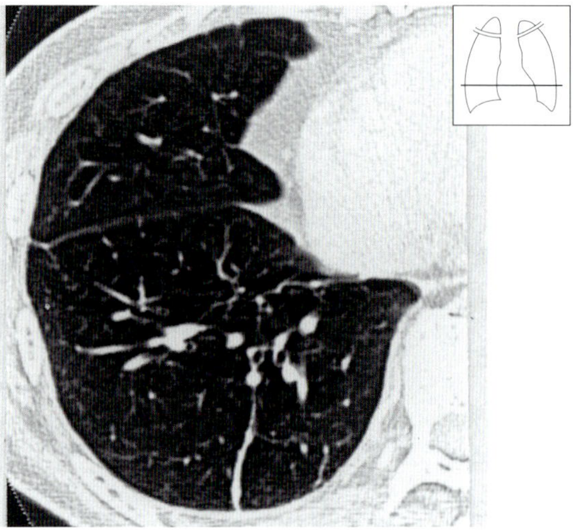

Figure 8. **Chest CT: Pneumonia scar in the right S^{10}b region**

Asymptomatic, found on a regular checkup.

A chest radiograph shows a linear shadow traversing the length of the right lower lung field.

A chest CT shows a linear shadow reaching the pleura in the right lower lobe S^{10}b region. The shadow appears to originate from B^{10}b. With this slice only it seems to be an atelectasis in a specific segment, but with other slices combined, you can see that this is a nonanatomical collapse. Generally, in the healing process of pneumonia, initial consolidation completely disappears in most cases.

Sometimes, however, as in this case, it shrinks to form a linear shadow for an extended period of time until it becomes permanent. Often it can happen that a linear shadow is discovered in a medical checkup without any subjective episodes of respiratory infection. The radiological term used for this is parenchymal band, which is in fact a scar. It is said that it is a comparatively frequently observed pathology that occurs with diseases such as asbestosis, pulmonary tuberculosis and following pleurisy, but it has been reported to occur also in normal lungs.

Case 3 Plate atelectasis

64-year-old female

Asymptomatic, found on a medical checkup.

A plain lateral chest radiograph shows a linear shadow (→) close to and parallel with the diaphragm.

With chest CT it is somewhat difficult to interpret this kind of horizontal, linear shadow, for spread of the lesion coincides with CT slice angle. Actually, in this case only a slight degree of vascular convergence and ground glass opacity are observed in left S^5 region (→). This finding, along with scarring in right S^5, suggests inflammatory origin of this linear shadow.

Since it was first reported in 1935, various names have been proposed for this kind of lesion, such as plate-like atelectasis, discoid atelectasis and linear atelectasis. In many cases it appears as linear shadows 1 to 3 mm wide and 4 to 10 cm long in the basal area of the lung. Its etiology is diverse, many cases being caused by impaired diaphragmatic movement. That is to say, it often occurs

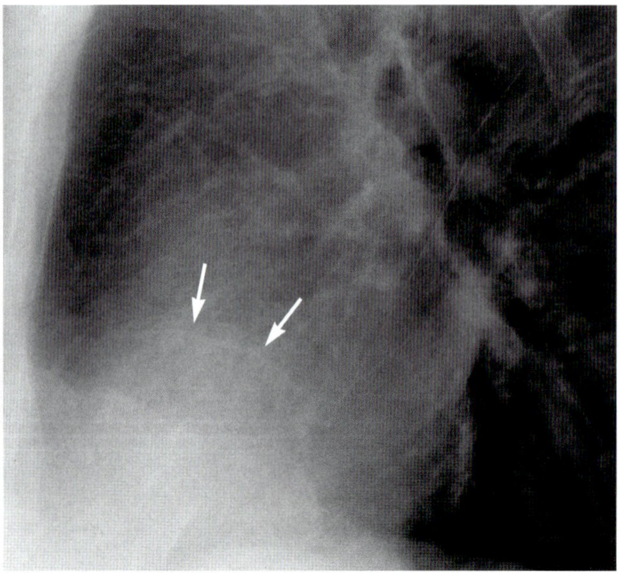

Figure 9. **Chest radiograph (lateral view): Plate atelectasis**

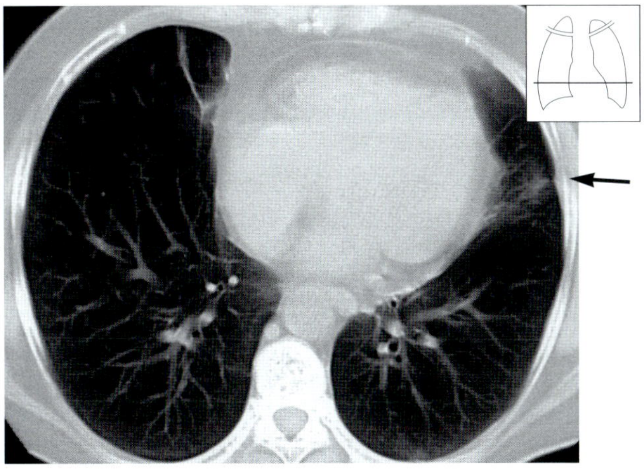

Figure 10. **Chest CT**

following abdominal surgery, with intraperitoneal infections and other situations. Also airway obstruction with excessive secretions due to inflammation resulting in the collapse of lung parenchyma and other mechanisms has been postulated. As can be seen in this case, the spread is not related to segments, and it rarely remains for a long time.

Case 4 Pulmonary infarction

57-year-old male

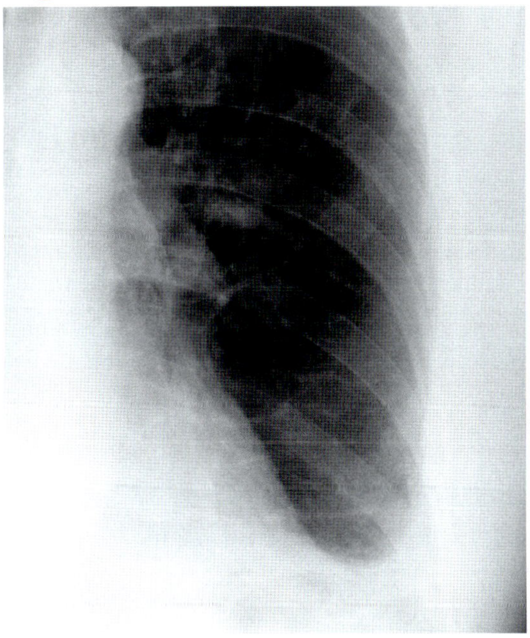

Figure 11. **Chest radiograph**: Left side pleural effusion and ground glass opacity, linear shadow (Kindly provided by Dr. Masashi Sato, Assistant Professor, Department of Radiology, Nippon Medical School)

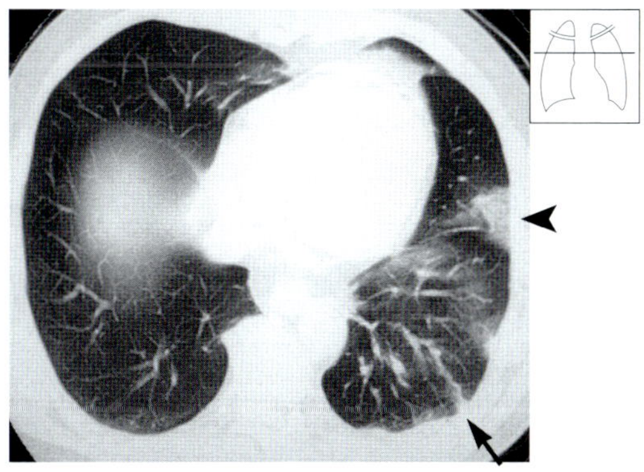

Figure 12. **Chest CT: Lung window setting**

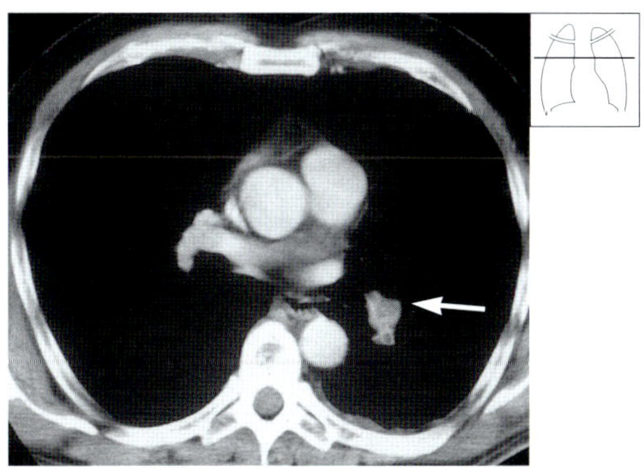

Figure 13. **Chest CT: Mediastinal window setting**

Visited the hospital because of sudden chest pain and dyspnea. Blood examination revealed increased WBC count, and also elevated serum CRP and LDH levels. Blood gas analysis showed hypoxemia accompanied by hyperventilation.

A plain chest radiograph taken on admission (*Fig. 11*) shows left pleural effusion and ground glass opacity and linear shadow in the left lower lung field.

A CT in the lung window setting (*Fig. 12*) shows a funicular shadow (→) reaching to the pleura, a hemispherical mass (➤) and patchy ground glass opacity.

A CT in the mediastinal window setting (*Fig. 13*) shows filling defect (→) in the left pulmonary artery, which suggests thrombus formation leading to the diagnosis of pulmonary infarction.

Pathologically, pulmonary infarction is hemorrhagic necrosis of the lung parenchyma resulting from a sudden obstruction in a pulmonary artery at the peripheral level. Plain chest radiograph findings of pulmonary infarction include diaphragm elevation, a mass shadow in contact with the pleura (Hampton's hump), and ground glass opacity or consolidation while it sometimes appears as a linear shadow as in this case. Except for Hampton's hump (which is not frequently encountered), the diagnostic specificity of these findings is low, making it difficult to differentiate between infarction and pneumonia or other pulmonary diseases with plain chest radiograph only.

For the diagnosis of pulmonary thromboembolism, including pulmonary infarction, perfusion scintigram was thought indispensable for verifying perfusion defect. Recently, contrast-enhanced CT has come to be used widely because of its accessibility and high diagnostic specificity.

Case 5 Cardiac failure
61-year-old female

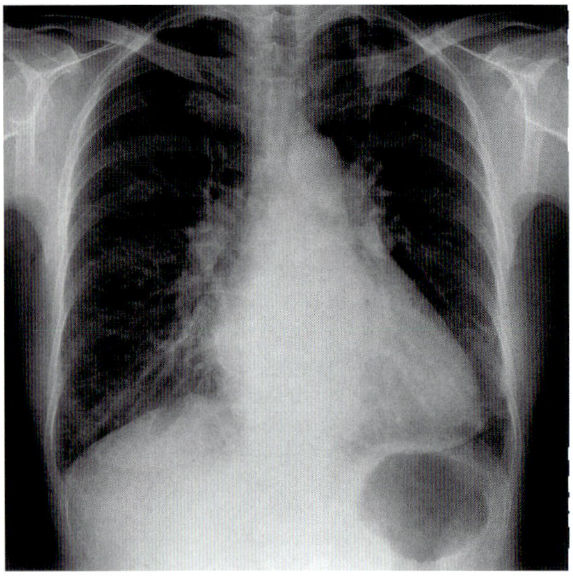

Figure 14. **Chest radiograph: Kerley's B lines**

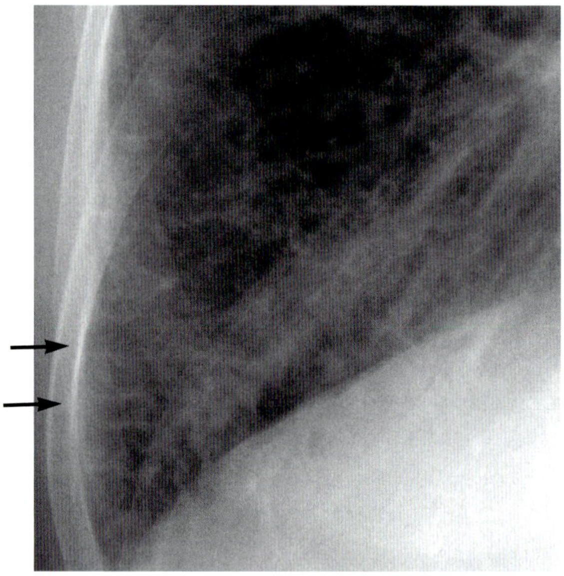

Figure 15. **Chest radiograph: Kerley's B lines (magnified view)**

Consulted us for palpitations and dyspnea lasting 2 weeks.

A plain chest radiograph shows cardiac enlargement and indistinct pulmonary blood vessels (the tumor in the left lung apex is a complication of lung cancer). In the magnified view of the right costophrenic angle region, there are multiple 1 to 2 cm long horizontal linear shadows (→) reaching the chest wall. These are typical Kerley's B line (septal line) findings.

Taking it together with cardiac enlargement, cardiac failure was suspected. An ECG showed tachycardia/atrial fibrillation, and an echocardiograph showed mitral regurgitation and left atrial enlargement, making the diagnosis of cardiac failure conclusive.

The findings of Kerley's B lines are said to be an expression of interlobular septal thickening, which in addition to cardiac failure, appears in lymphangitic carcinomatosis, acute eosinophilic pneumonia and interstitial pathologies in general. This finding appears more often in the right lower lung field, appearing in lower areas partly due to the influence of gravity, and partly because, compared to the left side, there are fewer factors preventing observation.

Case 6 Giant bulla
47-year-old male

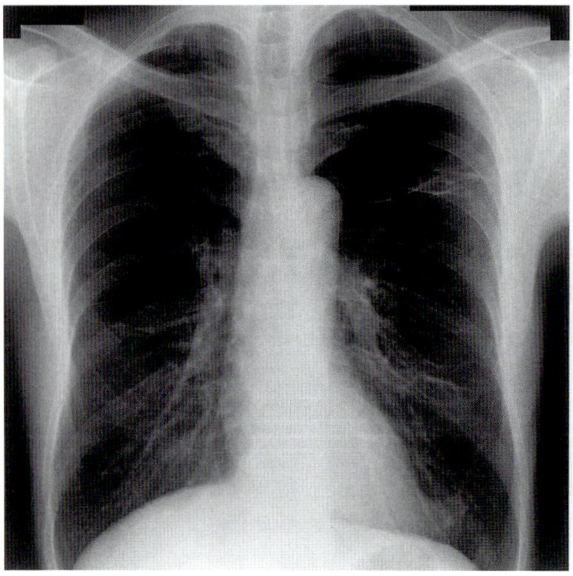

Figure 16. **Chest radiograph: Giant bulla**

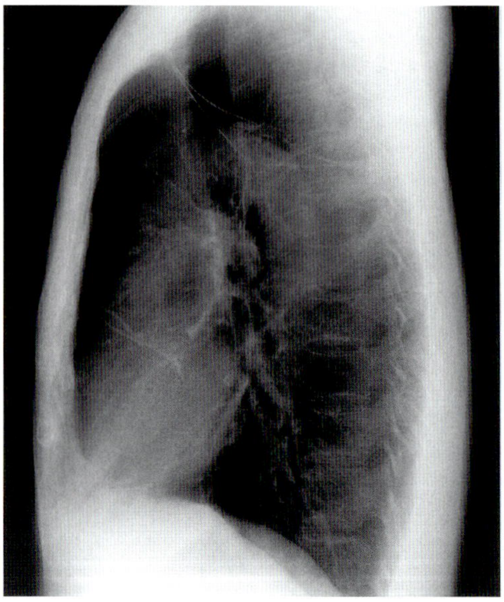

Figure 17. **Chest radiograph**

Consulted us for a linear shadow in the left upper lobe and an enlarged avascular area above it detected on a medical checkup.

A plain chest radiograph (*Fig. 16*) shows multiple linear shadows from the aortic arch to the chest wall, and above them an avascular area, so-called giant bulla.

The same findings can be interpreted from a lateral chest radiograph (*Fig. 17*).

A chest CT shows extensive emphysematous changes in the right lung, and almost no normal lung architecture on the left, which has become a single space, indicating a giant emphysematous cyst. There are no symptoms but the patient has been a heavy smoker with a smoking history of 40/day for 30 years. Regarding pulmonary function, a mild decrease in %VC was seen. Left untreated, the giant bulla would increase in size and exert pressure on normal lung which could obstruct pulmonary ventilation. Resection of the left upper lobe was conducted under thoracoscopy. Postoperative course was favorable and vital capacity was restored 142%.

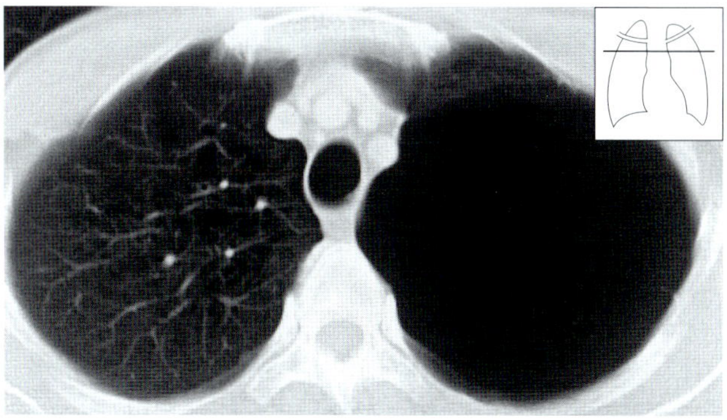

Figure 18. **Chest CT**

Case 7 Pneumomediastinum

27-year-old female

Consulted us for an asthmatic attack brought on by upper respiratory tract infection.

A plain chest radiograph shows linear shadows (→) following the aorta. This is mediastinal emphysema (pneumomediastinum). An improvement was seen with treatment for asthma only. Mediastinal emphysema is caused by the leakage of air into the mediastinum, and a wide range of causal factors are known such as acute increase in intra-alveolar pressure (asthma, sports that involve breath holding), *Pneumocystis* pneumonia, tracheal and bronchial damage and esophageal rupture (spontaneous, tumor, etc.). Accompanying symptoms are often chest pain and subcutaneous emphysema of the neck.

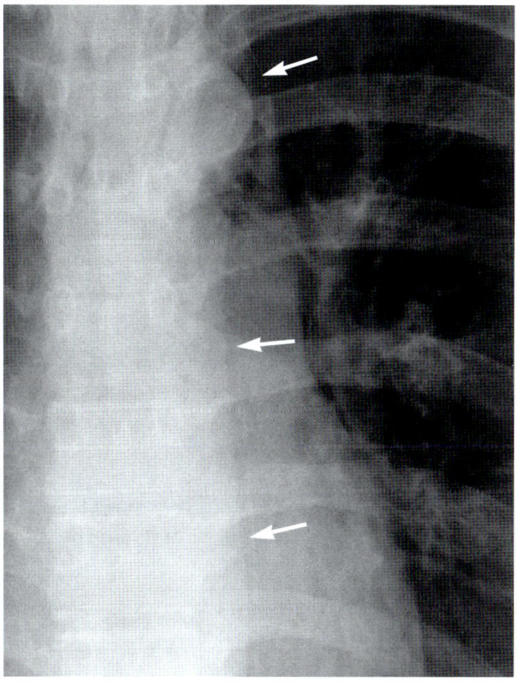

Figure 19. **Chest radiograph: Mediastinal emphysema (pneumomediastinum)**

Nonpathological linear shadows

The following are two examples of linear shadows that, although not disease-related, can easily mislead inexperienced doctors.

1. Azygos fissure / 36-year-old male

"Abnormal shadow" detected on a medical checkup.

A plain chest radiograph (*Fig. 20*) shows tear-drop shaped nodular shadows (→) near the right superior mediastinum, and an arc-shaped shadow (➤) continuing on from there reaching the apical pleura.

A chest CT (*Fig. 22*) indicates that a blood vessel from the posterior chest wall passes through the lung joining the superior vena cava. This is an anomalous azygos vein, corresponding to the tear-drop shadows in the plain radiograph. Higher up, linear shadows continue (*Fig. 21*). This is a kind of dysplasia in which an azygos vein enters the lung during lung formation, and is referred to as azy-

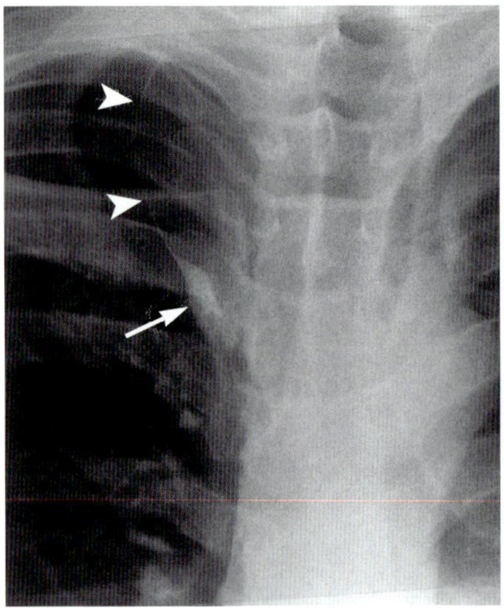

Figure 20. **Chest radiograph: Azygous fissure**

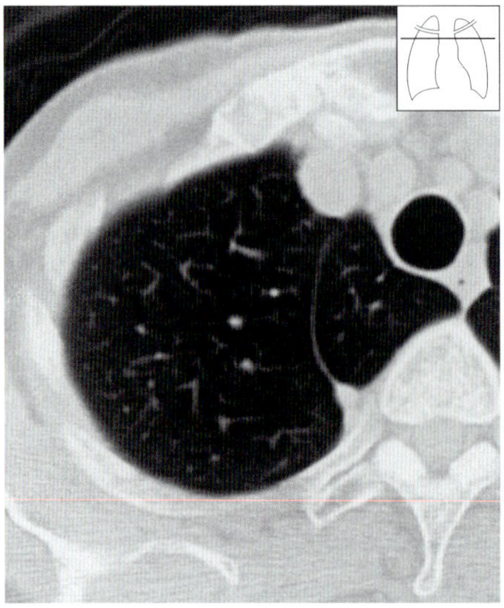

Figure 21. **Chest CT**

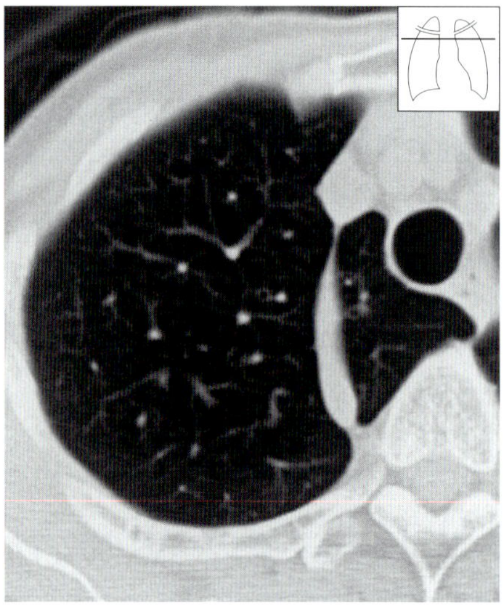

Figure 22. **Chest CT**

gos fissure. This azygos fissure is composed of four layers of pleura, which envelops the azygos vein. The inner side of the interlobular fissure is an accessory lobe called an azygos lobe. This is observed in 0.5% of all chest imagings. It poses no clinical problems.

2. Shadows due to the sternum / 35-year-old male

A plain chest radiograph (*Fig. 23*) shows the entire outline (→) of the manubrium of the sternum. It is shaped like the home plate in baseball. It is rare to be able to see the entire outline of the manubrium in regular plain radiograph but it should be understood that it is roughly this shape and located in this position. This is because it sometimes occurs that the right border of the manubrium appears clearly in plain chest radiographs. On such occasions, it is difficult to differentiate it from SVC or the winding, protruding right brachiocephalic arteries. In this region of plain chest radiographs physicians are required to pay the utmost attention to the detection of lymph node swelling and so lines should be identified one at a time. The possibility of involvement of the right border of the sternum should also be borne in mind.

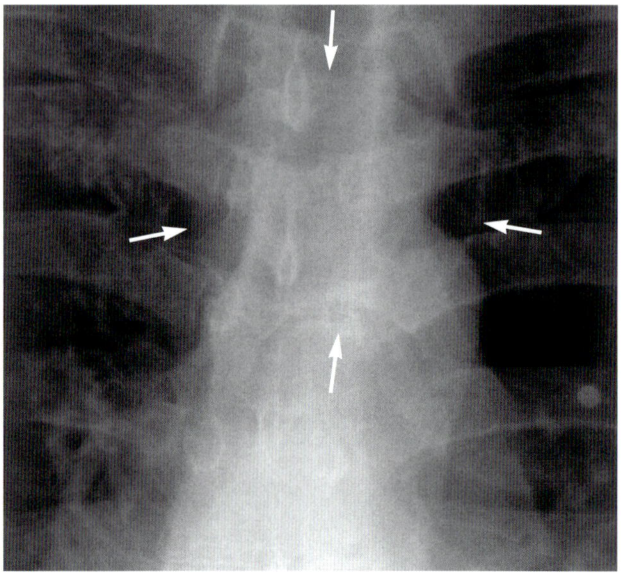

Figure 23. **Chest radiograph: Sternum**

Chapter 4

Radiographs of intrapulmonary lesions with decreased radiolucency

14. Hilar shadow

[Pattern classification IV-G]

●Author — Atsuko Kurosaki

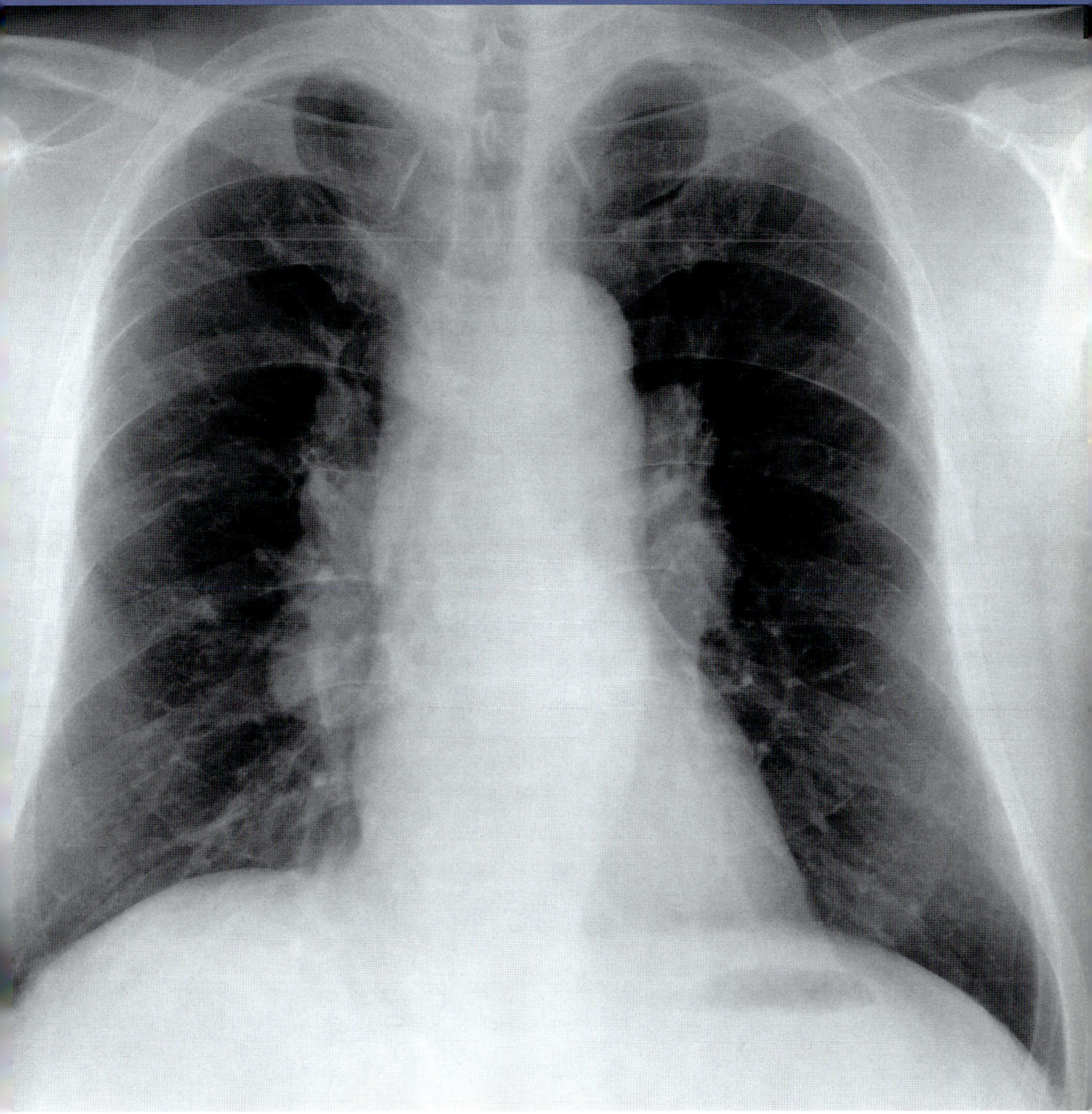

Keywords of this section

Hilar shadow
Sarcoidosis
Hilum
Hilum (hilus) convergence sign
Teratoma
Hilum (hilus) overlay sign
Hilar lung cancer
Tracheal/bronchial amyloidosis
Malignant lymphoma
Scimitar syndrome
Hypogenetic lung syndrome
Hilum (hilus) bifurcation sign

Hilar shadow

Atsuko Kurosaki
Department of Diagnostic Radiology, Toranomon Hospital, Tokyo, Japan

The hilum is the exit for the blood vessels and bronchi from the mediastinum to the lungs. Hilar shadows are composed mainly of left and right bronchi and their branches, left and right pulmonary arteries and their branches, and superior pulmonary veins. Hilar enlargement can be caused by factors such as pulmonary artery enlargement, hilar lymph node swelling and pulmonary or mediastinal lesions overlaying the hilum. This section describes how to differentiate between these factors using chest radiographs. Explanations are also provided concerning CT and MRI, which are frequently necessary.

Case 1 54-year-old male

Chief complaint: Asymptomatic
Medical history: Unremarkable
Occupation: Company employee (office work)
Family history: Mother, hypertension
Present illness:
Examined after a medical checkup revealed enlarged bilateral hilar shadows, and was admitted for detailed examination.
Findings on admission: No findings of note observed
Laboratory data on admission:
TP 6.5, Alb 3.7, T-Bil 1.1, UN 12, Cr 0.9, Na 140, K 3.7, AST 23, ALT 28, LDH 148, CK 35, ESR 4, CRP 0.1, ACE 26.8, Lysozyme 17.7, WBC 5200, Hb 15.9, Ht 44.9, PLT 313 x 1000.

Chest radiograph: Frontal view (P. 149) shows bilateral symmetrical hilar enlargement. They have distinct borders and a potato-like shape. The lungs appear normal. Even in a lateral view (*Fig. 1*) hilar lymph node enlargement (→) can be seen as tumor-like shadows with sharp borders.

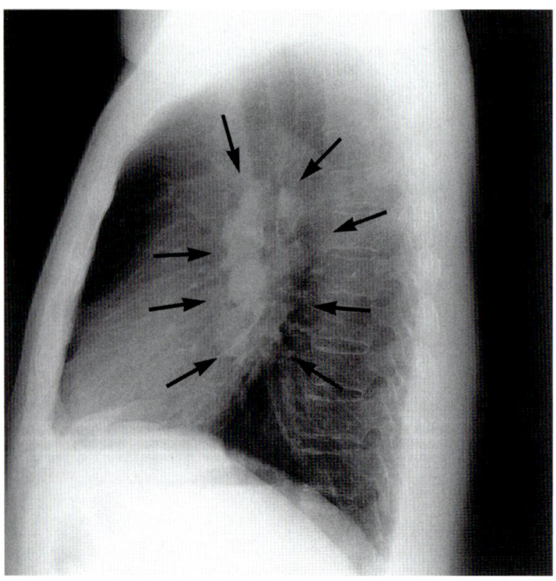

Figure 1. **Chest radiograph**

Chest CT (*Figs. 2–5*): Lymph node enlargement (→) can be observed in paratracheal, para-aortic, subcarinal, and subaortic regions, and bilateral hila. Each of the lymph nodes has a smooth border. No abnormality can be seen in pulmonary parenchyma.

Course after admission:
At bronchoscopy, the right superior truncus and truncus intermedius spurs are blunted. A transbronchial lung biopsy (TBLB) sample from right bronchi B^3 and B^8 revealed epithelioid granuloma (→) and sarcoidosis was diagnosed (*Figs. 6, 7*).

Other findings:
Abdominal ultrasound examination: No abnormality
A gallium scintigram (^{67}Ga-citrate) (*Fig. 8*) showed intense bilateral hilar accumulation (→).
Brain CT: No abnormality
Echocardiogram: No abnormality
Electrocardiogram: Premature ventricular contraction
Myocardial scintigram (^{201}Tl-Cl): Reduced nonuniformity of anterior septum and inferior posterior wall incorpo-

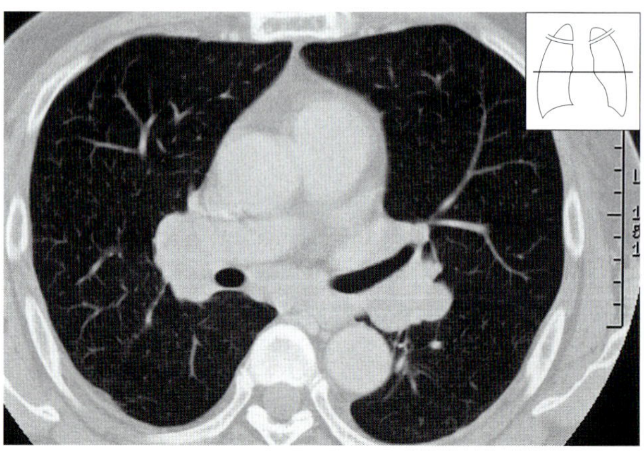

Figure 2. **Chest CT: Lung window setting**

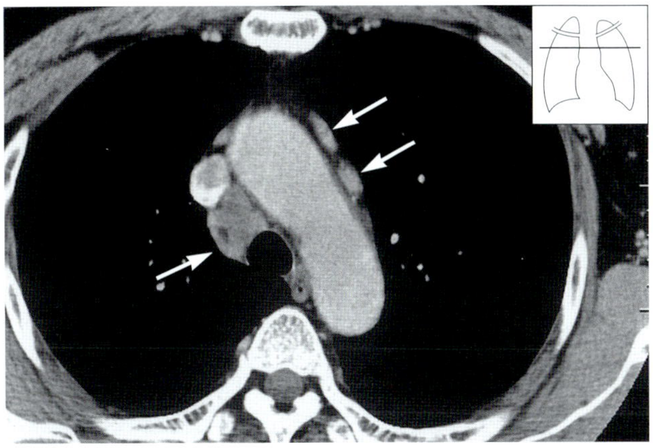

Figure 3. **Chest CT: Mediastinal window setting**

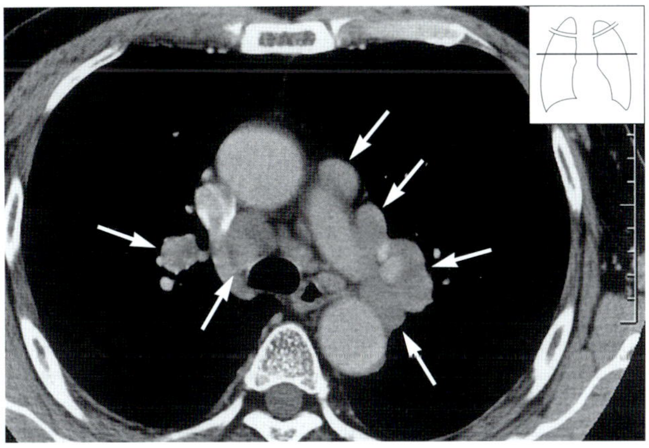

Figure 4. **Chest CT: Mediastinal window setting**

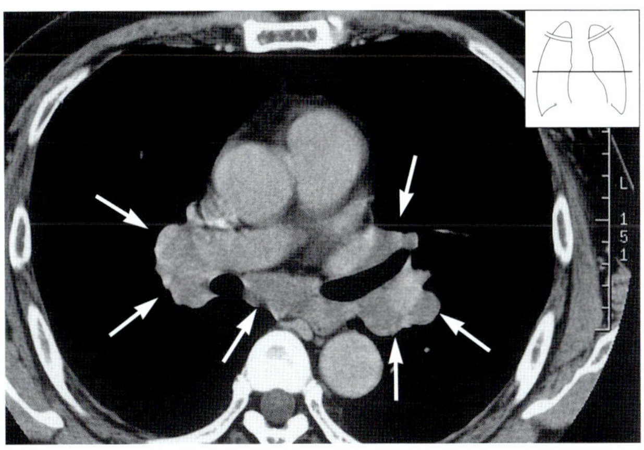

Figure 5. **Chest CT: Mediastinal window setting**

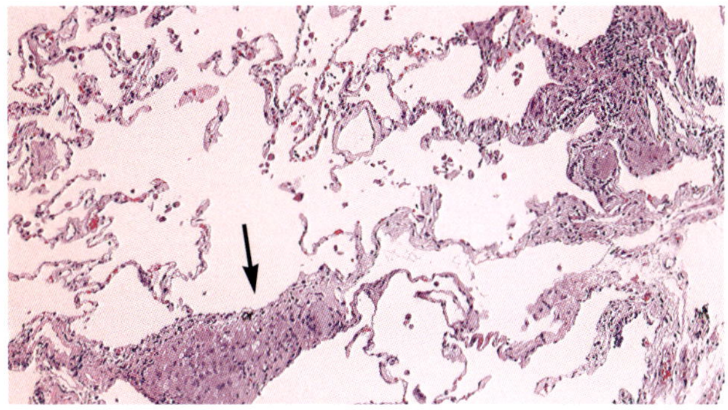

Figure 6. **Histological picture**

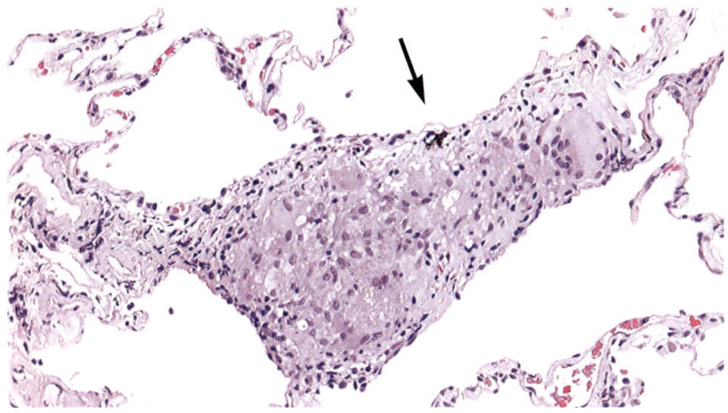

Figure 7. **Histological picture**

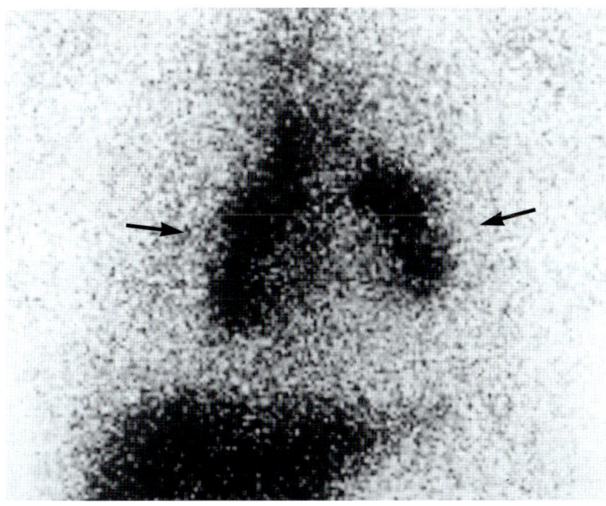

Figure 8. **Gallium scintigram**

ration, suggesting myocardial damage
Myocardial biopsy: No abnormality
Eye: No abnormality
Upper gastrointestinal series: No abnormality

Sarcoidosis

Sarcoidosis is a systemic disease of unknown cause characterized by formation of noncaseating epithelioid cell granuloma in multiple organs. Pulmonary lesions including mediastinal and hilar lymph node lesions are observed in over 90% of cases. For classification in chest radiographs, the system developed by DeRemee[1] (*Table 1*) is often used but in most cases of sarcoidosis, lymph node enlargement occurs at some point during the course of the disease.

During the natural course of many cases, lymph node enlargement subsides within a few years (within 2 years for 70% of cases). The disease develops preferentially in bilateral hila (BHL) and the right paratracheal region, but is accompanied at the same time by Bottalo's lymph nodes. In cases of unilateral hilar lymph node enlargement showing a strong tendency towards adhesion, diseases other than sarcoidosis (malignant lymphoma, cancer metastasis, etc.) should be considered.

At TBLB, pulmonary parenchymal lesions are present in

90% of cases, even if imaging studies show no abnormality. The lesions exist along pulmonary lymphatics. Consequently, in HRCT they show as changes in bronchovascular bundles, pulmonary veins, interlobular septa and pleura. In other words, there are nonuniform bronchovascular bundle thickening, extensive interstitial and peribronchiolar granular lesions, large and small nodules, increased ground glass opacity, and mass lesions with contraction.

Stage 0	Normal radiograph
Stage I	Lymph node enlargement
Stage II	Lymph node enlargement and pulmonary parenchymal abnormality
Stage III	Pulmonary parenchymal abnormality

Table 1. **Classification of sarcoidosis by chest radiograph**

Hilum

The hilum (*Fig. 9*) is the exit for the blood vessels and bronchi from the mediastinum to the lungs, and is composed of main left/right bronchi and their branches, left and right pulmonary arteries and their branches, and the superior pulmonary veins. Establishing the normal size of the hilum is difficult but in general, the diameter of the right descending pulmonary artery along the intermediate bronchus should be 10 to 16 mm in males and 9 to 15 mm in females. The position of the pulmonary arteries also differs slightly, with the left one being 1 to 2 cm higher than the right.

The causes of hilar enlargement include pulmonary artery enlargement, hilar lymph node enlargement and pulmonary or mediastinal lesions overlaying the hilum (*Table 2*).

Causes of hilar enlargement

1. Causes of pulmonary artery enlargement
   Bilateral: Pulmonary hypertension (congenital heart disease with accompanying left to right shunt, cor pulmonale, left heart failure, mitral stenosis)
   Unilateral: Pulmonary embolism, pulmonary artery stenosis, idiopathic pulmonary artery enlargement, pulmonary aneurysm cancer, congenital pericardial defect
2. Hilar lymph node enlargement
   Bilateral: Neoplastic (lymphoma, metastatic tumor, leukemia), Inflammatory (sarcoidosis, tuberculosis, fungal infection, silicosis, others.)
   Unilateral: Neoplastic (lung cancer, lymphoma, metastatic tumor), Inflammatory (primary tuberculosis, fungal infection, viral infection, others.)
3. Pulmonary or mediastinal lesions overlaying the hilum
   Pulmonary or mediastinal tumor (benign, malignant), pneumonia, pulmonary abscess and pulmonary parenchymal lesions such as atelectasis.

Causes of small hilum

Bilateral: Pulmonary artery stenosis, defect, and displacement (congenital heart disease with cyanosis)
Unilateral: Pulmonary artery stenosis, lung hypoplasia, pulmonary embolism, atelectasis, Swyer-James syndrome

Table 2. **Diseases causing hilar abnormality**

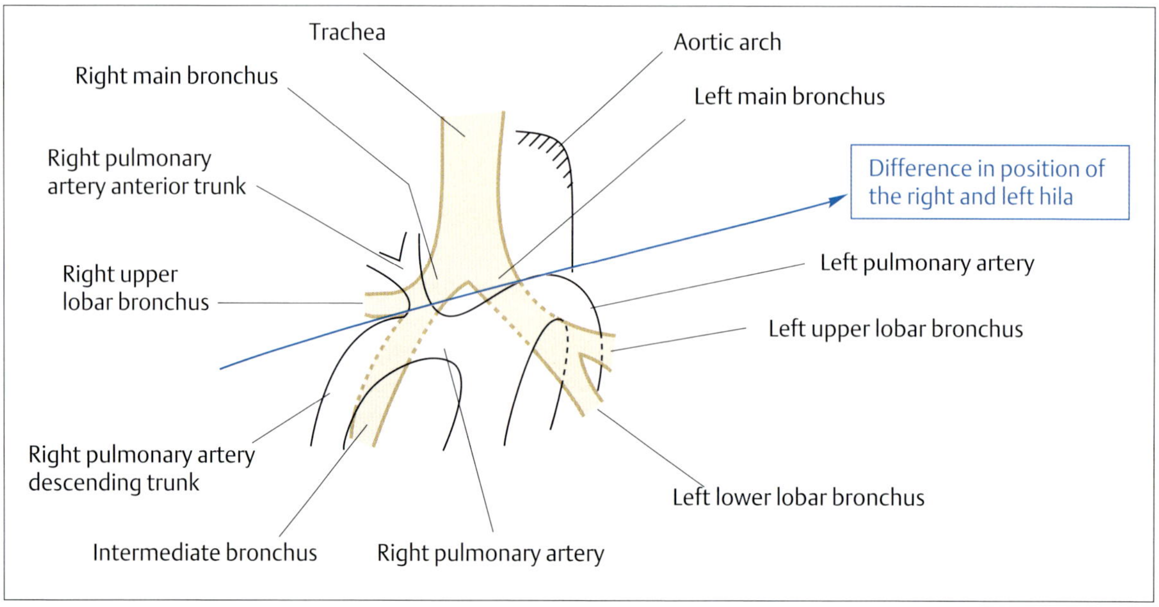

Figure 9. **Scheme of the hilum**

Case 2 Primary pulmonary hypertension
50-year-old female

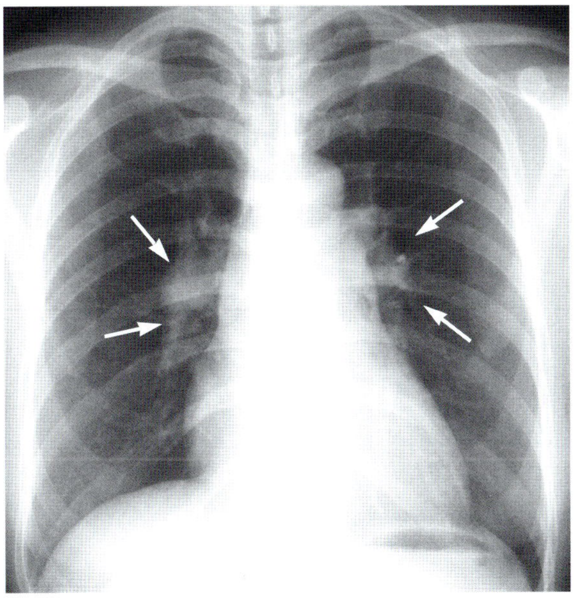

Figure 10. **Chest radiograph**

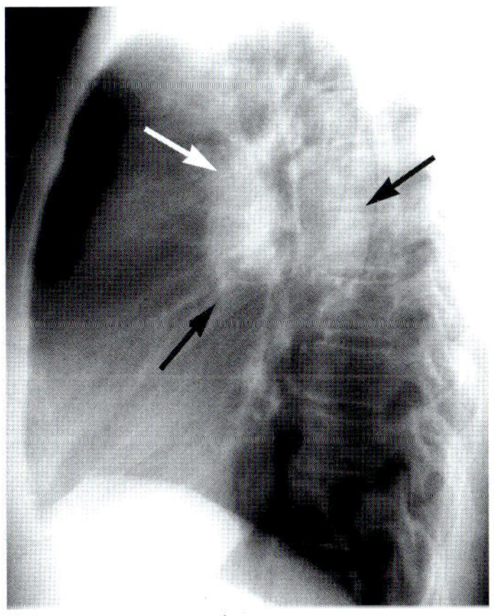

Figure 11. **Chest radiograph**

Chief complaint: Shortness of breath on exertion

Chest radiograph: findings: Frontal view (*Fig. 10*) shows bilateral hilar enlargement (➞). The convergence of pulmonary vessels uniformly facing the enlarged hilar image (hilum convergence sign) can be confirmed, and hilar enlargement could be due to pulmonary artery enlargement. Peripheral pulmonary vessels are similarly fewer, and the lung field periphery appears lucent. Even on a lateral view (*Fig. 11*), an enlarged hilum (➞) is clearly seen without potato-like appearance.

CT findings (*Figs. 12, 13*): Contrast-enhanced CT with mediastinal window setting shows clear enlargement from the undivided pulmonary artery to the left and right pulmonary arteries (➞), but no filling defect suggesting thrombus can be seen. In the lung window setting (*Fig. 13*), there are no abnormalities in pulmonary parenchyma, and lung attenuation is uniform.

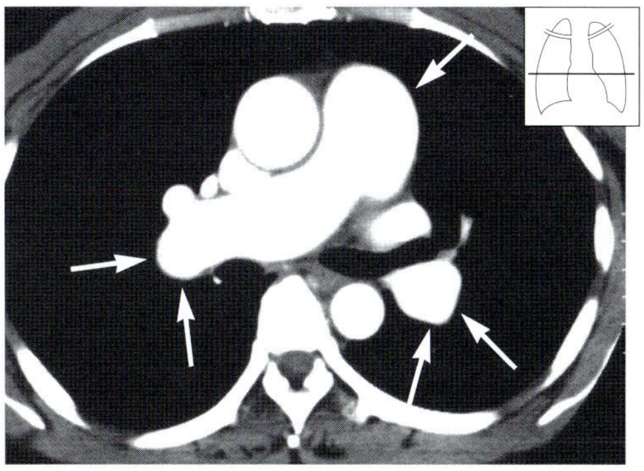

Figure 12. **Chest CT: Mediastinal window setting**

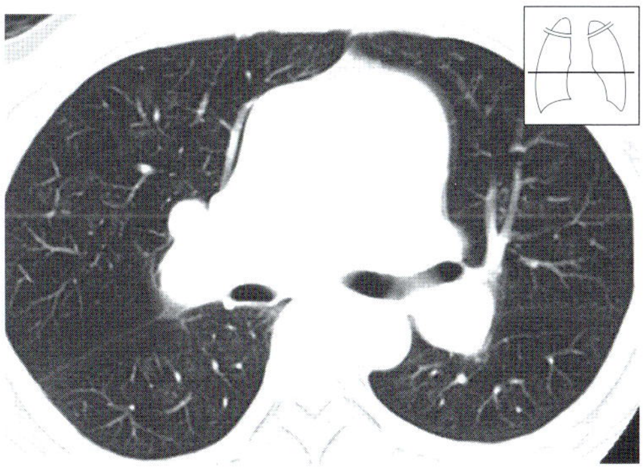

Figure 13. **Chest CT: Lung window setting**

Primary pulmonary hypertension

Primary pulmonary hypertension is a generic term for severe precapillary pulmonary hypertension of unknown cause. At chest radiograph, it characteristically shows as an enlarged bilateral hila with a uniform reduction in bilateral pulmonary peripheral branches. At CT, enlargement of central pulmonary arteries is also clear, with no accompanying filling defect and no lung abnormalities.

It is important to differentiate between this disease and chronic thromboembolic pulmonary hypertension. Points for differentiation include the same radiographic findings of hilar enlargement due to enlarged central pulmonary arteries, but the reduction of peripheral pulmonary arteries is nonuniform. Contrast-enhanced CT also shows the same enlargement of central pulmonary arteries, but there are filling defects indicative of thrombi and since areas of reduced blood flow result in decreased lung attenuation in the lung window setting, contrast between areas of normal perfusion and decreased perfusion produces a mosaic pattern.

Case 3 Teratoma
14-year-and-4-month-old female

Chief complaint: Left anterior chest pain

Chest radiographs (*Figs. 14, 15*): There is a mass (➞) measuring 8 cm in diameter in the left hilar area (*Fig. 14*). The left border is distinct and smooth, and the hilar vessels overlaid by the tumor shadow can be seen (hilum overlay sign), indicating possible mediastinal tumor. The left border of the descending aorta in preserved, excluding the possibility of a posterior mediastinal lesion. Lateral view (*Fig. 15*) shows decreased retrosternal radiolucency (➞).

Chest CT (*Figs. 16–18*): On the left side of the anterior

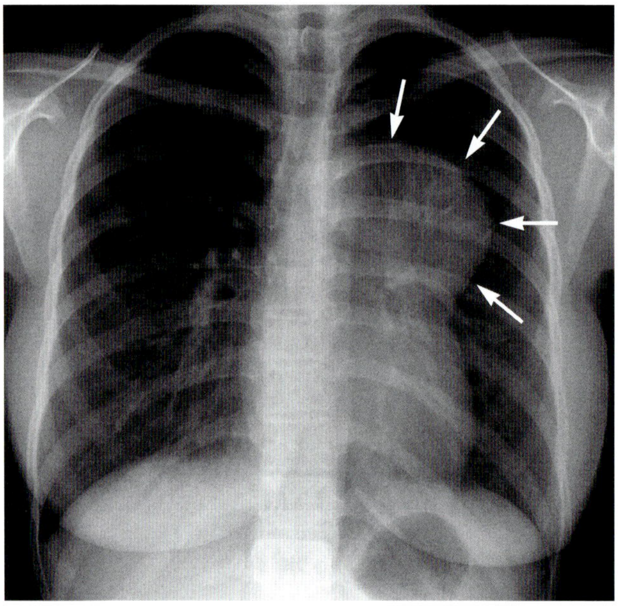

Figure 14. **Chest radiograph**

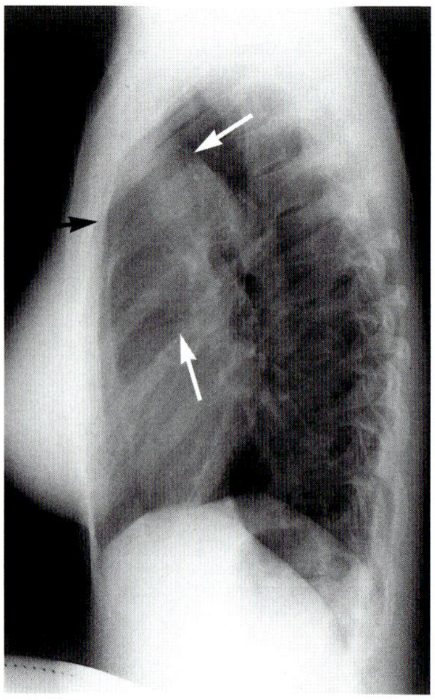

Figure 15. **Chest radiograph**

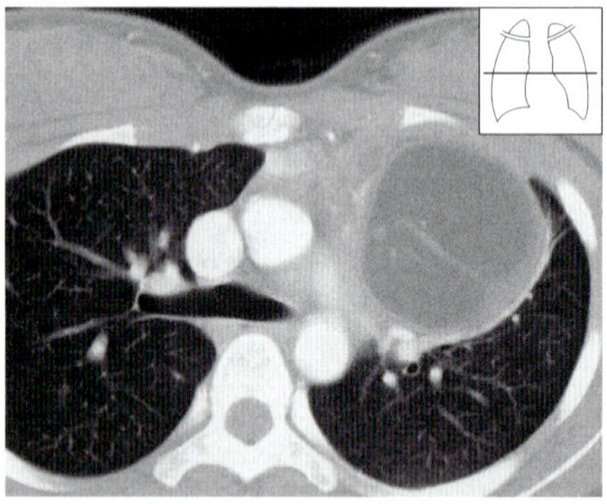

Figure 16. **Chest CT: Lung window setting**

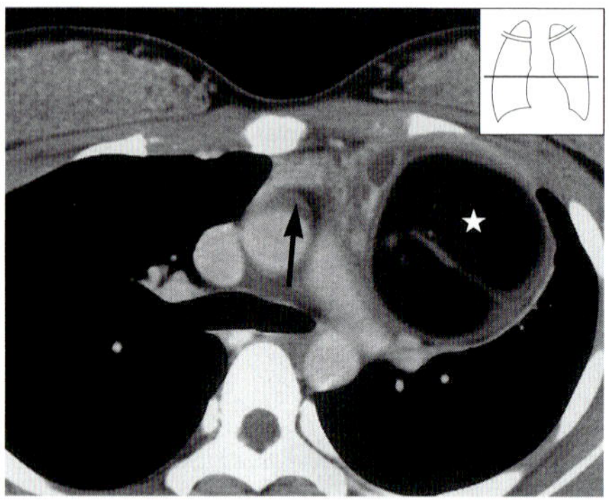

Figure 17. **Chest CT: Mediastinal window setting**

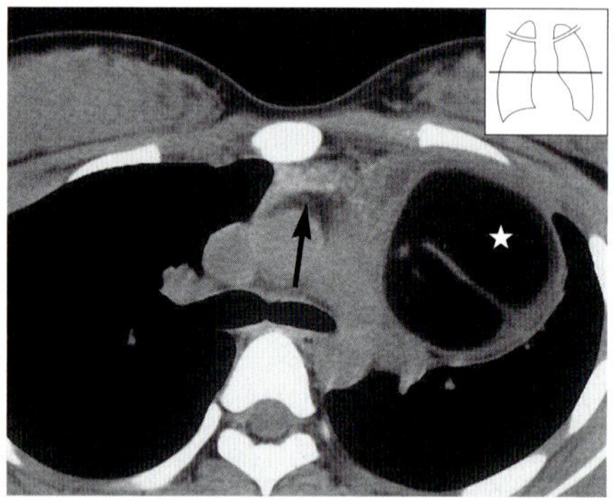

Figure 18. **Chest CT: Mediastinal window setting**

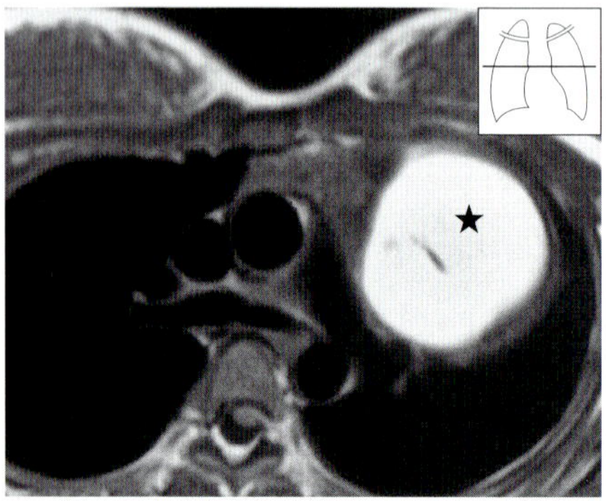

Figure 19. **T1-weighted MRI**

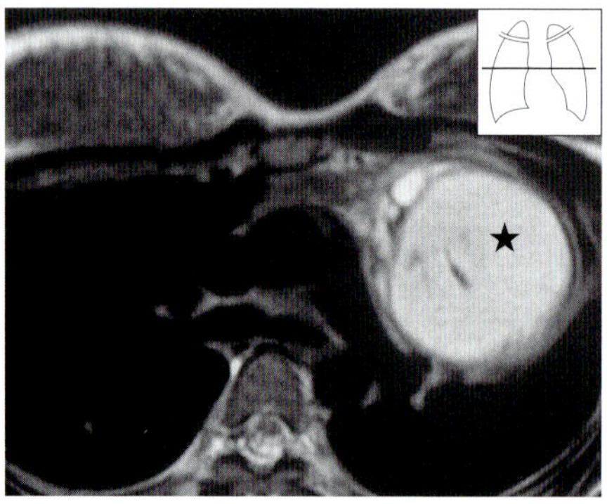

Figure 20. **T2-weighted MRI**

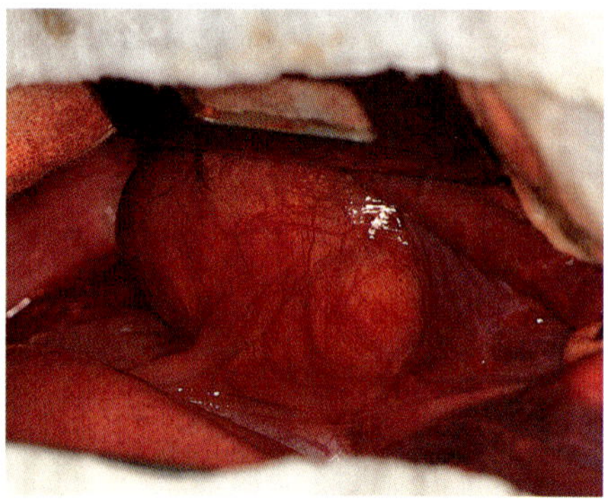

Figure 21. **Photograph during surgery**

mediastinum, there is an 8 x 6 cm tumor extending from the aortic arch to the ventral side of the left pulmonary artery. It is composed mainly of fatty tissue (☆), but the border is layered with a reinforcing capsule-like structure. It appears to be connected to the thymus (➞).

Thoracic MRI (*Figs. 19, 20*): As with CT, a spherical tumor is present at the anterior mediastinum. The same degree of very high intensity (★) as the subcutaneous fatty tissue is indicated for most of the lesion in T1 and T2-weighted images. A T2-weighted image shows a low intensity band following the border of the tumor, which could indicated a capsule.

Preoperative diagnosis: Mature teratoma of the anterior mediastinum

Operation (*Fig. 21*): There is a fist-size anterior mediastinal tumor connected to the thymus. The mediastinal pleura covering the tumor was milky-white and thick, and had firmly adhered to the lung and the left phrenic nerve. There was a small amount of bloody pleural effusion.

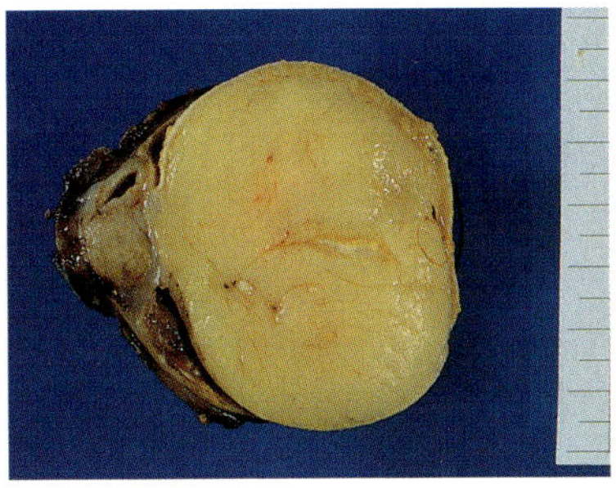

Figure 22. **Macroscopic findings: Bisected gross specimen**

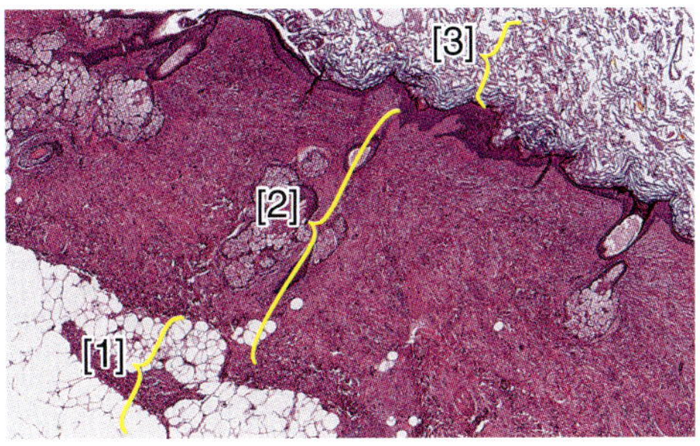

Figure 23. **Histological picture**

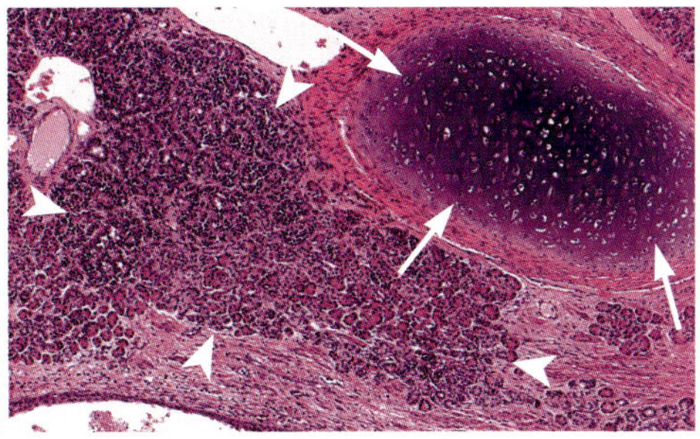

Figure 24. **Histological picture**

Pathological diagnosis: Mature teratoma

The anterior mediastinal tumor (*Fig. 22*) is 7 x 7 x 4.5 cm in size and an elastic hard, spherical cystic lesion. There is a pedunculated yellow tumor in the internal space, with keratinized material adhering to the surface. Small cyst aggregation is present in the cyst wall.

A histological picture (*Fig. 23*) shows that most of the solid components protruding into the internal space are composed of mature fatty tissue ([1]). The surface is abundant dermal tissue composed of keratinized epithelium and sebaceous glands ([2]), with a covering of additional keratinized material ([3]). At the adhesion site of the pedunculated tumor there is also a mixture of cartilage tissue (*Fig. 24*) (➞), tubes derived from ciliated epithelium, gastrointestinal tract tissue, pancreatic tissue and other tissue (➤). Chronic inflammation is seen in the pancreatic tissue. Most of the cyst walls are composed of hyalinized collagen fiber, with thymus tissue in the surrounding area also excised.

Teratoma

Teratoma is a tumor consisting of ectoderm, mesoderm, and endoderm of various quantities and degrees of differentiation. The tissue in a mature teratoma, which is derived from these three types of germ cells, can be of any kind found in the body, and may have reached a point of maturity where it can be identified, in which case it is benign. In immature teratomas, the tissues derived from the three types of germ cells may be mixed. None shows differentiation or organic structure. Some immature teratomas may take a malignant course.

Mediastinal teratomas account for 16 to 24% of all mediastinal tumors, making it a disease of comparatively high frequency. Many mature teratomas are unilocular or multilocular cystic lesions, reflecting the structural components of the three types of germ cells. Accordingly, if fat, teeth, bone and fluid are detected, a diagnosis is straight forward. It is said that fat, teeth and bone respectively can be identified in roughly half the cases. CT and MRI are used for diagnosis, and in cases of cystic lesions, clues to diagnosis include fatty density, bone or teeth. Immature teratomas are rare, and appear as inhomogeneous solid masses with irregular borders.

Case 4

Hilar lung cancer

61-year-old male

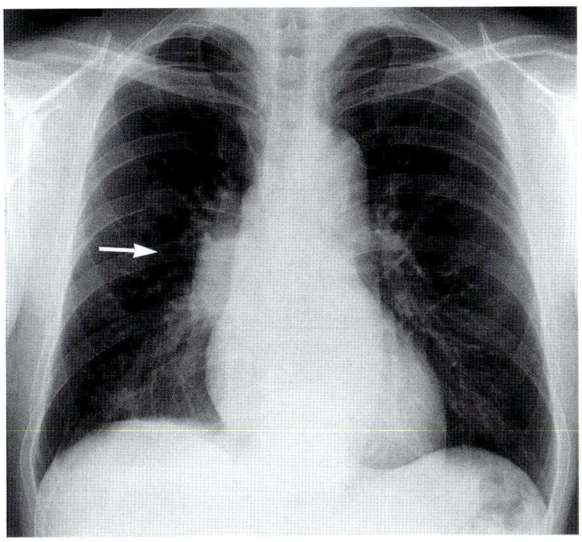

Figure 25. **Chest radiograph**

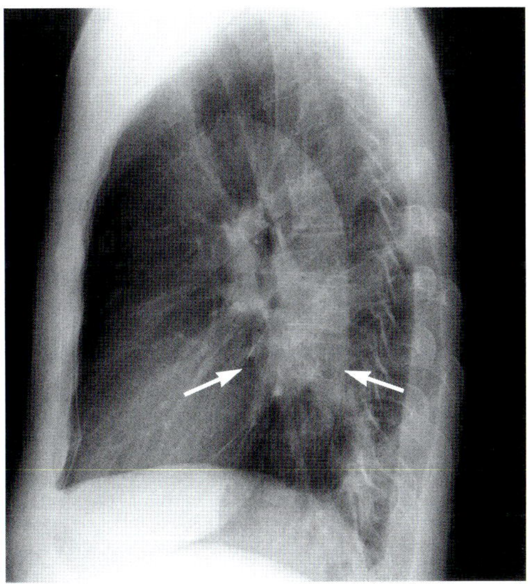

Figure 26. **Chest radiograph**

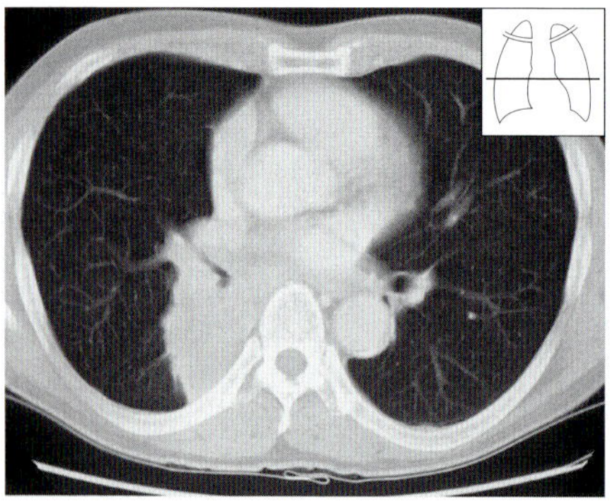

Figure 27. **Chest CT: Lung window setting**

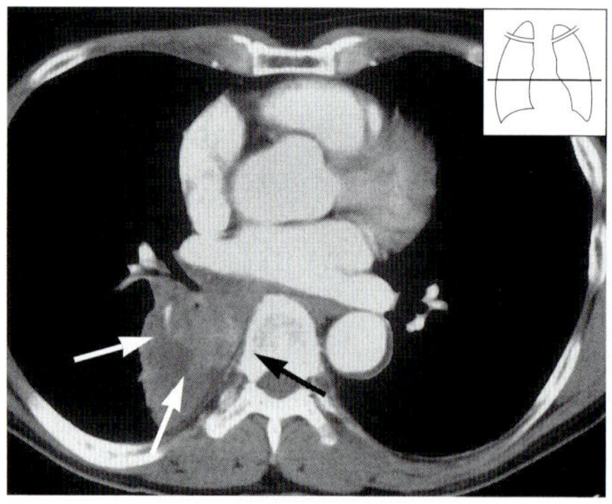

Figure 28. **Chest CT: Mediastinal window setting, early-phase**

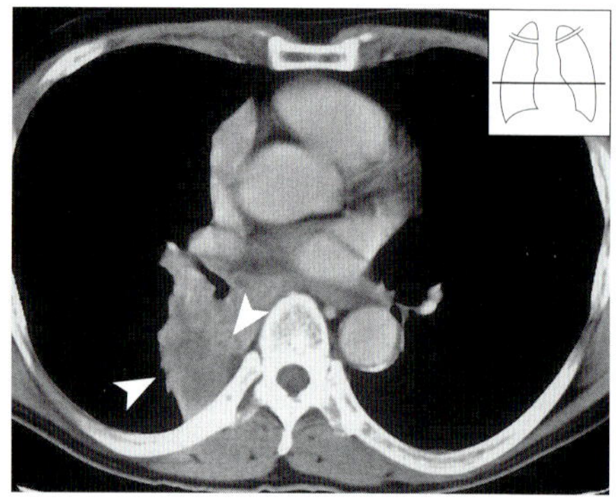

Figure 29. **Chest CT: Mediastinal window setting, delayed-phase**

Chief complaint: Cough

Chest radiograph findings: Frontal view (*Fig. 25*) shows enlargement in the right hilar region (→). It is difficult to follow inside but the intermediate bronchus gradually becomes narrower, and the lower lobar bronchus cannot be identified. There is reduced radiolucency in the right lower lung and A^8, which should run towards the right costophrenic angle, can also not be confirmed. At the right costophrenic angle there is an oblique linear opacity that could indicate downward displacement of the major fissure, suggesting reduced volume of the lower lobe. Lateral view (*Fig. 26*) shows that on the slightly caudal level of bronchial bifurcation, there is a roughly 6 cm tumor shadow overlaying the spine (→). About a third of the rear of the right diaphragm is indistinct (positive silhouette sign).

Chest CT (*Fig. 27*): There is a roughly 8 cm tumor at the orifice of the right B^6, causing obstruction of the lower lobar bronchus and circumferential stenosis of the intermediate bronchus. With dynamic CT, a contrast-enhanced early-phase image (*Fig. 28*) shows strong enhancement of a tumor (roughly 4 cm in diameter) in the central area supplied by the bronchial arteries (→). On a delayed-phase image (*Fig. 29*), strongly enhanced atelectasis (roughly 4 cm in diameter) can be clearly seen in the periphery supplied by the pulmonary arteries (➤).

Case 5 Tracheal/bronchial amyloidosis

63-year-old male

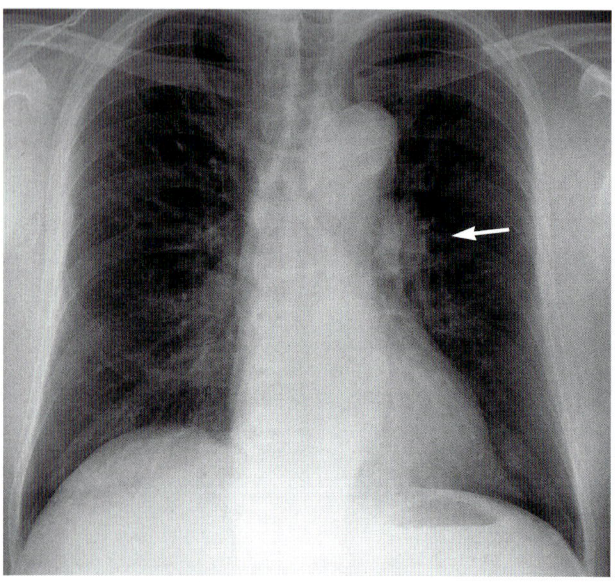

Figure 30. **Chest radiograph**

Chief complaint: Cough

Chest radiograph (frontal view) (*Fig. 30*): The left hilum is enlarged (→).

Chest CT (*Figs. 31–33*): There is a soft tissue lesion (→) at the left inferior trunk. Punctate calcification can be seen within the tumor (➤).

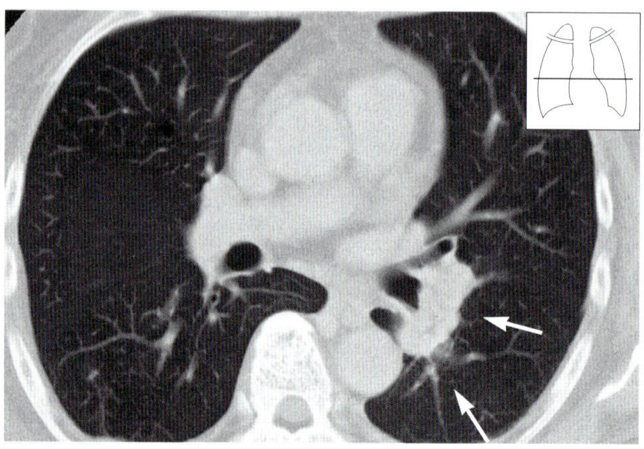

Figure 31. **Chest CT: Lung window setting**

Bronchoscopy (*Figure 34*): There is obstruction at the orifice of left B^6 which is filled with fragile tissue. Amyloid deposition was demonstrated with TBLB.

Amyloidosis

Amyloidosis is a disease of unknown cause characterized by the deposit in various organs of the body of a specific protein (amyloid) with a fibrous structure. It is often deposited in the liver, spleen and kidneys, with rare cases of

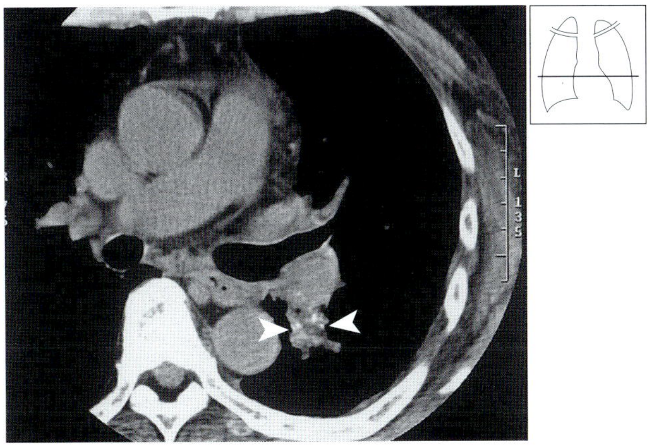

Figure 32. **Chest unenhanced CT: Mediastinal window setting**

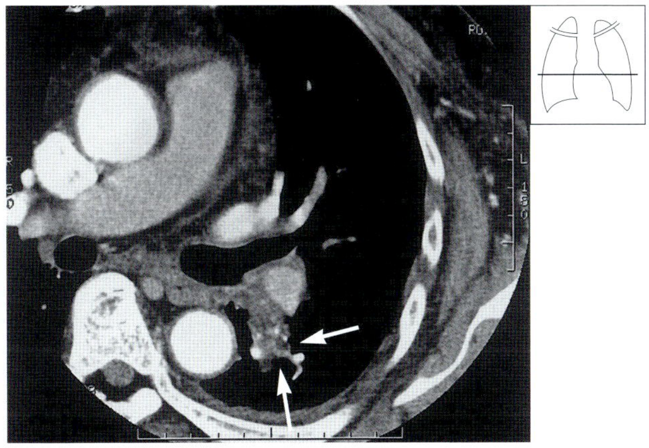

Figure 33. **Chest enhanced CT: Mediastinal window setting**

deposition in the lungs and bronchi. However, thoracic amyloidosis is an important disease for the differential diagnosis of tumorous lesions and diffuse pulmonary diseases. Fraser classifies thoracic amyloidosis into the tracheobronchial form, nodular parenchymal form and the diffuse interstitial form. The tracheobronchial form is the most frequent, associated with symptoms resulting from respiratory manifestations (cough, dyspnea, wheeze, etc.). The nodular parenchymal form manifests as 1 to 10 cm nodular lesions in the pulmonary parenchyma, and needs to be differentiated from other pulmonary tumorous lesions. The diffuse interstitial form is a condition in which amyloid is diffusely deposited in alveolar walls, perivascular regions and other interstitial tissue. Symptoms are cough or dyspnea and in general the prognosis is poor.

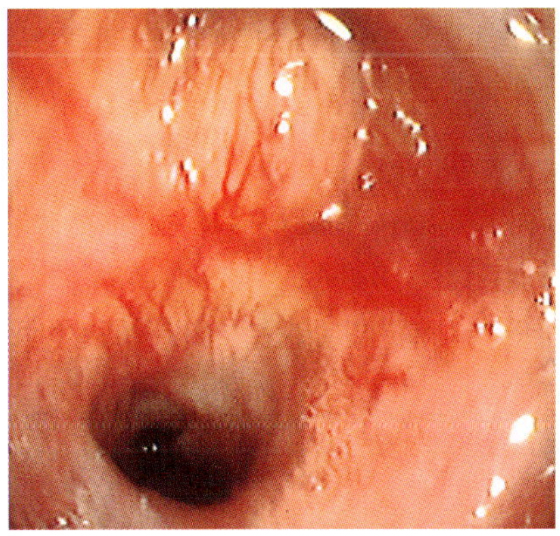

Figure 34. **Bronchoscopy**

Case 6 Malignant lymphoma

23-year-old male

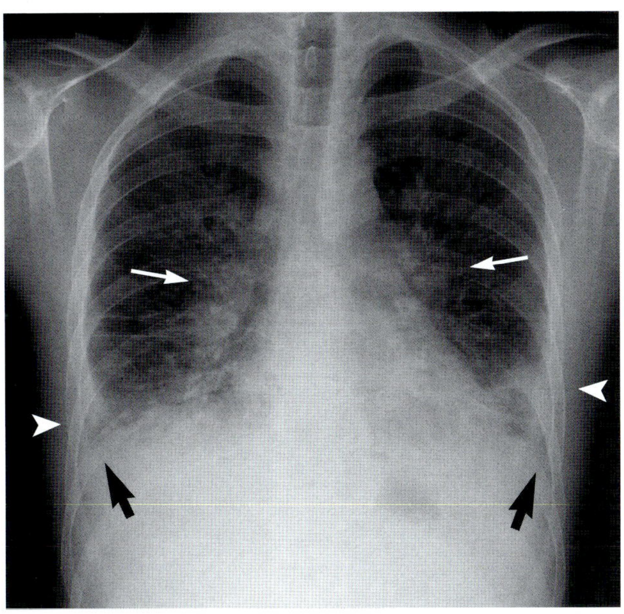

Figure 35. **Chest radiograph**

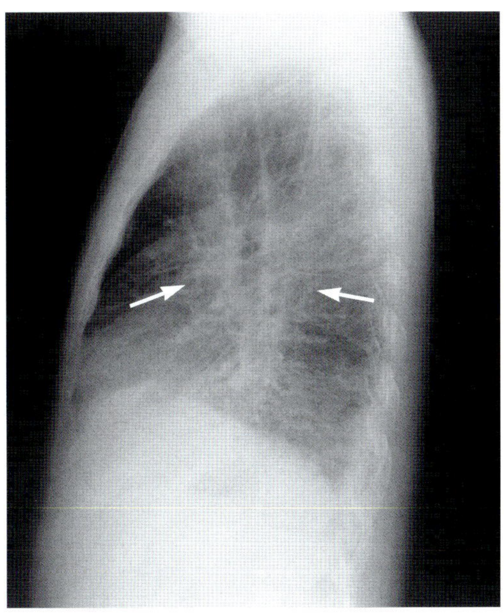

Figure 36. **Chest radiograph**

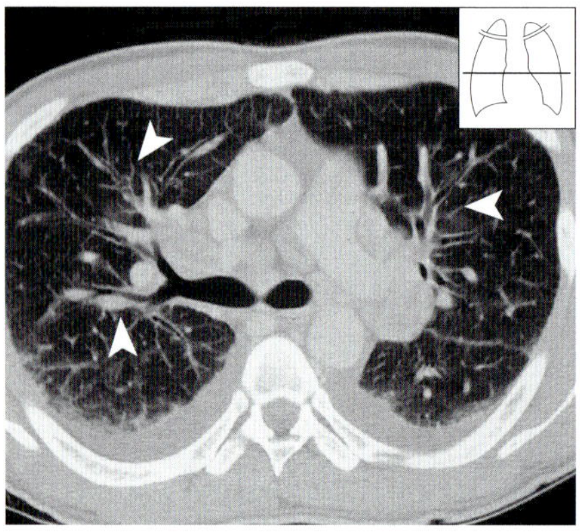

Figure 37. **Chest CT: Lung window setting**

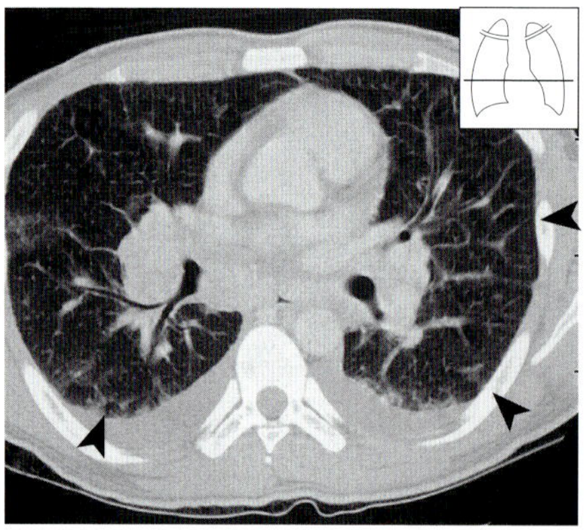

Figure 38. **Chest CT: Lung window setting**

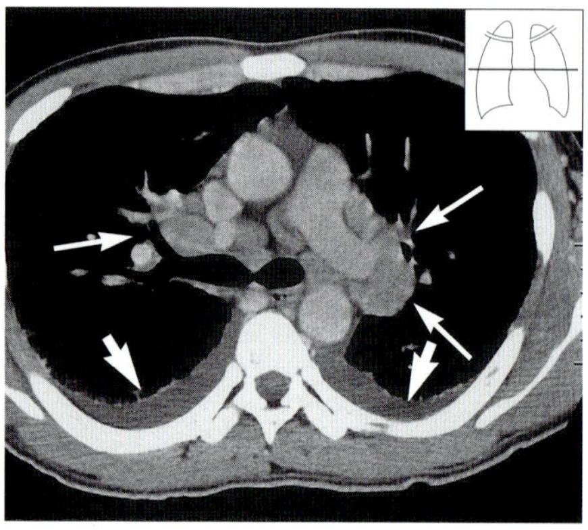

Figure 39. **Chest CT: Mediastinal window setting**

Chief complaints: Dyspnea, fever, weight loss

Chest radiograph (*Figs. 35, 36*): There is bilateral hilar enlargement (on both frontal and lateral views ➛), reticular shadows in the middle lower lung (➤) and bilateral pleural effusion (➔).

Chest CT (*Figs. 37–40*): There is conspicuous mediastinal and hilar lymph node enlargement (➛), with a moderate amount of bilateral pleural effusion (➔). Interlobular interstitial thickening (black ➤) and bronchovascular bundle thickening (white ➤) can also be seen.

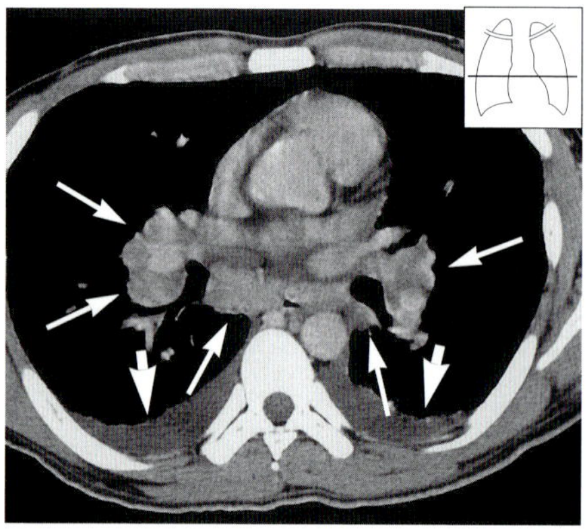

Figure 40. **Chest CT: Mediastinal window setting**

Malignant lymphoma

Malignant lymphoma is frequently accompanied by intrathoracic lesions. At the initial presentation, the frequency of intrathoracic involvement is 67% in Hodgkin's disease and 43% in non-Hodgkin's lymphoma (Filly).[2] Mediastinal and hilar lymph node enlargement is the most common with some reports indicating that it accounts for roughly half of all cases. There are comparatively few cases of pulmonary parenchymal lesions, but the image findings vary widely and include bronchovascular bundle thickening, interlobular interstitial thickening, increased ground glass opacity, miliary shadow, pneumonia-like shadows and nodules.

Case 7 Scimitar syndrome

30-year-old male

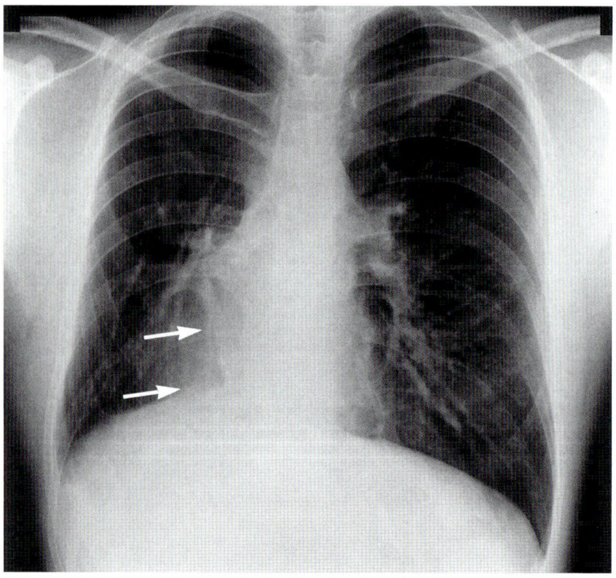

Figure 41. **Chest radiograph**

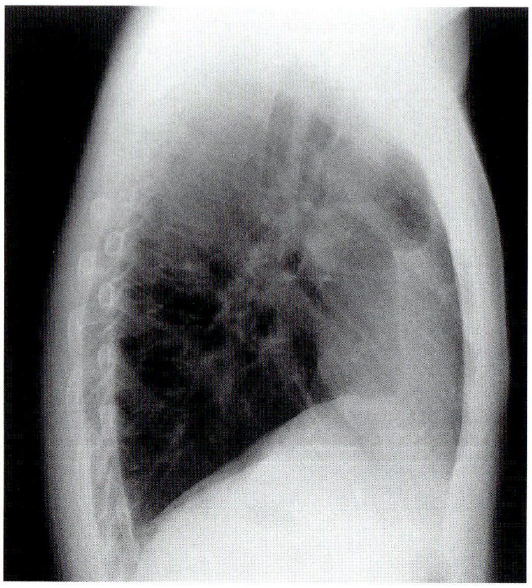

Figure 42. **Chest radiograph**

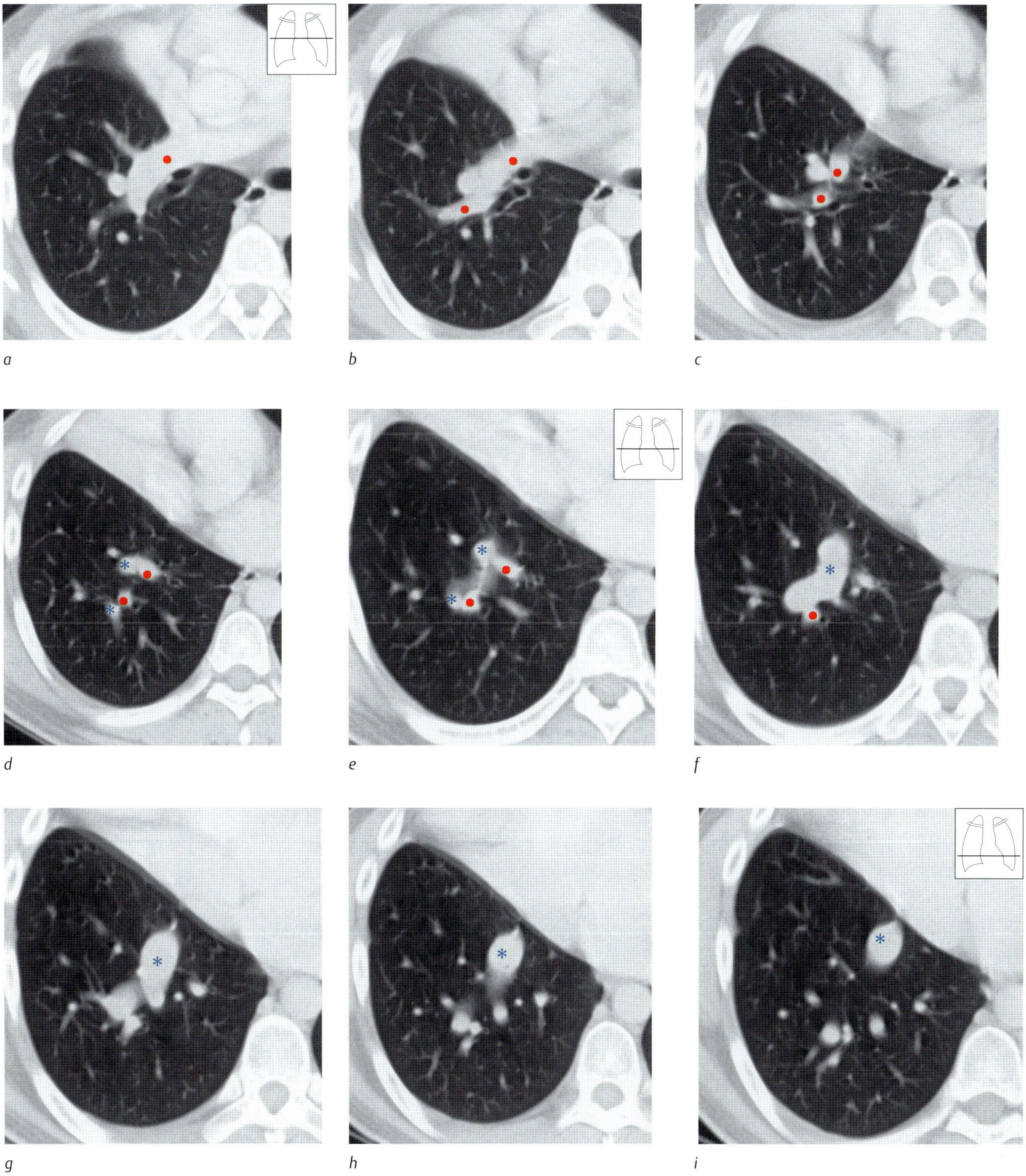

Figure 43 a–i. **Chest CT: 5 mm-thick slice at 5 mm intervals**

Chief complaint: Asymptomatic
Chest radiographs (*Figs. 41, 42*): The right thorax is smaller. Blood vessels are sparse in the right upper lung. An arc-like band shadow pointing inwards and then following a downward course is seen in the right lower lung. The right heart border is obscured.

Chest CT (*Figs. 43, 44*): The right lung is hypoplastic, and consists of a single lobe that could be equivalent to the lower lobe. The right pulmonary artery (●) bifurcates from the main pulmonary artery. The right pulmonary vein (*) descends obliquely slightly towards the mediastinum, and drains into the inferior vena cava. In 3D-CT (*Fig. 44 a–b*), the right pulmonary vein (➞) can be clearly seen following a downward course.

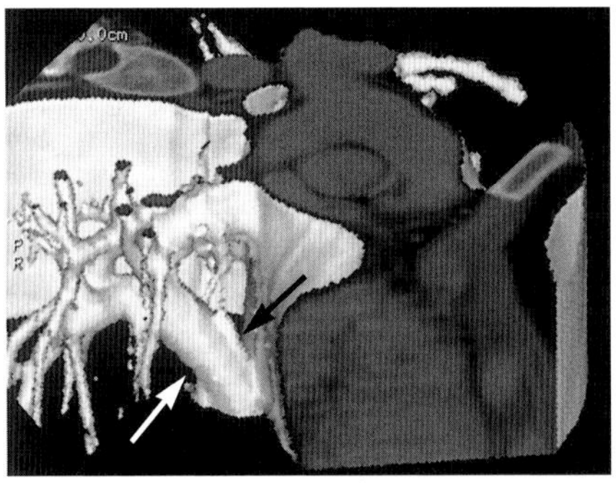

a

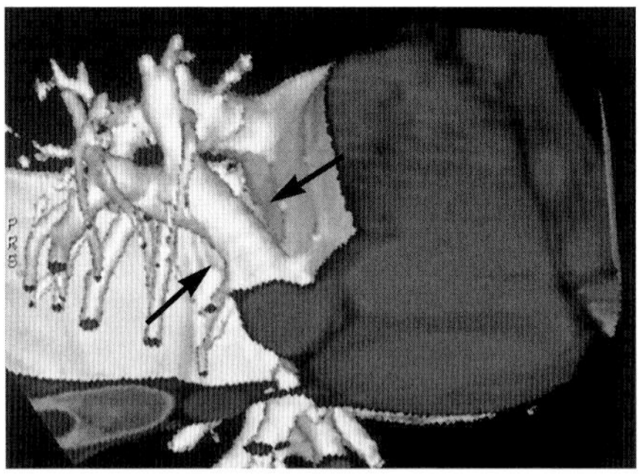

b

Figure 44 a–b: **3D-CT**

Scimitar syndrome (hypogenetic lung syndrome)

Scimitar syndrome is characterized by hypoplasia of the right lung and right pulmonary artery, abnormalities of the right bronchi, and anomalous pulmonary venous drainage to the inferior vena cava from the right lung. The course of this abnormal drainage resembles the shape of a scimitar. The area drained by an anomalous vein ranges from a segment to the right whole lung. The degree of right lung hypoplasia also differs widely. In this case, this was also accompanied by displacement of the heart to the right with counter-clockwise rotation, and right diaphragm elevation.

Scimitar: A curved sword mainly used by Arabs and Turks. The edge is rounded outward.

Conclusion

The hilum is the exit for the blood vessels and bronchi from the mediastinum to the lungs, and is composed of main left and right bronchi and their branches, left and right pulmonary arteries and their branches, and superior pulmonary veins.

The causes of hilar enlargement include pulmonary artery enlargement, hilar lymph node enlargement and pulmonary or mediastinal lesions overlaying the hilum. Hilum (hilus) bifurcation sign, hilum (hilus) convergence sign and hilum (hilus) overlay sign are useful for conducting differential diagnosis of the hilar region on radiographs.

Hilum (hilus) bifurcation sign, hilum (hilus) convergence sign

The cause of hilar enlargement is differentiated by the signs of either blood vessel enlargement or lymph node or other tumor shadows. If it can be confirmed that pulmonary vessels are concentrated towards a continuous, enlarged hilum, hilar enlargement could be due to enlargement of the pulmonary artery (Case 2) (*Figs. 10, 11*). Vascular branching seen within an enlarged hilum could indicate the presence of a mass.

Hilum (hilus) overlay sign

When a mass is seen to overlay the hilum on a frontal chest radiograph and the hilar shadow can just be seen within it, it could be a mediastinal tumor rather than cardiomegaly. (Case 3) (*Figs. 14, 15*)

As mentioned earlier, however, since the hilum is composed of many organs and tissues, it is difficult to ascertain the cause of hilar enlargement using only radiographs, and in many cases contrast-enhanced CT and MRI are required. First, using CT and/or MRI enables lesion localization. Second, it provides a wide range of information related to internal structure such as whether the lesion is solid or cystic, whether there is any contrast enhancement or not, and intravascular details in the case of vascular lesions. Third, it enables confirmation of specific factors such as calcification and fat, which is useful for definite diagnosis. These modalities should be used effectively to reach a correct diagnosis.

References

1) DeRemee RA: The roentgenographic staging of sarcoidosis. Historic and contemporary perspectives. Chest 83:128-133, 1983
2) Filly R, Bland N, and Castellino RA: Radiographic distribution of intrathoracic disease in previously untreated patients with Hodgkin's disease and non-Hodgkin's lymphoma. Radiology 120: 277-281, 1976

Chapter 5

Radiographs of mediastinal lesions with decreased or increased radiolucency

Mediastinal lesions

[Pattern classification V]

●Author — Masayoshi Kuwabara

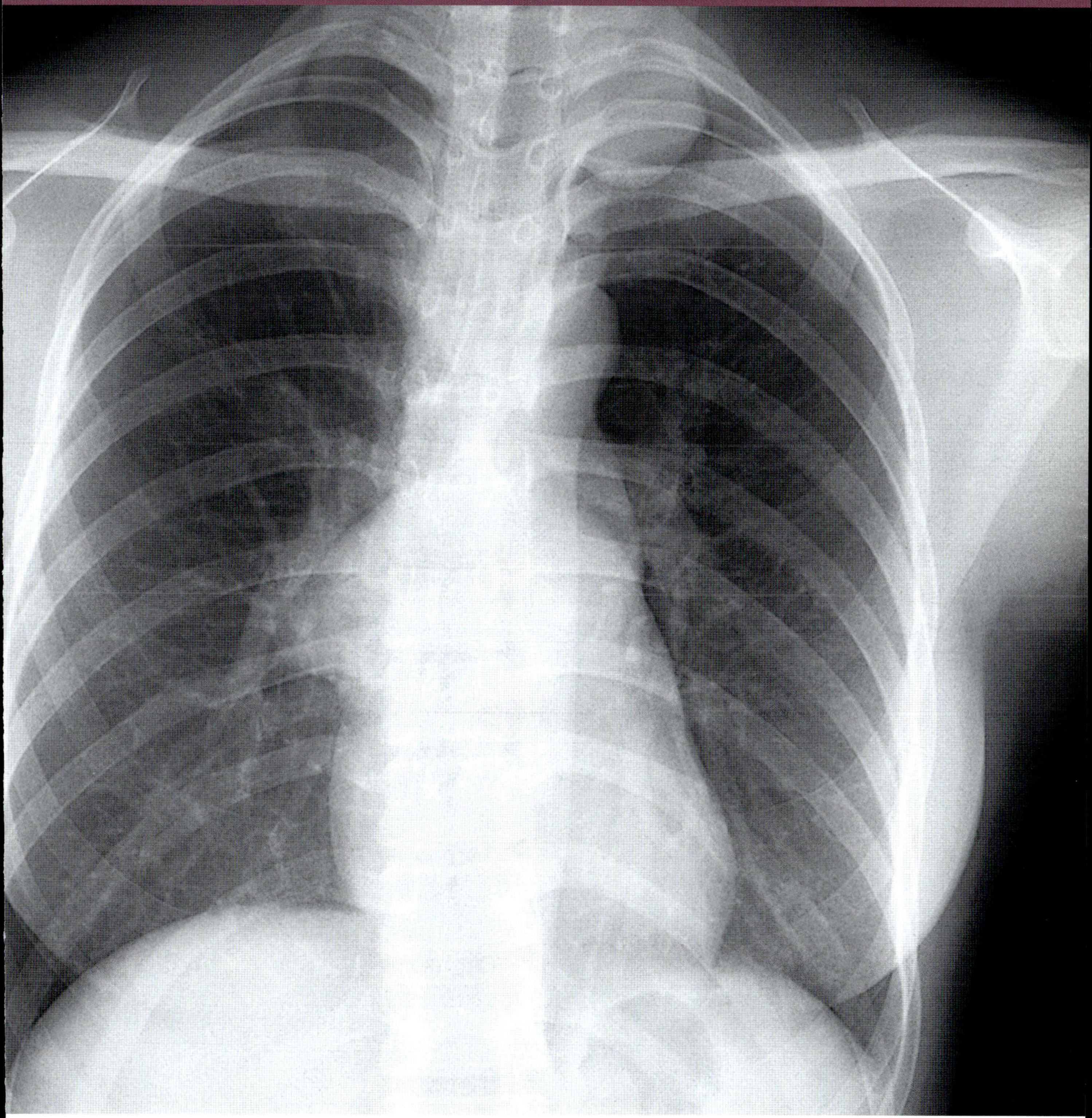

Keywords of this chapter

Von Recklinghausen's disease
Double contour shadow
Mediastinal classification
Fraser's classification
Calcification shadow
Felson's classification
Heitzman's classification
Superior mediastinum
Anterior mediastinum
Middle mediastinum
Posterior mediastinum
Tumor shadow
Hilum overlay sign
MR angiography

Mediastinal lesions

Masayoshi Kuwabara
Director of the Lung Cancer and Chest Diseases Center, Kusatsu General Hospital, Shiga, Japan

For mediastinal lesions, the role of plain chest radiographs is to detect abnormal shadows and their localization. In general, differential diagnosis of mediastinal lesions with plain chest radiographs alone is difficult, with CT examination being required for the next diagnostic step. In addition to the shape of the shadow and surrounding conditions, CT examination provides information concerning tumor attenuation differences and whether there is calcification, and if so, its distribution, thereby enabling differential diagnosis. With MRI examination, which provides even higher contrast resolution than CT, exceptional signal strength also enables diagnosis of hemorrhage, cystic and solid diseases. Furthermore, sagittal and coronal MRI section of lesions provide useful information regarding tumor invasion and other factors.

Case 1 31-year-old female

Chief complaint: None
Medical history: 20 operations (mainly orthopedic surgery) for multiple neurofibromas (Von Recklinghausen's disease) from the age of 13
Family history: Mother, neurofibromatosis
Smoking history: None
Present illness:
From the age of about 13, the patient had 20 operations for neurofibromatosis of the trunk and in the extremities. When she was 16, she underwent surgery for resection of a right posterior mediastinal tumor (neurofibroma). At the age of 30 she underwent surgery for resection of a tumor of the spine/cauda equina, left thigh leg tumor, left neck tumor and right calf tumor (all neurofibromas). At that time, a mediastinal tumor was detected and the patient was observed over an extended period. The examination this time was conducted after the tumor shadow was seen to enlarge.
Physical findings on admission:
Height 161.5 cm, weight 50 kg, café-au-lait spot (-), surgical scars in 20 locations on the trunk and extremities.
Laboratory data on admission:
Blood/biochemical examinations: No abnormalities, no tumor marker (CEA, CYFRA, ProGRP) abnormalities.

Chest radiograph findings: A plain posteroanterior chest radiograph (P.161) shows a 4 x 3.5 cm spherical shadow with homogeneous density and sharply defined border in the left superior mediastinum. No calcification shadow can be seen. Also seen are a cardiac contour, double contour shadow, and a mass lesion protruding into the lung side partially from the right ventricular segment of the heart shadow.

Chest CT findings (*Figs. 1 a–b*): At the level of the clavicle, a 4 x 3.5 cm spherical shadow (➞) can be seen in the posterior part of the left superior mediastinum, with a sharp border and slightly low attenuation. No calcification is observed.

At the left atrium level, a gourd-shaped tumor can be seen in the bilateral posterior mediastinum, with left atrial compression from the dorsal to the ventral side (➤). The border with the cardiac contour is sharp.

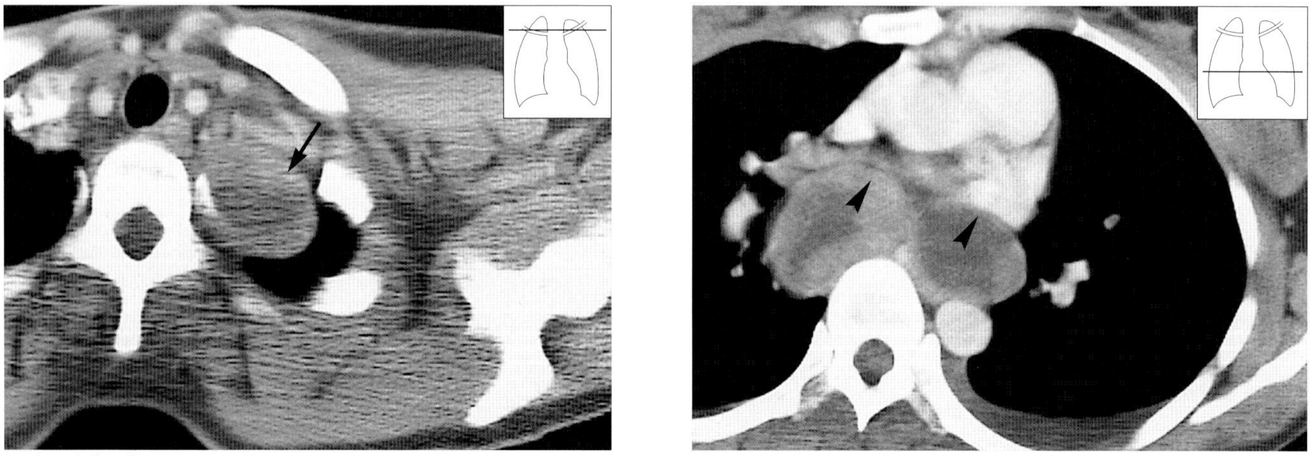

a. Clavicle level

b. Left atrium level

Figure 1 a–b. **Chest CT**

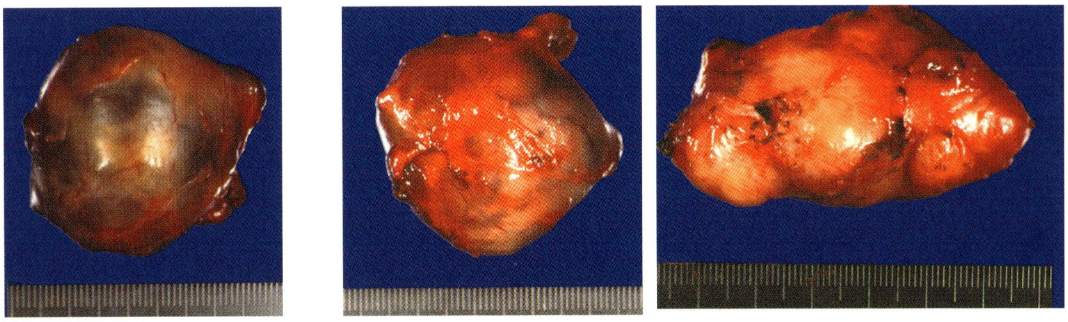

Figure 2 a–c. **Macroscopic pictures** *a.* Left superior mediastinal tumor *b.* Right posterior mediastinal tumor *c.* Left posterior mediastinal tumor

Diagnosis

After diagnosis of a mediastinal tumor associated with Von Recklinghausen's disease, a one-step operation was performed. First, extirpation of the tumor in the left superior mediastinum was conducted with a left thoracotomy. The tumor had a capsule, the surrounding tissue was peeled off easily, and the tumor was extirpated. Next, from the left the posterior mediastinal tumor was peeled off the pericardium and posterior mediastinum, and then with a right thoracotomy, from the right the tumor was peeled off from the pericardium and posterior mediastinum and extirpated *(Figs. 2 a–c)*.

Pathological findings: Histological findings indicating Antoni type A palisading pattern and cyst formation were observed, and neurilemmoma was diagnosed. No findings of malignancy were seen (histological findings).

Postoperative course: Postoperative plain chest radiograph and chest CT showed that the tumor shadows had disappeared and the heart had returned to its original position (➞).

Conclusions of this case: Mediastinal tumors accompanying Von Recklinghausen's disease

Von Recklinghausen's disease is a hereditary disease characterized by café-au-lait spots and multiple neurofibromas. The disease is frequently accompanied by mediastinal tumors, with malignant neurilemmomas in particular being the most frequent. In this case, pathologically no malignant findings were seen but there are reports of cases changing from benign to malignant. As a result, observation over an extended period is required.

Points concerning interpretation of chest radiographs: It was noticeable that in the chest radiograph, there were two abnormal shadows, a cardiac double contour shadow and tumor shadow in different mediastinal regions. There was the possibility that one or other of the shadows could possibly be overlooked. Taking this as a basic principle when interpreting chest radiographs, it is necessary to proceed with checking of the anatomical elements

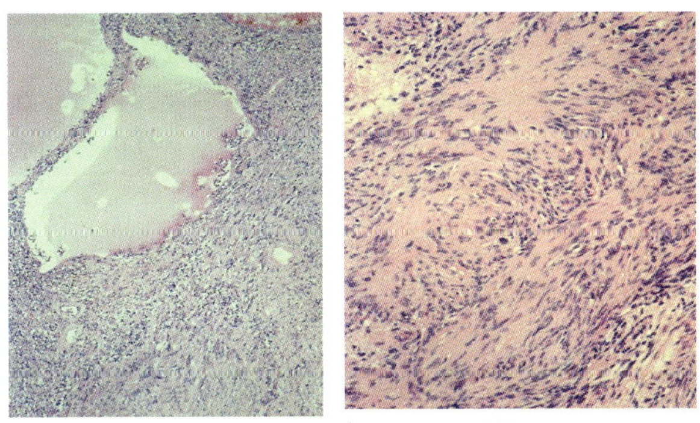

a. HE stain, x 40 *b.* HE stain, x 100
Figure 3 a–b. **Histological findings**

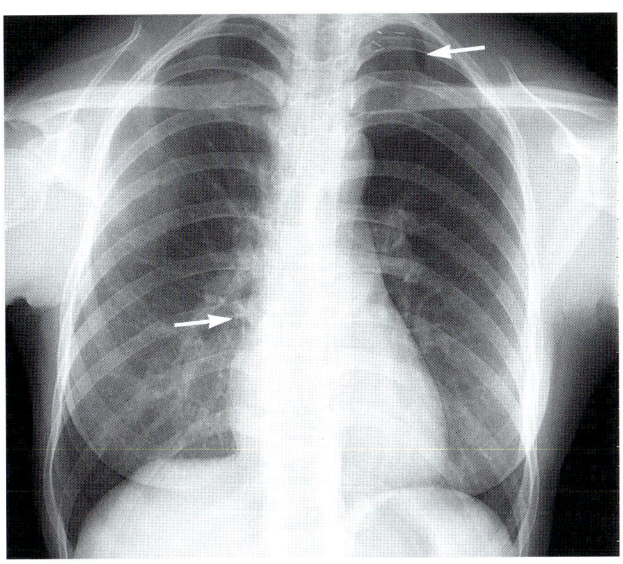

Figure 4. **Chest radiograph**

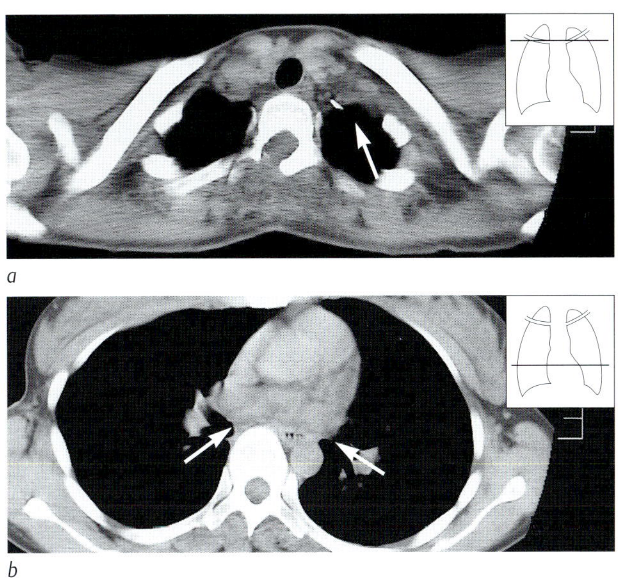

Figure 5 a–b. **Chest CT: postoperative**

extremely carefully. CT findings of neurogenic tumors are homogeneous, generally spherical or elliptical shadows with sharply defined borders, and occasionally patchy calcification shadows can be observed. In malignant cases, the borders of tumors with surrounding organs are indistinct, a finding indicating that tumor infiltration into surrounding organs is highly possible.

Mediastinal compartments and common locations of mediastinal tumors

Mediastinal lesions, particularly mediastinal tumors, have common locations depending on their histological type. Knowing this is a useful tool when considering diagnosis. Fraser divided the region of the mediastinum into the four compartments of superior mediastinum, middle mediastinum, anterior mediastinum and posterior mediastinum. Felson, on the other hand, divided it into the three compartments of anterior mediastinum, middle mediastinum and posterior mediastinum, while Heitzman includes anatomical elements for more detailed compartments. In this chapter the widely used classification by Fraser has been adopted. The compartments' relationship with anatomical regions and tissue elements is indicated in the figure.

These anatomical compartments are the sites of origin for mediastinal tumors. The superior mediastinum is often the region of neurogenic tumors (Case 1), thymomas and intramediastinal (intrapleural) goiters (Case 2); the anterior mediastinum is often the region of thymomas (Cases 3, 4), related germ cell tumors (Case 7), mediastinal teratomas (Case 5) and lymphomas; the middle mediastinum is often the region of bronchogenic cysts, pericardial cysts (Case 6) and lymphomas; and the posterior mediastinum is often the region of neural tumors (Case 8) and bronchogenic cysts (Case 9).

CT examination is the most effective method for diagnostic imaging of mediastinal lesions. In addition to showing the shape of the shadow, CT provides information concerning tumor attenuation differences, calcification distribution conditions, border conditions and the relationship with surrounding organs, the contrast-enhanced effect and other details that are the criteria when considering differential diagnosis of diseases including benign and malignant diseases *(Table)*.

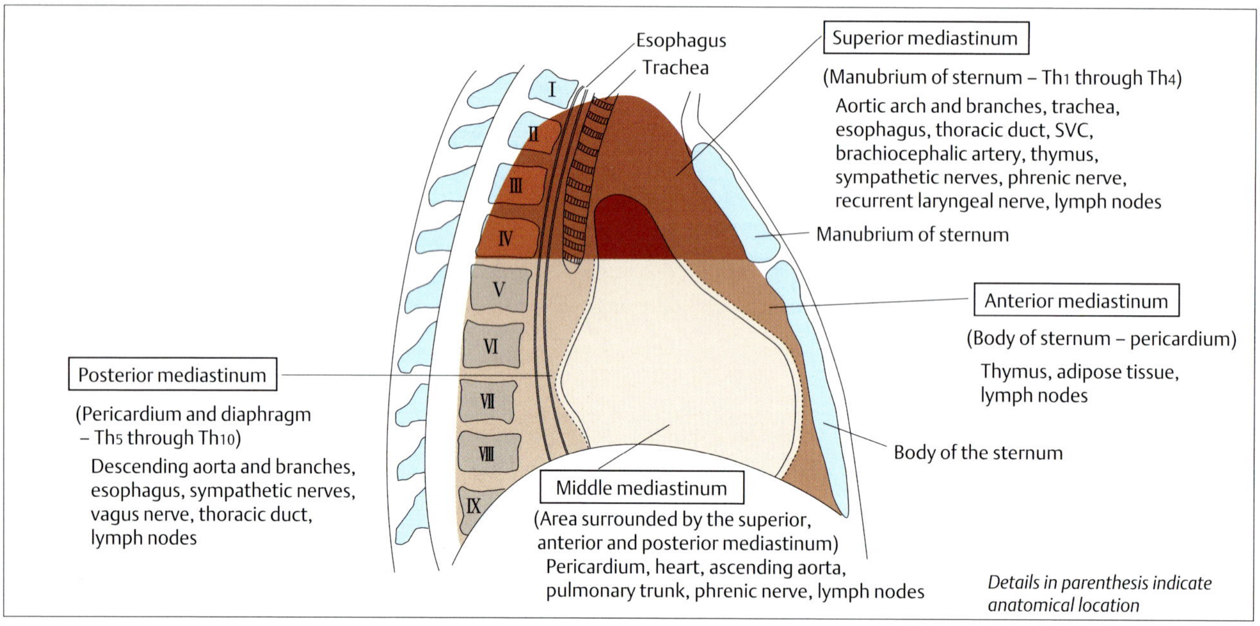

Figure 6. **Schematic illustration of mediastinal compartments and anatomical elements (Fraser's division)**

	Internal uniformity	Internal nonuniformity	Distinct border	Indistinct border	Contrast-enhanced effect	Calcification
Thymoma	○	△	○	○ (Malignant)	△	△ (Patchy, ring shaped)
Teratoma		○	○	○ (Malignant)		△ (Tooth-like, bone-like)
Neural tumor	○		○			△
Bronchogenic cyst	○ (Low density)		○		○ (Border)	
Pericardial cyst	○ (Low density)		○		○ (Border)	
Lymphoid tumor	○			○ (Malignant)		
Germ cell tumors		○		○		△
Intrapleural goiter		○	○			○ (Spot shaped, nodular)
Lipoma	○ (Low density)					

Table. **Differential diagnosis of mediastinal tumors with CT findings**

○: Usually, △: Sometimes

Case 2 Intramediastinal (intrapleural) goiter
56-year-old female

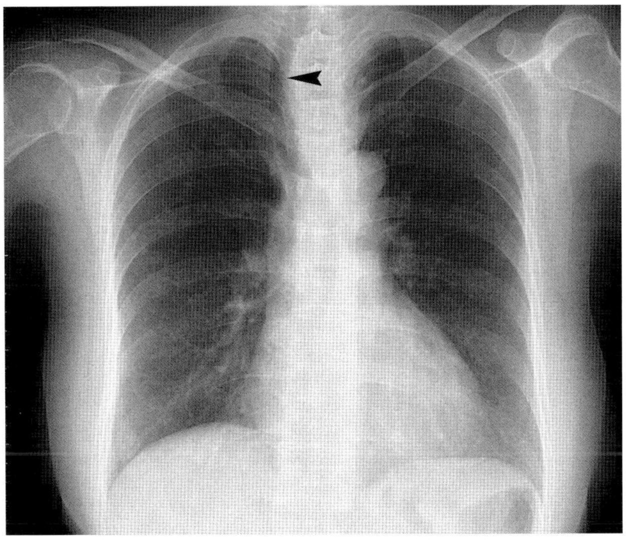

Figure 7. **Chest radiograph**

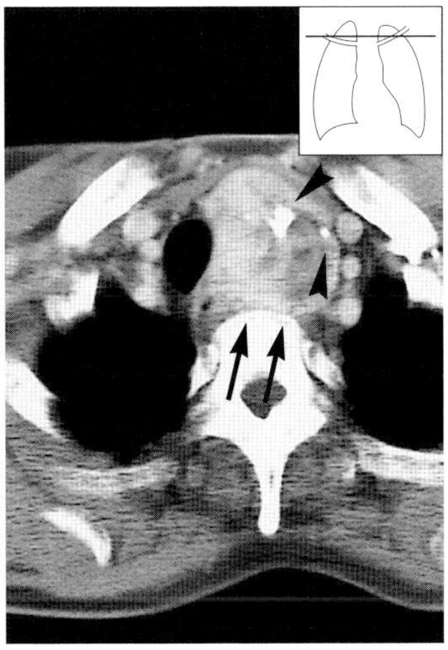

Figure 8. **Chest CT**

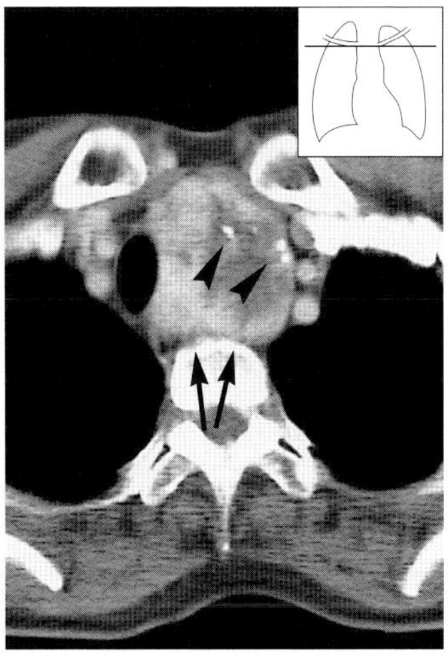

Figure 9. **Chest CT**

Chief complaint: None
Chest radiograph findings: A tumor shadow can be observed on the left side of the trachea, with pressure on the tracheal shadow displacing it to the right (➤).

Chest CT (contrast-enhanced) findings: A tumor shadow can be observed on the left side of the trachea (➞). The tumor shadow is uneven and nodular shadows and calcification can be seen (➤). Slices on other levels show that the tumor shadow continues from the thyroid gland. The tumor shadow is also contrast-enhanced at its margin. A diagnosis of intramediastinal (intrapleural) goiter was established and the tumor was removed.

Case 3 Thymoma
66-year-old female

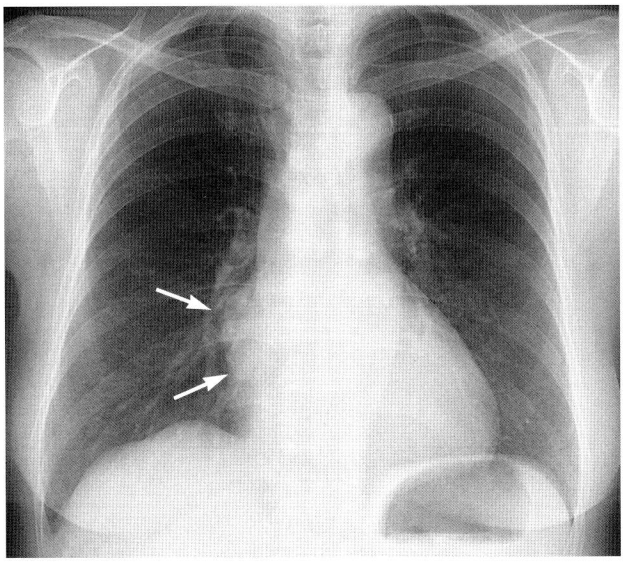

Figure 10. **Chest radiograph**

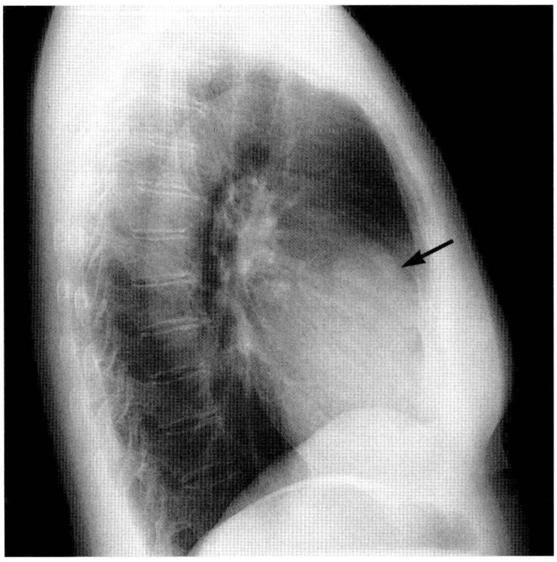

Figure 11. **Chest radiograph**

Chief complaint: None
Chest radiograph findings: A shadow projecting outwards at the right ventricular segment (2nd border) of the heart border (➞) can be seen. The border is distinct. The right second border of the heart has a double contour.

The lateral chest radiograph shows a cardiac contour overlaid by a spherical shadow in the anterior mediastinum (➞).

Chest CT findings: In the anterior mediastinum, on the right anterior side of the ascending aorta a tumor shadow can be seen with a sharply defined border and even

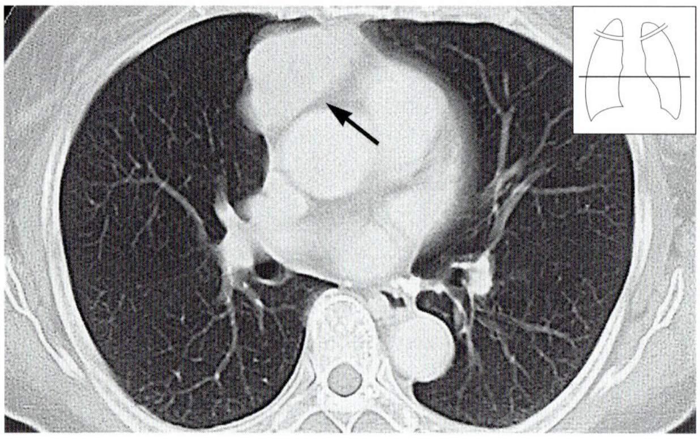

Figure 12. **Chest CT**

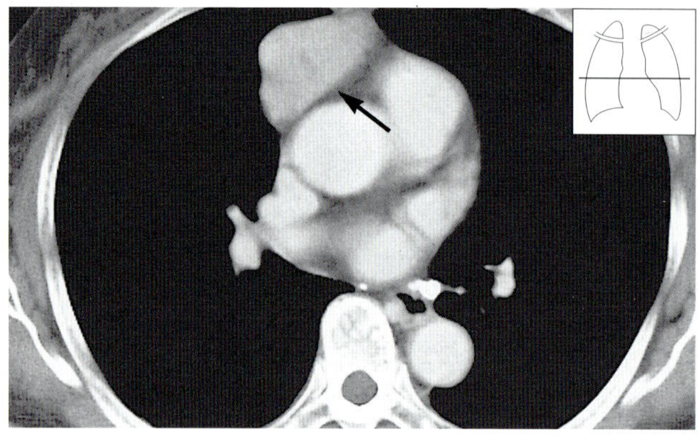

Figure 13. **Chest CT**

attenuation (→). It was diagnosed as a thymoma.

Chest CT (*Fig. 12*): In the lung window setting, care should be taken because part of the cardiac contour may be misdiagnosed (→).

Chest CT (*Fig. 13*): In the mediastinal window setting, a localized shadow that is clearly different from the cardiovascular system can be seen on the right anterior side of the ascending aorta (→).

Case 4 Thymoma (with pure red cell aplasia)

48-year-old female

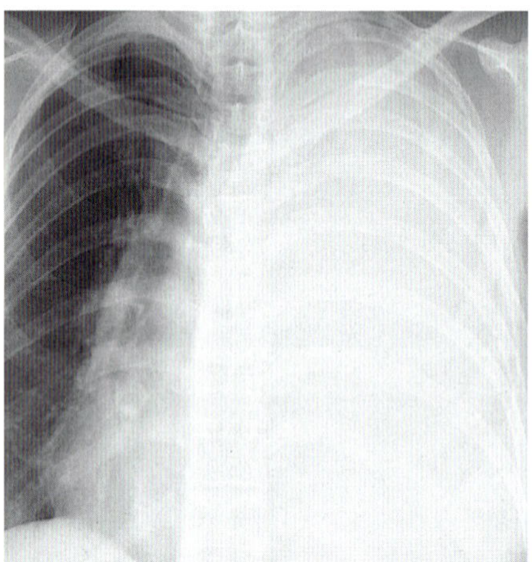

Figure 14. **Chest radiograph**

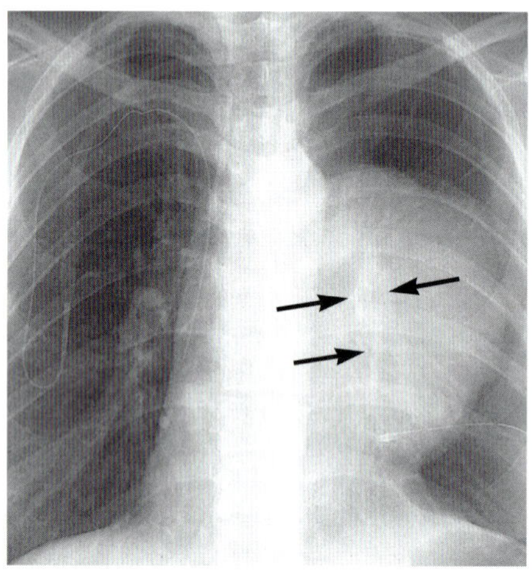

Figure 15. **Chest radiograph: After drainage of pleural effusion**

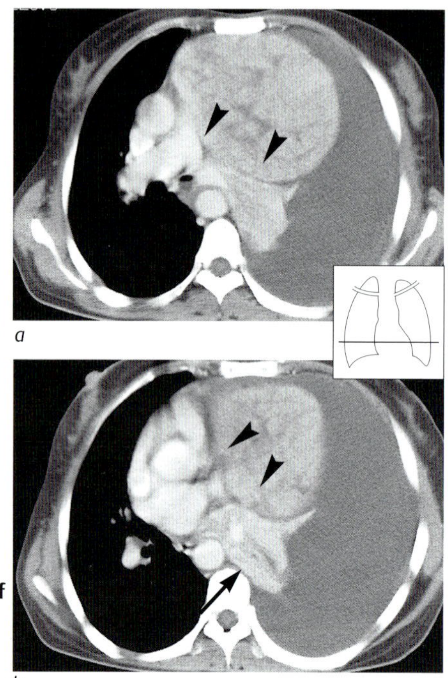

a

b

Figure 16 a–b. **Chest CT: Contrast-enhanced CT**

Chief complaint: Dyspnea on exertion

Received a medical examination by a home doctor for dyspnea on exertion. Chest radiograph showed left pleural effusion, and the patient was referred to a medical specialist. The patient had severe anemia.

Chest radiograph findings: Opacity can be seen in the left lung, and the mediastinum is shifted to the right. This is a finding of pleural effusion. After drainage, a large mass shadow can be seen protruding outwards from the left hilum. Pulmonary markings can be clearly seen running inside the shadow (→) (Hilum overlay sign).

Chest CT findings: A large volume of pleural effusion in the left lung and a large mass shadow in the anterior mediastinum can be seen. The mass shadow is putting pressure on the heart from the right dorsal side, but the border with blood vessels is distinct (➤). Severe collapse of the left lung on the left dorsal side can be seen (→).

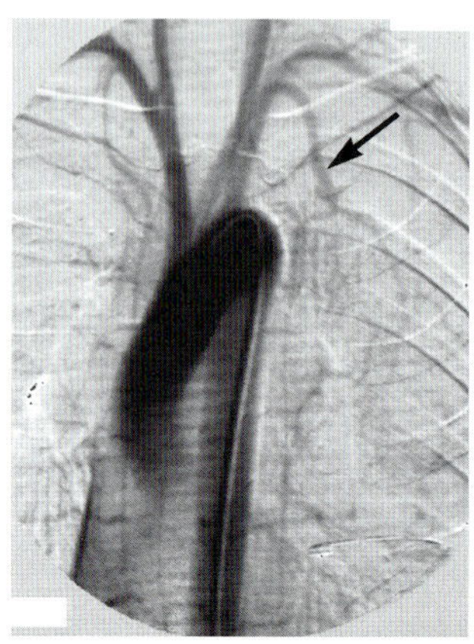

Figure 17. **Conventional angiography**

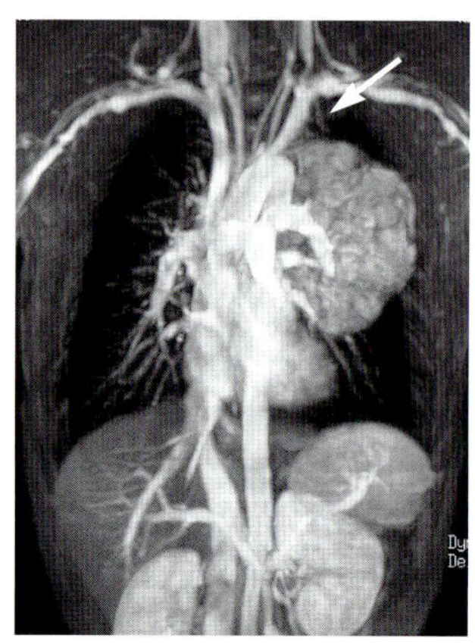

Figure 18. **MR angiography**

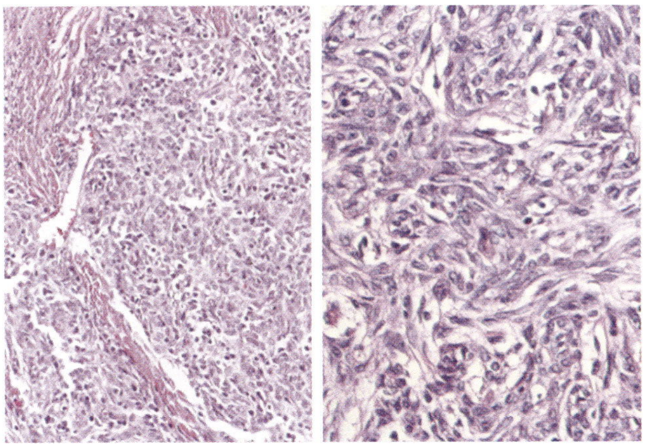

a. HE stain, x 40 *b.* HE stain, x 100

Figure 19 a–b: **Histological findings**

Because the mass shadow is also highly contrast-enhanced, MR angiography and conventional angiography were conducted. The findings showed a well-developed left internal thoracic artery running inside the tumor (→). At the time of surgery this left internal thoracic artery was treated first to avoid massive bleeding.

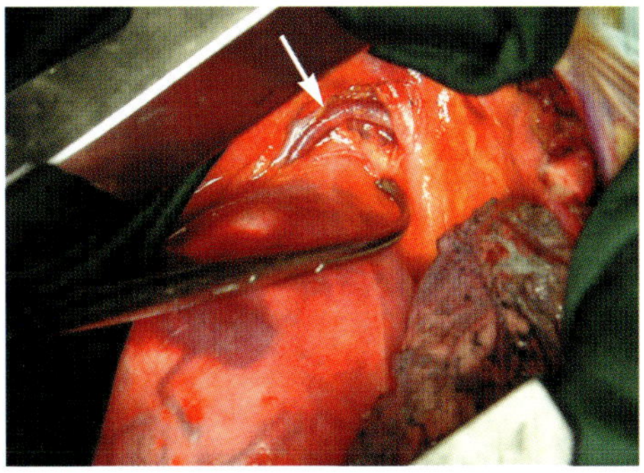

Figure 20. **Surgical findings**

Surgical findings: A well-developed internal thoracic artery (→) bifurcating from the left subclavian artery can be seen following the tumor. The tumor was diagnosed as a thymoma.

Case 5 Mediastinal teratoma

39-year-old female

Chief complaint: None

Chest radiograph findings: Widening of the superior mediastinal shadow can be seen, with the trachea slightly shifted to the right (→).

Chest CT findings: A tumor shadow can be seen in the anterior part of the superior mediastinum (→). The tumor shadow is uneven, and CT values suggesting soft tissue, adipose tissue and bone were seen. The border with blood vessels is distinct. With surgery, a mature type of mediastinal teratoma was diagnosed.

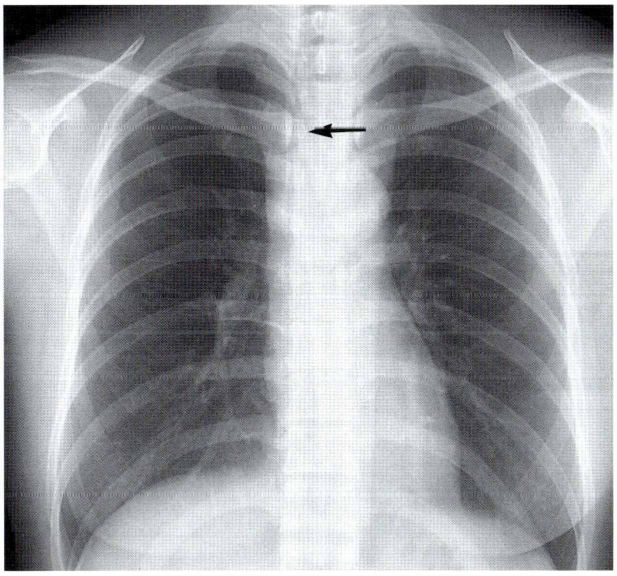

Figure 21. **Chest radiograph**

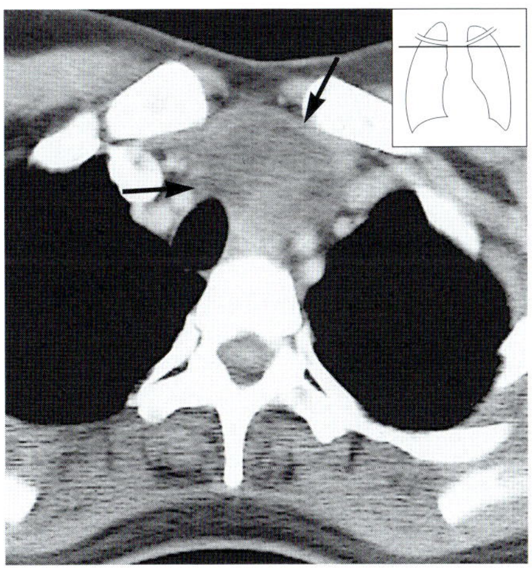

Figure 22. **Chest CT**

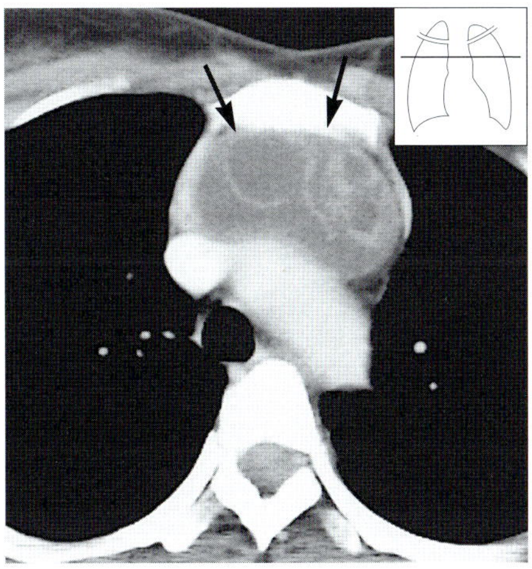

Figure 23. **Chest CT**

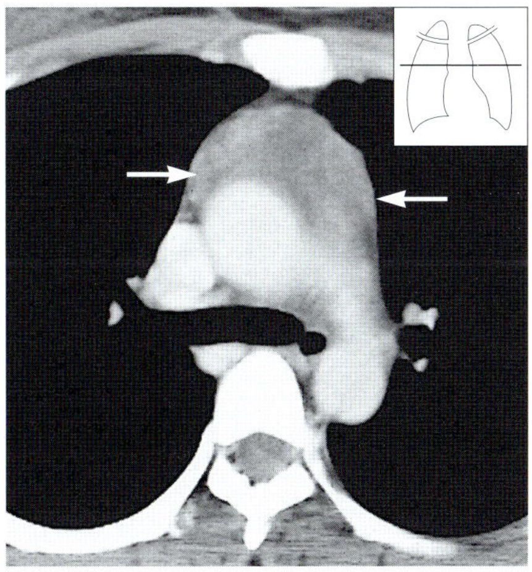

Figure 24. **Chest CT**

Case 6 Pericardial cyst
23-year-old male

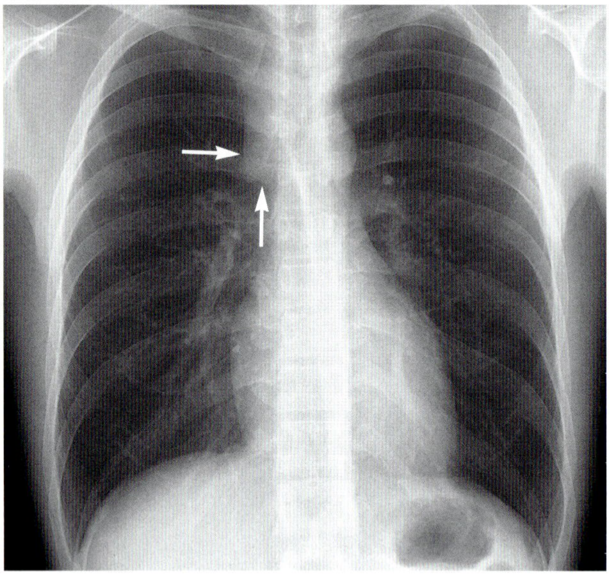

Figure 25. **Chest radiograph**

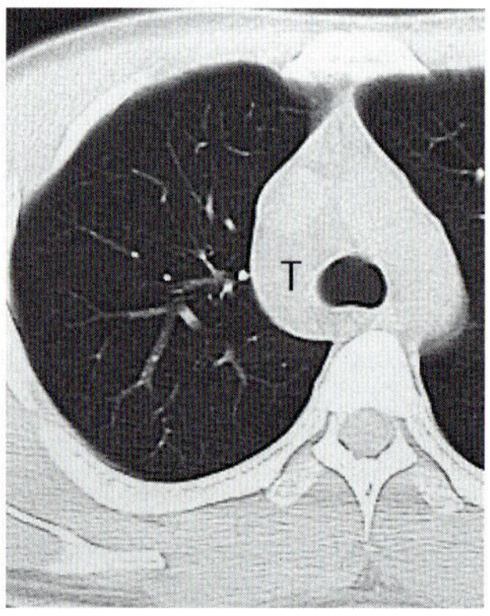

Figure 26. **Chest CT**

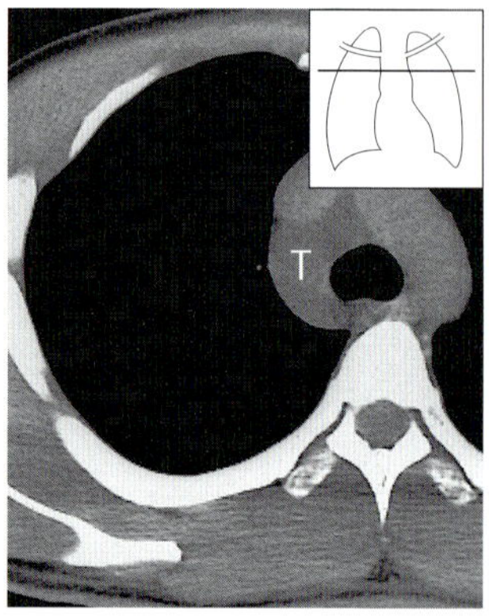

Figure 27. **Chest CT**

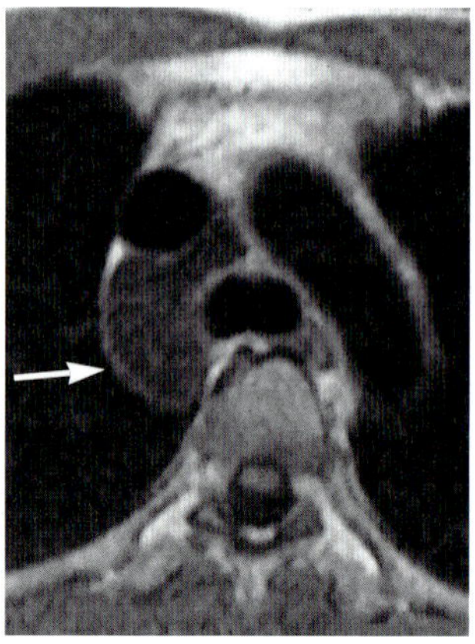

Figure 28. **T1-weighted MRI**

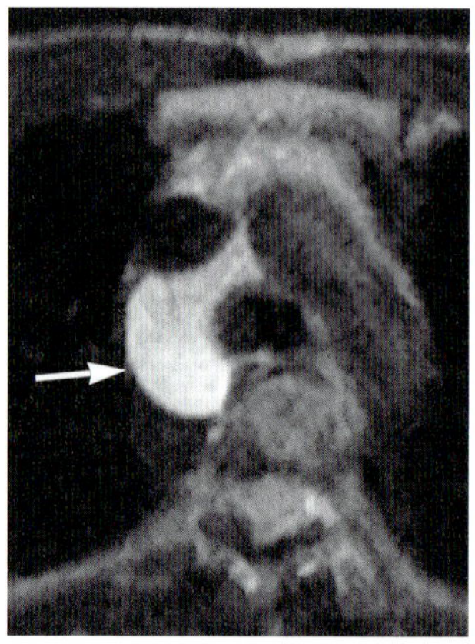

Figure 29. **T2-weighted MRI**

Chief complaint: None
Chest radiograph findings: A sharply defined and homogeneous tumor shadow can be seen protruding into the right side of the superior mediastinum (→). No tracheal shifting can be seen.

Chest CT findings: A low attenuated, even tumor shadow (T) can be seen on the right wall of the trachea in the superior mediastinum.

Chest MRI findings: From a T1-weighted MRI indicating a low signal and a T2-weighted MRI indicating a high signal, a cystic disease was suspected. With surgery under thoracoscopy, a pericardial cyst was diagnosed.

Case 7 Germ cell tumor (seminoma)
22-year-old male

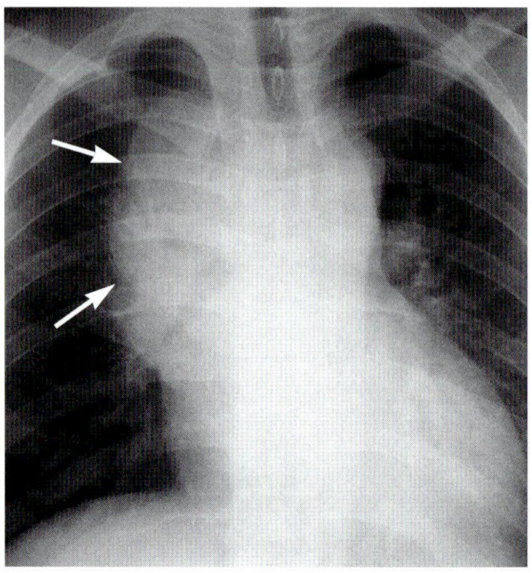

Figure 30. **Chest radiograph**

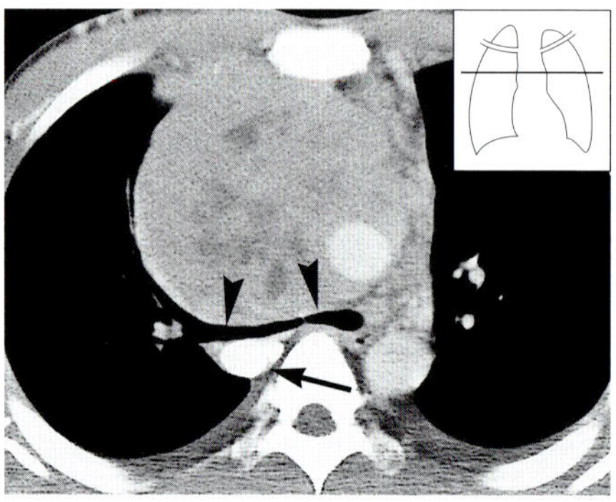

Figure 31. **Chest CT: Tracheal bifurcation level**

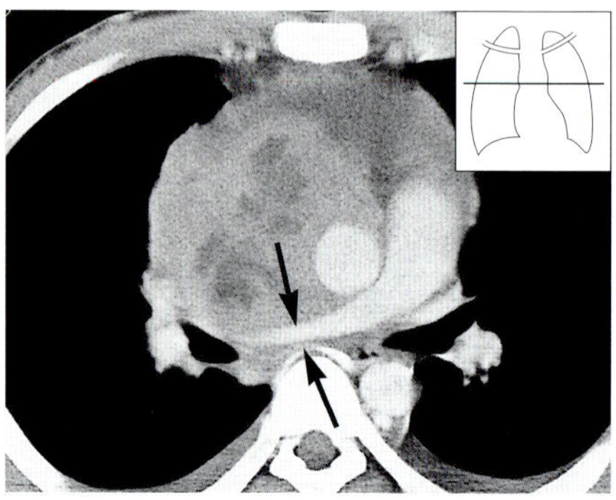

Figure 32. **Chest CT: Right pulmonary artery level**

Chief complaint: Dyspnea on exertion
Chest radiograph findings: A large mass shadow can be seen protruding outwards from the right hilum/superior mediastinum. An enlarged cardiac contour can also be seen.

Chest CT findings: At the tracheal bifurcation level (*Fig. 31*), a large mass shadow can be seen in the anterior mediastinum, putting pressure on the dorsal side of the left and right main bronchi (➤). The superior vena cava (SVC) is also almost blocked, and the azygos vein is enlarged to act as a bypass (→). The border with the chest wall is indistinct, pointing to suspected tumor infiltration.

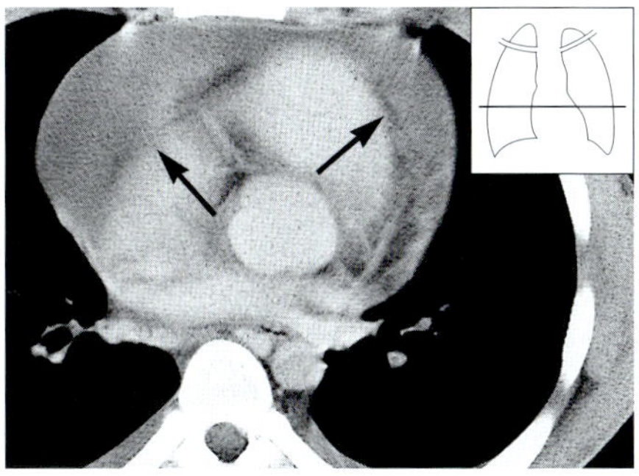

Figure 33. **Chest CT: Inferior pulmonary vein level**

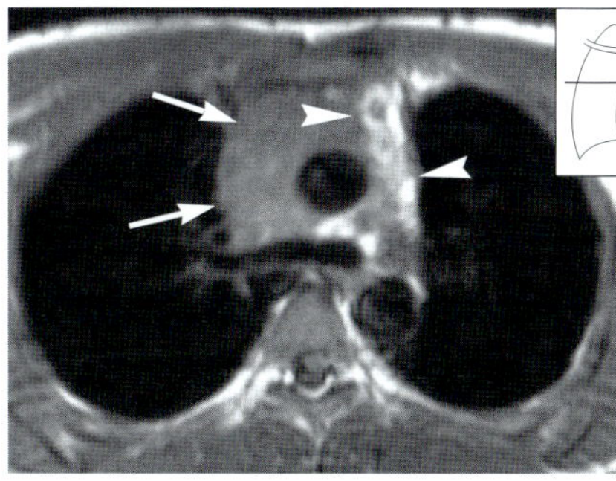

Figure 34. **T1-weighted MRI**

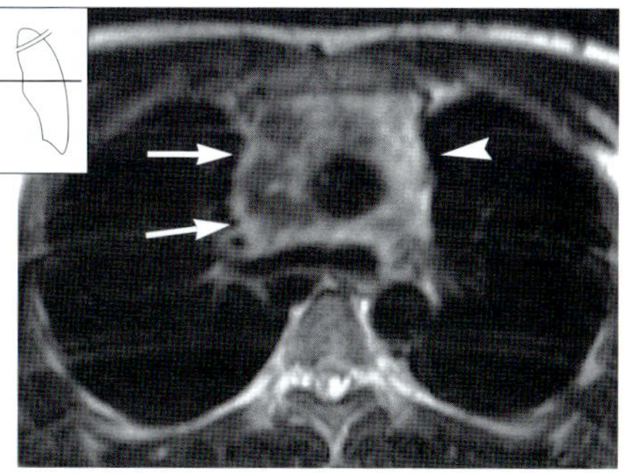

Figure 35. **T2-weighted MRI**

At the right pulmonary artery level (*Fig. 32*), pulmonary artery stenosis due to the tumor can be seen (➞).

At the inferior pulmonary vein level (*Fig. 33*), pericardial fluid can be seen (➞). The tumor shadow is uneven, and after a needle biopsy it was diagnosed as a seminoma.

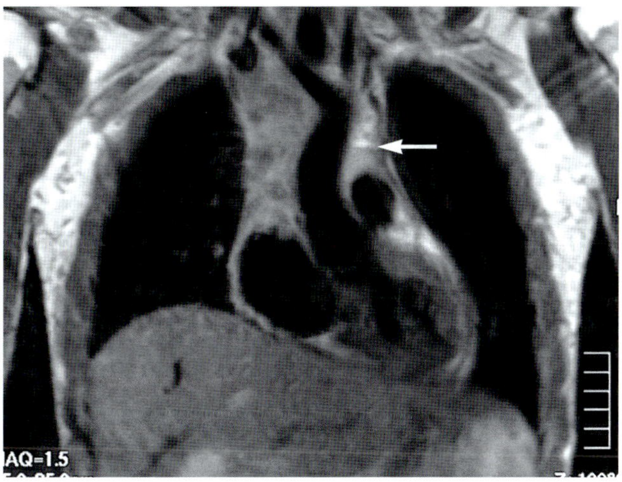

Figure 36. **MRI at the same time: Coronal section**

MRI after one course of chemotherapy: In a T1-weighted image (*Fig. 34*), the size of the tumor shadow is reduced but it appears to enclose two-thirds of the ascending aorta's surroundings (➞). On the left side of the ascending aorta a high signal can be seen that could be adipose tissue, and it can be seen that the tumor and ascending aorta are not directly touching (➤).

In a T2-weighted MRI (*Fig. 35*), a low signal on the right side of the ascending aorta indicating a tumor can be seen. A low signal on the left side of the ascending aorta could indicate adipose tissue.

An MRI taken at the same time (*Fig. 36*) (coronal section, Gd-DTPA contrast-enhanced): A T1-weighted MRI shows a tumor in the right superior mediastinum. The tumor is localized and touching from the ascending vena cava, ascending aorta, right brachiocephalic trunk and trachea to the main bronchi. The high signal on the left of the ascending aorta (➞) indicates no direct infiltration from the tumor to the aorta.

Case 8 Neurilemmoma

22-year-old female

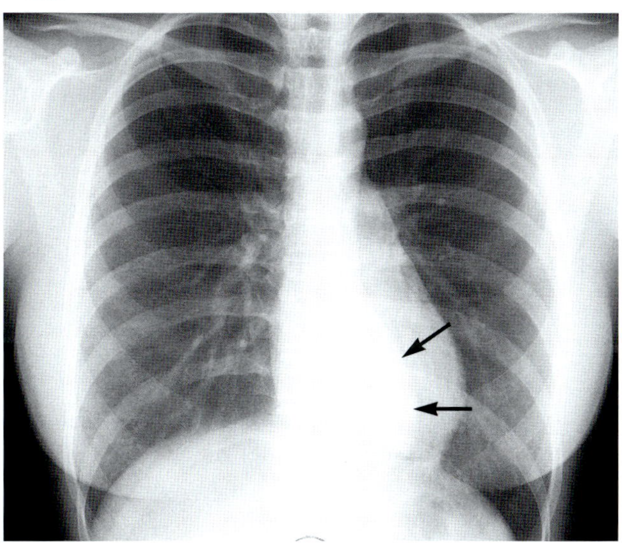

Figure 37. **Chest radiograph**

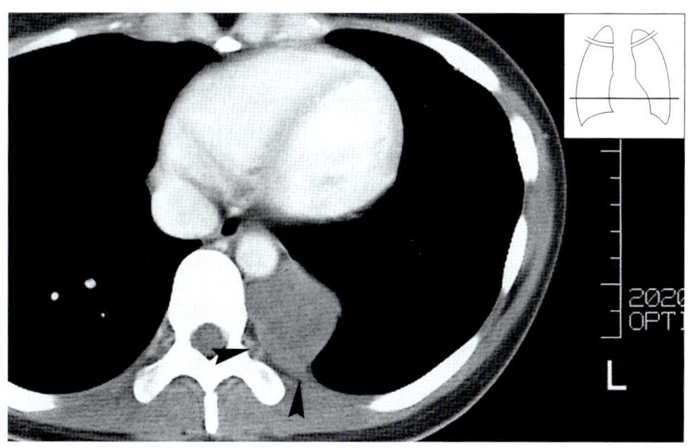

Figure 38. **Chest CT**

Chief complaint: None

Chest radiograph findings: A mass shadow on the outer side of the descending aorta can be observed overlaying the cardiac contour in the left lower lung field (➞). The left border of the descending aorta is distinct, and there is no connection with the shadow.

Chest CT findings: A spherical shadow with distinct border and even density can be seen on the left of the thoracic vertebrae obliquely posterior to the descending aorta (➤).

T1-weighted MRI findings: The signal strength inside

the tumor is the same as that for muscle. The signal strength is also high in a T2-weighted MRI (→), and is suspected to be adipose tissue.

T2-weighted MRI findings: A high signal is indicated in most of the inside of the tumor shadow but one low signal part can be seen.

Sagittal section MRI findings: Using a contrast medium (Gd-DTPA), a T1-weighted MRI shows an enhanced uneven tumor shadow in the posterior mediastinum. The top of the tumor shows as a high signal (→), indicating suspected adipose tissue.

From the tumor's occupied area and CT and MRI findings, the diagnosis was suspected solid neurogenic tumor, which was extirpated. This was neurilemmoma with accompanying cyst and hemorrhage.

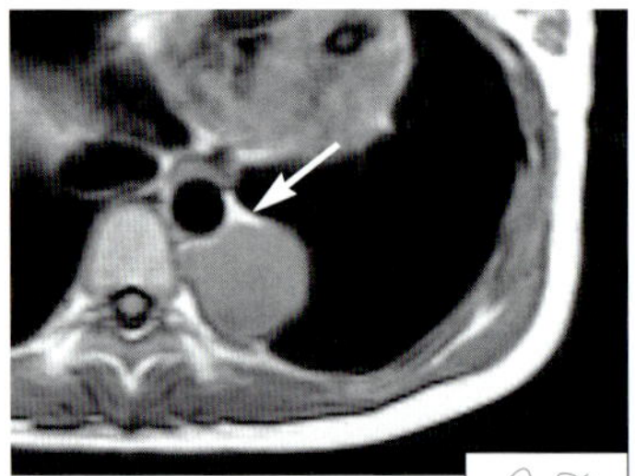

Figure 39. **T1-weighted MRI**

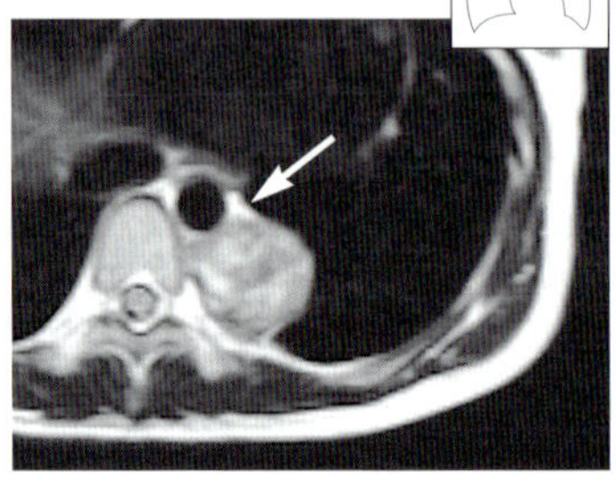

Figure 40. **T2-weighted MRI**

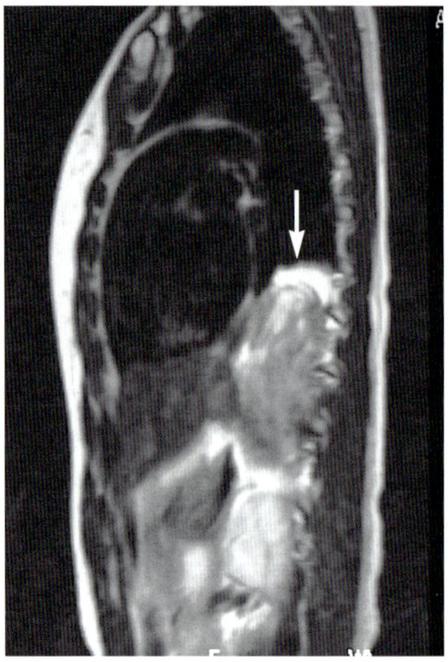

Figure 41. **Sagittal section MRI**

Case 9 Bronchogenic cyst

38-year-old male

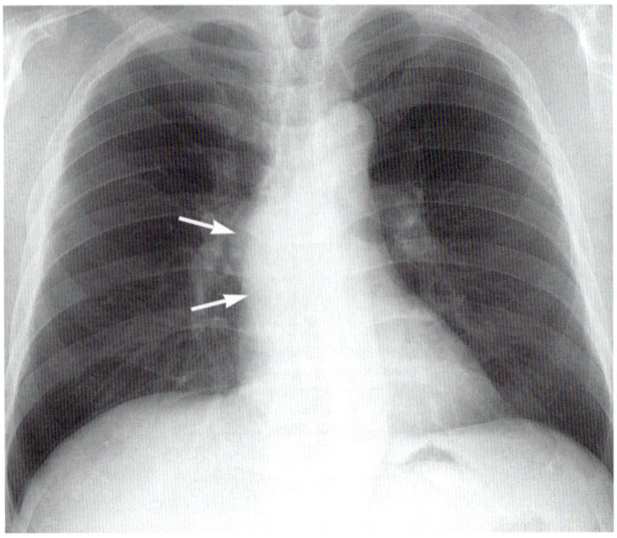

Figure 42. **Chest radiograph**

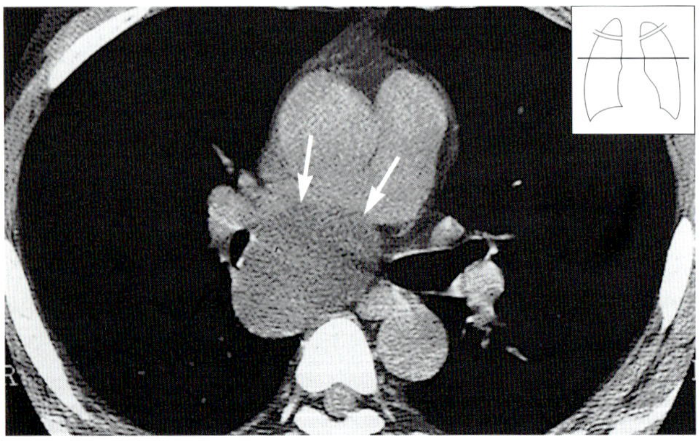

Figure 43. **Chest CT**

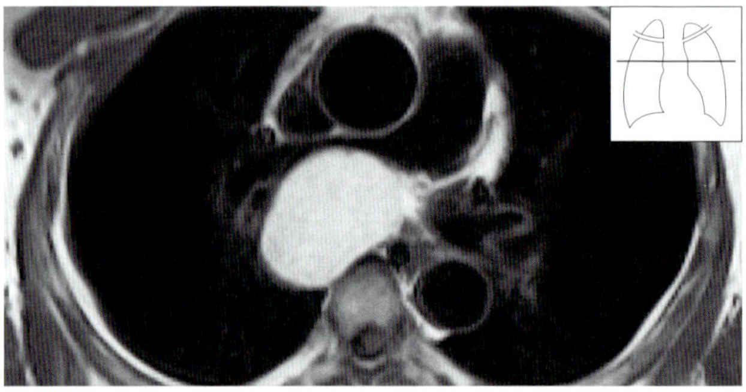

Figure 44. **T1-weighted MRI**

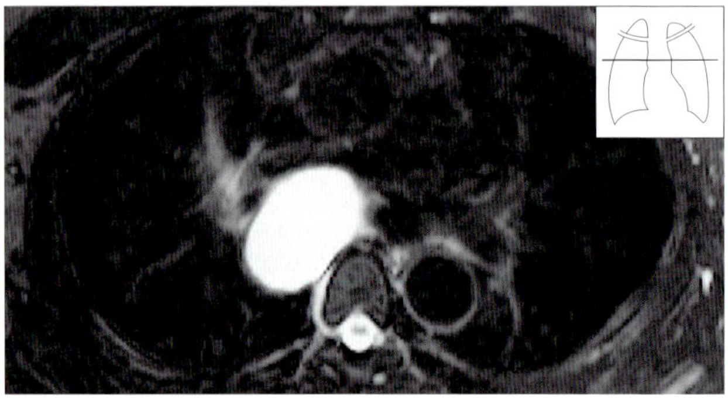

Figure 45. **T2-weighted MRI**

Chief complaint: None

Chest radiograph findings: A mass shadow can be seen protruding outwards at the ascending aortic segment (→). The border is distinct.

Chest CT findings: An even tumor shadow, with a distinct border, can be seen on the right anterior side of the thoracic vertebrae in the posterior mediastinum (→).

MRI findings: On T1-weighted and T2-weighted MRI, signals are high, but they are comparatively higher in the T2-weighted MRI than T1-weighted MRI. From these MRI and CT findings, a bronchogenic cyst with a sticky, protein-dense fluid was suspected and extirpated. It was diagnosed as a bronchogenic cyst.

Case 10 Mediastinal and subcutaneous emphysema
19-year-old male

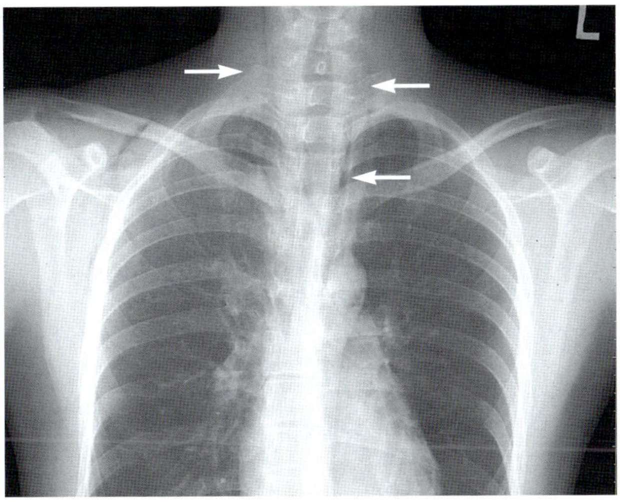

Figure 46. **Chest radiograph**

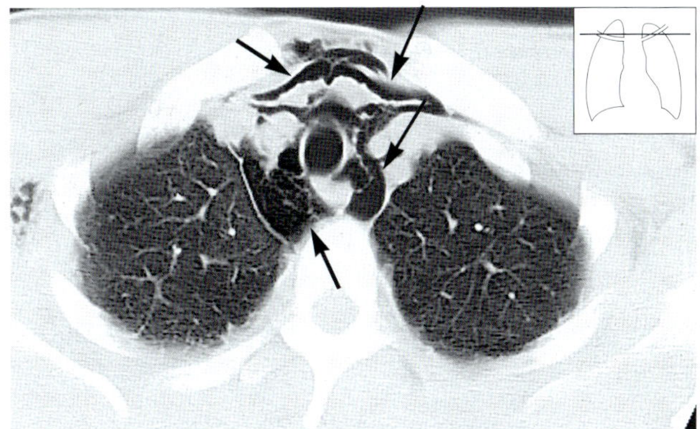

Figure 47. **Chest CT**

Chief complaint: Dyspnea
Chest radiograph findings: An air-contrasted shadow can be seen in the mediastinum and subcutaneous tissue. The air-contrasted shadow in the subcutaneous tissue extends as far as the neck. No pneumothorax is seen.

Chest CT findings: An air-contrasted shadow can be seen in the mediastinum consisting of air layers surrounding the trachea, blood vessels and esophagus.

Case 11 Acute mediastinitis
42-year-old male

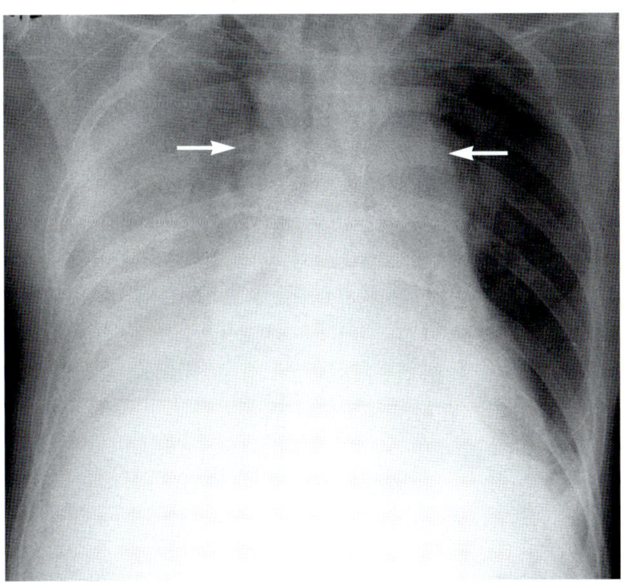

Figure 48. **Chest radiograph: Portable AP projection**

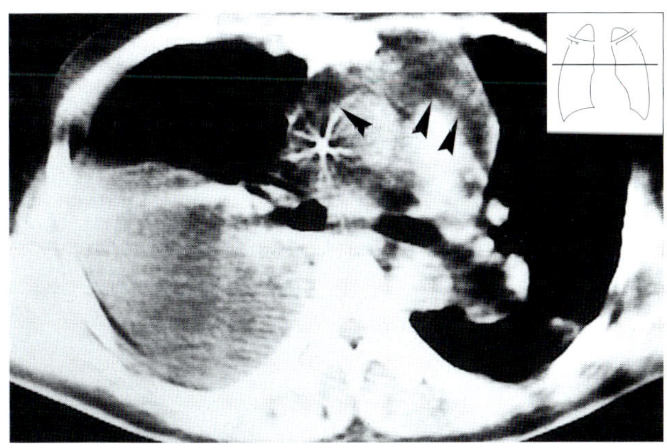

Figure 49. **Chest CT**

Chief complaints: Fever, dyspnea
Chest radiograph findings: Widened mediastinum (➞) and a large volume of pleural effusion on the right side can be seen.

Chest CT findings directly below the area of tracheal bifurcation: Diffuse soft tissue-like shadows can be seen on the ventral side of both main bronchi in the anterior mediastinum (➤). A large volume of pleural effusion can be seen in the right pleura.

Diagnosing mediastinal diseases with chest radiographs

Diagnosing localization of tumors is possible with chest radiographs. Major imaging findings indicating mediastinal abnormality are (1) tumor shadows projecting outwards from a central shadow (heart and aorta shadows) in posteroanterior radiographs, (2) widening mediastinal shadow (Cases 5, 11), (3) tracheal/bronchial compression and/or shift (Case 2), and (4) shadows accompanied by calcification and/or air. If these findings are indicated, lateral chest radiographs are extremely useful for localization diagnosis of mediastinal disease (Case 3).

Differential diagnosis

Using plain chest radiographs for the differential diagnosis of mediastinal diseases other than teratoma and intramediastinal goiter, where calcification is seen, and mediastinal emphysema accompanied by air (Case 10), is generally difficult. Furthermore, the above-mentioned findings also apply to atelectasis, hiatus hernia, aortic aneurysm, mediastinal type lung cancer and other diseases. With atelectasis, increased radiolucency in other lobes of the affected side and/or decreased pulmonary volume is seen, and with hiatus hernia there are accompanying gas imaging inside the cardiac contour and mass legion with a double contour shadow, features that enable differential diagnosis. However, differential diagnosis of aortic aneurysm and mediastinal type lung cancer is difficult. The next diagnostic step required is CT examination. Aortic aneurysm can be differentiated with contrast-enhanced CT, while mediastinal type lung cancer can be differentiated by the relationship between the mediastinal pleura and the tumor.

Diagnosing mediastinal diseases with chest CT

CT is exceptionally good for imaging diagnosis of mediastinal diseases. In addition to the shape of the shadow, CT provides information concerning tumor attenuation differences, calcification distribution conditions, border conditions and the relationship with surrounding organs, the contrast-enhanced effect and other details that are the criteria for differential diagnosis of benign and malignant diseases.

In CT of mediastinal tumors, benign tumors generally show as spherical or elliptical shadows with sharply defined borders that enable easy differentiation from surrounding organs. With malignant tumors, the tumor follows an organ's insterstitium and proliferates until it infiltrates the organ itself. As a result, the boundary with the organ becomes indistinct and the tumor shows as a mass lesion with a distorted shape (Case 7). In the same way, mediastinitis (Case 11), mediastinal hematoma and sclerosing mediastinitis are intramediastinal diseases that show as diffuse shadows. The episodes and MRI of mediastinal hematoma, the sudden onset of accompanying fever and severe inflammatory findings of mediastinitis, and in the case of sclerosing mediastinitis, the compression and obstruction of surrounding organs as fibrosis progresses but with no infiltration of the organs, enable differentiation of these diseases from malignant tumors. Characteristic findings of diseases also help with differentiation. These include internal uniform low attenuation with cystic diseases, CT values as low as those for adipose tissue with lipoma, and nonuniformity and calcification inside the shadow as well as the shape and distribution with teratoma, which sometimes shows as tooth-like or bone-like shadows, and intramediastinal (intrapleural) goiter, which sometimes shows as punctate or nodular calcifications. Calcification is sometimes seen with thymoma, but in many cases the calcification is patchy or ring-shaped. All of these findings should be taken into consideration during diagnosis.

Using MRI

This chapter focused on descriptions of lesions seen in plain chest radiographs and CT, but for diagnosing mediastinal lesions, analyzing contrast between soft tissues with MRI is an even more useful than CT. In general, for air and blood vessels and calcification and fibrosis, there is either no signal or a low signal in both T1-weighted and T2-weighted MRI. For adipose tissue, the signal is high in both T1-weighted and T2-weighted MRI, medium in T2-weighted MRI, and with hemorrhage shows as a wide range of other signals. For subacute hemorrhage and cysts with high protein density fluid, the signal is high in both T1-weighted and T2-weighted MRI, and for solid diseases and cystic diseases the signal is low in T1-weighted MRI and high in T2-weighted MRI. These indications are the criteria for imaging differential diagnosis. Furthermore, since sagittal and coronal images of any desired part of the lesion can be taken, useful information such as the relationship with surrounding organs and the progress of infiltration can be obtained.

References

- Yoshito Matsubara, Rikuro Hatanaka, Masayoshi Kuwabara, Sadao Ikeda, Takeshi Funatsu: Abnormal Shadows on Mediastinal and Chest CT – 3D Anatomy CT Atlas – 1st Ed., 435–470, Kinpodo Inc., Kyoto, 1995
- Masayoshi Kuwabara et al.: A Case of Mediastinitis Due to Esophageal Diverticulum Rupture. The Japanese Journal of Thoracic and Cardiovascular Surgery, 38: 1351–1355, 1990
- E. R. Heitzman: The Mediastinum, 2nd Ed. Springer-Verlag, Berlin, 1988

Index of Radiograph, CT, and other Pictures Classified by Diseases

ch: Chapter, Fig(s): Figure(s)